The Truth About

PROSTATE HEALTH

PROSTATE CANCER

Prevention • Cancer Life Extension

Charles B. Simone, M.D.

Princeton Institute
PrincetonInstitute.com
Princeton, NJ 08654

First Edition

Cover design: Charles B Simone, M.D.
3 Dimensional Prostate Treatment Plan graciously supplied
by the Lawrence Livermore National Laboratory in
California, USA

Library of Congress Cataloging-in-Publication Data

Simone, Charles B.
    The Truth About Prostate Health – Prostate Cancer,
Prevention • Cancer Life Extension / Charles B. Simone,
M.D.
                        Includes bibliographical references and index.

ISBN 0-9714574-2-5
        1.Prostate – Cancer – Prevention. Popular Works I. Title
        2.Prostate – Cancer – Life Extension
        3.Prostate – Diseases – Popular Works. I. Title
        4.Antioxidants – Therapeutic use.
        5.Cancer – Nutritional Aspects and Diet therapy.
        6.Cancer – Risk factors. I. Title

        RC280. S53 2004   01-14177
        616.99'4052 – dc20   CIP

Table of Contents

Part Four. Prostate Cancer: Detection to Conventional Treatment

Part Five. Simone Ten Point Plan for Prostate Disease Prevention and Cancer Life Extension

To my family

****
****

"It is impossible for anyone to begin to learn what he thinks that he already knows."

Epictetus

****
****

A paradigm shift occurs as exceptions, often startling changes. "Such changes, together with the controversies that almost always accompany them, are the defining characteristics of scientific revolutions."

Thomas Kuhn

Introduction

All men should strive to attain optimum prostate health because the incidence of benign prostate disease and prostate cancer is rising at alarming rates. Eight of ten men develop benign prostate disease; one in every six men in the United States will develop prostate cancer, and the odds are getting worse.

Cancer is the most feared of all diseases. People immediately associate cancer with dying. Unlike some other killer diseases, cancer usually causes a slow death involving pain, suffering, mental anguish, and a feeling of hopelessness. It now affects two of every five Americans. The number of new cancer cases has been increasing over the past nine decades; the accelerated rise in lung cancer, for example, is alarming. According to the U.S. Bureau of the Census, 47 people out of every 100,000 died of cancer in 1900, making it the sixth leading cause of death. Today, 212 people out of every 100,000 will die of cancer, ranking it second.

In 1971, the United States declared war on cancer with the following statement from President Nixon: "The time has come in America when the same kind of concentrated effort that split the atom and took man to the moon should be turned toward conquering this dread disease." In that year, 337,000 people died of cancer, and about $250 million was spent on cancer research.

Since then, billions of dollars have been invested in cancer research. Approximately $104 billion is spent on cancer treatment each year: about $35 billion for direct health care, $12 billion in lost productivity due to treatment or disability, and $57 billion in lost productivity due to premature death.[1] Each month, it seems, new therapies are trumpeted. Some show promise, others fizzle quickly. So intense is the concern to find "the cure for cancer" that more money is collected each year than can actually be spent responsibly on meaningful research. More of these funds should be directed to cancer prevention than the National Cancer Institute's current allocation of less than 5 to 7 percent.

Despite the enormous effort to combat cancer, the number of new cases of nearly every form of cancer has increased annually over the last century as shown in Table 1 and Figure 1. From 1930 to the present, despite the introduction of radiation therapy, chemotherapy, and immunotherapy with biologic response modifiers, despite CT scans, MRI scans, and all the other new medical technology, lifespans for people with almost every form of cancer except cervical cancer and lung cancer have remained constant, which means that there has been no significant progress in treatment for cancer including prostate cancer.[2] See Figure 2. The incidence of stomach cancer has gone down probably due to the advent of refrigeration in the 1930s and the consequent removal of carcinogenic chemicals as food preservatives. The National Cancer Institute and American Cancer Society set an unrealistic goal of a 50 percent reduction in cancer mortality by the year 2000.[3-9] Looking at the almost vertical rise in Figure 1 in the number of new cancer cases each year, I predicted in 1994 that the goal could not be attained. It was not.

Table 1. United States Cancer Incidence				
	1900	1962	1971*	2005
Total Cases	25,000	520,000	635,000	1,368,200
Leading Cancers				
Prostate	N/A	31,000	35,000	231,230
Breast	N/A	63,000	69,600	217,440
Lung	N/A	45,000	80,000	186,550
Colon/Rectum	N/A	72,000	75,000	146,940
Uterus	N/A	N/A	N/A	51,000

*President Nixon declared war on cancer. N/A = Not available. Data from US Bureau of Vital Statistics and *CA – A Cancer Journal for Clinicians*

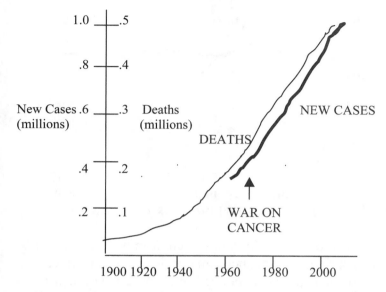

Figure 1. Cancer deaths and new cases. Note the rise in new cancer cases and cancer related deaths despite billions of dollars in research.

The chilling prospect remains: two of every five Americans will develop cancer, and the majority of them will die from it.

Cancer research and treatment are extremely complex fields of study because the exact nature of the single cancer cell is so elusive. Cancers are many diseases with many different causes. We cannot expect miracle cures just because so much money has been poured into cancer research. At the same time, we should not expect miracles from "cancer-cure" facilities that take money from cancer patients desperate to try any treatment in hope of another chance at life.

After collating the existing cancer data, I found that 80-90 percent of all cancers are produced as a result of dietary and nutritional factors, lifestyle (smoking, alcohol consumption, lack of exercise, etc.), chemicals, and other environmental factors.[10] This information has now been corroborated by major agencies: the National Academy of Sciences,[11] the U.S. Department of Health and Human Services,[12] the National Cancer Institute,[13] and the American Cancer Society.

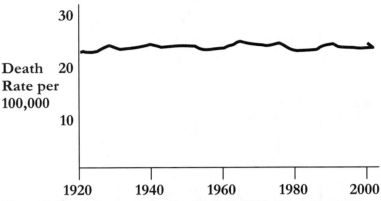

Figure 2. Prostate cancer death rate 1920-2005. *CA–A Canc J Clin.*

Since nutrition, lifestyle, and the environment are the most common risk factors for cancer, many of these cancers can be eliminated or substantially reduced in number if you can identify the risk factors pertinent to you and modify them accordingly. Many people have the fatalistic attitude that anything and everything can cause cancer, and believe there is no use in trying to do anything about it. That attitude is unwarranted and fosters even more apathy. Everything does not cause cancer.

The public's perception of cancer causes and cancer "cures" comes mainly from the news media that portrays cancer risks quite differently from what scientists have actually shown to be cancer risks.[16] By reviewing over 1,100 newspaper, magazine, and television news stories between 1972 and 1992, media representatives cited the risks they believed to be the leading factors in causing cancer: manmade chemicals such as food additives and pesticides, pollution, hormone treatments, and radiation. When members of the American Association for Cancer Research were asked the same question, they cited the following as the major risk factors for causing cancer: tobacco, diet, and sunlight. Here again, it is easier for people to complain about risk factors perceived to be important and over which they have no control, rather than take on the responsibility to modify risk factors over which they have total control. People do, in fact, have total control over the leading causes of cancer.

The type of diet we eat today and its preparation are major risk factors in the development of certain cancers, risk factors that can definitely be modified. Nutrition is a very complex topic - one that is not well understood by the public or even by many physicians. Americans need to know the role that nutrition plays in major diseases.

Diet and nutrition appear to be factors in 60 percent of women's cancers and 40 percent of men's cancers as well as about 75 percent of cardiovascular disease cases. Tobacco is a factor in about 30 percent of human cancers. Other known risk factors associated with the development of cancer include alcohol, age, immune system deficiencies, chemicals, and drugs. You have total control over most of these risk factors, including the major two: diet and tobacco. The cancers most closely associated with nutritional factors are cancers of the prostate, breast, colon, rectum, and endometrium.

Having one or more of the risk factors does not mean that cancer will necessarily develop. It simply means that a person exposed to risk factors has a greater than normal chance of developing cancer.

Physicians in our country too often wind up treating the cancer rather than the whole cancer patient. Much has been learned since 1981 about the role of nutrition, the immune system, and the patient's mental state in the healing process. Because these issues are not properly addressed by the medical community, many patients with advanced tumors seek questionable treatment. At great financial and emotional cost to themselves and their families, they resort to quack remedies, get-healthy-quick schemes, and practitioners and "health" centers that claim to reverse or eliminate chronic diseases easily and quickly.

It is *your* responsibility to learn about the risk factors involved in cancer development, and specifically prostate cancer, and then modify those risk factors accordingly. In order to prevent cancer, you should devise your own anticancer plan based on risk factor modification. In addition, your family, and particularly your children, should be taught about risk factor modification. If nutritional and other risk factors are modified, the benefit will be evident in all people, but especially in the young and in the succeeding generations. Obviously, there are some risk factors, like air and water that you cannot directly control; therefore, your community must devise plans to modify environmental factors.

We must eliminate or modify all known risk factors so that we will eventually be able to prevent cancer and heart disease. Nutritional factors and tobacco smoking, for example, are major risk factors, which, if modified or eliminated, can dramatically reduce the number of cancer as well as heart disease patients. Our health-care system emphasizes expensive medical technology and hospital care. It does not emphasize preventive medicine and health education. *It is your responsibility to learn about risk factors and then modify them.* Good health does not come easily, you must work for it.

You have almost total control over the destiny of your health and the health of your family! Do something about it.

I am convinced that if everyone would follow Dr. Simone's plan early enough in life and take it seriously, we would make major strides toward putting the cancer doctors out of work and approach the legacy of health that is within our reach.

Robert A. Good, Ph.D., M.D.
Former President and Director, Memorial Sloan-Kettering Cancer Hospital, New York City 1980

PART ONE

Prostate Disease Today

1

The Scope of Prostate Disease

One man in six will develop prostate cancer during his lifetime. In the United States, it is the most common cancer detected. The number of new cases of prostate cancer in the United States is about 230,600.[1] Total deaths from prostate cancer are estimated to be 29,900. African American men are more likely to develop prostate cancer than white men and they fare worse because the cancer is more advanced at the time of diagnosis. There are about 520,000 cases of prostate cancer worldwide accounting for almost 10% of all male cancers in the world. The number of new cases of prostate cancer increases every year. About 85% of patients are older than 65.

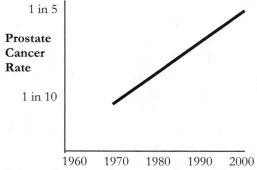

In 1960, the number of prostate cancer cases was low, but those odds have gotten worse with each year. By 1980, the rate had risen to one in ten men and kept zooming: in 1990 one in eight, in 2000, one in six developed prostate cancer.

Figure 1. Odds that a man develops prostate cancer in the US.

Table 1. Risk of Developing Prostate Cancer By Age in US	
Birth to 39:	1 in 12,833
Ages 40 – 59:	1 in 44
Ages 60 – 79:	1 in 7
Ever, Birth to Death :	1 in 6

CA- A Cancer J for Clinicians. Jan/Feb 2004; 54:24.

The number of new cases and death rate per 100,000 men in the United States varies by race and ethnicity (Table 2). African-Americans have more new cases and a higher death rate compared to all other groups in the US – alarming numbers.

Table 2. New Cases and Death Rate in US by Race and Ethnicity		
	New Cases/100,000	Death Rate/100,000
All Races	170	33
White	164	30
African American	272	73
Asian/Pacific Islander	100	14
American Indian/Alaskan Native	54	22
Hispanic-Latino	137	24

When mortality figures are examined from 1930 onward, no change is seen in survival for men with prostate cancer, which means there has been no change in the life span of men affected with prostate cancer since 1930. And the number of prostate cancer deaths goes up every year.

Since lifespans have not changed appreciably since 1930 for prostate cancer patients despite all of our treatments (Figure 2 Introduction), it is important to understand the role nutrition and other risk factors play in the development of prostate cancer so that you can modify them. Most risk factors for prostate cancer and benign prostate disease can be modified. For example, a high-fat, low-fiber diet, tobacco use, alcohol use, etc can be modified. Your genetics cannot be directly modified, but genetics play only a small role in the development of prostate cancer – less than 7 percent. Age is another risk factor that cannot be modified.

Table 3.	Estimated New Prostate Cancer Cases by State				
Alabama	4,850	Louisiana	3,690	Ohio	8,620
Alaska	230	Maine	1,150	Oklahoma	2,620
Arizona	3,920	Maryland	4,080	Oregon	2,920
Arkansas	2,150	Massachusetts	5,700	Pennsylvania	12,010
California	23,160	Michigan	8,540	Rhode Island	1,000
Colorado	2,540	Minnesota	4,230	South Carolina	4,770
Connecticut	3,310	Mississippi	3,390	South Dakota	920
Delaware	690	Missouri	3,460	Tennessee	4,540
D.C.	620	Montana	1,080	Texas	13,540
Florida	17,090	Nebraska	1,460	Utah	1,080
Georgia	5,700	Nevada	2,000	Vermont	460
Hawaii	1,000	New Hampshire	1,000	Virginia	5,080
Idaho	1,080	New Jersey	7,930	Washington	4,850
Illinois	9,930	New Mexico	1,690	West Virginia	1,540
Indiana	5,390	New York	14,470	Wisconsin	3,850
Iowa	3,160	North Carolina	7,160	Wyoming	620
Kansas	2,690	North Dakota	540		
Kentucky	2,620				

Treatment has minimally improved survival. Most scientists/physicians are convinced, however, that the slight increase in life span is due largely to earlier detection of prostate cancer by the PSA. But let us not forget what five-year survival means as defined by the oncologist. If a patient lives five years and one day, that man is counted as a cure or survivor even though he has died. If, however, he lives one day less than five years, he is counted as a nonsurvivor.

As countries around the world have become more westernized especially in their dietary habits, the number of deaths from diet-related tumors has increased. When you examine the mortality from cancers in Japan, you find that tumors related to nutritional factors have increased dramatically in the last twenty-five years. Cancers of the colon and rectum, cancers of the breast, and prostate cancer all have increased dramatically. This trend is mainly seen in younger Japanese who are more likely to have adopted Western ideas and habits, especially dietary habits. Since prostate cancer is seen mainly in older men, the current global incidence rates of prostate cancer reflect dietary habits relatively unchanged by Western influences as shown in Table 4.

Table 4. Global Incidence Rate of prostate Cancer per 100,000	
USA African-American	137
USA White	101
Canada	65
Sweden	55
Norway	48
USA, Los Angeles Japanese-Americans	47
Zimbabwe (Harare)	29
England and Wales, UK	28
Uganda (Kyadondo)	28
Italy (Veneto)	27
Slovenia	21
USA, Los Angeles Chinese-Americans	20
Japan (Hiroshima)	11
India (Bombay)	8
China (Tianjin)	2

We still hear that if more money were given for the war on cancer and specifically prostate cancer, the magic bullet would be found. The Government Accounting Office showed that *prevention* of cancer is paramount in the battle against cancer since there is no clear strategy for improving survival. And even though the management of the disease has improved, life-span has not, and that is the primary objective of any treatment – to make the life span longer, improve survival. One major advance has come about: minimizing pain and suffering.

The *prevention* of all cancers, including prostate cancer, should be of primary importance. Less than 5 percent of the National Cancer Institute's budget is earmarked for prevention and of these studies, true prevention studies, unencumbered with other agenda, account for well under 2 percent. We are not winning the war against prostate cancer with the current conventional approach; therefore, we must prevent the disease.

Prostate diseases other than cancer also afflict many men today. It is estimated that 75 percent of all men develop benign prostate disease. We will consider benign prostate diseases in the next chapter.

2

Benign Prostate Syndromes and Erectile Dysfunction

Benign prostate syndromes include prostatitis (an inflammation of the prostate gland), and benign prostatic hyperplasia (BPH). A discussion of male reproductive health and erectile dysfunction will be included in this chapter as well. Before these conditions are reviewed, the anatomy and function of the prostate gland will be discussed. Please note, the word prostate is pronounced, PRA - STATE, and not PRA - STRAIGHT as is commonly done.

PROSTATE ANATOMY AND FUNCTION

Only men have prostate glands. It is a small organ that looks like a walnut weighing only about 20 grams (less than one ounce) and is located between the urinary bladder and the rectum. The prostate is composed of muscle and glandular tissue and encased by a thick fibrous capsule. Visualize the prostate gland as a donut with a hole in the middle through which passes the urethra, the tube that connects the urinary bladder to the penis. Urine passes out of the body via the urethra from the bladder to the tip of the penis. If the prostate gland enlarges, as commonly happens later in life, the donut hole gets smaller and thereby impedes the flow of urine out of the body causing pain and other symptoms discussed in the section entitled, benign prostatic hyperplasia.

The prostate gland produces a milk-like fluid that gets squeezed by muscular contraction into the urethra during orgasm. This prostatic fluid combines with sperm and other fluids manufactured in the seminal vesicles and glands of the urethra to form semen. These fluids nourish the sperm and transport it from the penis during ejaculation. The prostate supplies almost 90 percent of the ejaculate and all the propulsive power needed to expel the fluid.

The prostate fluid is increased and drips from the penis during sexual excitement. If ejaculation does not occur, the prostate swells and becomes painful, which in turn, transmits pain into the testicles. Ejaculation generally relieves this pain.

PROSTATITIS is an inflammation of the prostate gland caused by infectious organisms or noninfectious processes. Regardless of the cause, prostatitis is quite painful.

• **ACUTE INFECTIOUS PROSTATITIS** usually affects young men but may also occur in men who have a catheter in their penis (a soft tube inserted into the penis to drain urine from the bladder). Symptoms come on suddenly and include fever, chills, a tremendous urge to urinate, a pressure sensation in the bladder, burning in the urethra and tip of the penis when passing urine, frequent urination at night, painful ejaculation (that may temporarily relieve the prostate pain), and joint or muscle pain. The pain can radiate into the lower back, scrotum and rectum. These symptoms may be so severe that you may need to seek a physician immediately. Although infrequent, the infection can progress to the bladder and up to the kidneys.

Urine examination and a digital rectal examination performed by a physician can determine the diagnosis. Pus (white blood cells), bacteria or other organisms, and blood may be present in the urine. By inserting a gloved, lubricated finger into the rectum, the physician can feel a small portion of the surface of the prostate. The inflamed prostate characteristically feels tense or boggy. The examination itself may cause some pain because the prostate is swollen. It is not a good idea to massage the prostate gland in an attempt to squeeze out infected fluid because massaging can potentially seed the bloodstream with infectious organisms.

The infection may be caused by bacteria or non-bacteria, like Chlamydia trachomatis or Ureaplasma urealyticum. The physician reviews the laboratory analysis of the urine and decides upon the antibiotic for treatment. Within hours of antibiotic treatment, the patient feels better but must continue the treatment for 7 to 14 days to ensure eradication of the infection. Analgesic medication is given for pain relief, and sometimes, hospitalization may be required for severe infections.

• **CHRONIC INFECTIOUS PROSTATITIS** is a low-grade, smoldering infection. It is often present without symptoms until the organisms spill into the bladder causing painful urination, and the urge to urinate frequently or immediately. When the prostate gland is massaged for a specimen, bacteria will be seen. Unlike acute prostatitis the digital rectal examination is usually normal. If you do not have repeated bladder infections, you probably do not have chronic infectious prostatitis.

Antibiotics promptly relieve the acute bladder infection symptoms but the smoldering infection of the prostate is difficult to eradicate. Antibiotics do not penetrate the prostate gland very well so treatment is given for 12 weeks, and even then only about 60 percent of all cases are cured. In cases that are not cured, low-dose antibiotics over a prolonged period of time may be necessary.

• **PROSTATODYNIA** is simply a painful non-infected prostate gland. Antibiotics do not help. The pain radiates to the entire pelvis and between the scrotum and anus. Muscle spasms and other conditions affecting the musculo-skeletal system can also produce similar symptoms. An "alpha blocker" medication may be given to relax the muscle tissue in the prostate and thereby allow urination to proceed with less difficulty.

CAUSES OF PROSTATITIS
• Enlarged gland - benign prostatic hyperplasia (BPH).
• Recent bladder infection.
• Rectal intercourse.

- Anti-histamines and decongestants restrict the outflow of prostate fluid and thereby cause prostatitis. The only treatment is to allow time for the medicine to clear the body.
- Medical instrumentation like cystoscopy (rigid instrument inserted into the penis to exam the bladder) or catheter.
- Abnormal anatomy of urinary tract - rare.

PROSTATITIS TREATMENT
- Antibiotics are effective for infectious processes but are not effective for non-infectious processes.
- Drink lots of water, one glass every hour.
- Drink cranberry juice because it can change the pH of the urine and dislodge bacteria from the bladder wall allowing them to be washed away.
- Antioxidants, and the B vitamins are helpful
- A low-fat, high-fiber diet contributes to prostate health.
- Sitting in a hot tub of water for 20 minutes several times a day can relax the prostate muscles and allow prostatic fluid to drain out more easily.

BENIGN PROSTATIC HYPERPLASIA (BPH) is a non-cancerous enlargement of the prostate gland. BPH is common in all races and cultures. Ten percent of men between the ages of 25 and 30 have BPH. By age 60, almost 50 percent of men have BPH, and by age 85 the prevalence is 90 percent. By age 80, one in four men in the US will require treatment for BPH.

The prostate grows in spurts – during puberty and during ages 40 to 50 – as a result of hormonal changes, especially the conversion of testosterone to dihydrotestosterone (DHT) via the enzyme 5 alpha-reductase. DHT stimulates cellular growth within the prostate. Also, estrogen begins to rise as men age and further enhances DHT.

Symptoms of BPH include frequent urination, urinary urgency, weak urinary stream, and a sensation of incomplete bladder emptying. Mild to moderate symptoms should be treated with medicines. Surgery should be used only if a patient develops complications of BPH such as urinary retention, kidney failure, blood in the urine, bladder stones or repeated urinary tract infections. For almost a century transurethral resection of the prostate (TURP), the removal of some of the inside of the prostate, has been the standard treatment. TURP is second only to cataract removal as the most commonly performed surgery on men over age 65.   About 400,000 TURPs are performed each year costing the American taxpayer about $8 to $10 billion dollars.

EVALUATING SYMPTOMS.   A treatment is effective if it improves the patient's symptoms and improves the urinary flow. In 1992, the American Urological Association (AUA) **Symptom Index** was found reliable to objectively evaluate symptoms of an enlarged prostate.[1] Answer each question below by ranking the frequency of your symptoms from 0 to 5 as shown:

0 = not at all	3 = about half the time
1 = less than 1 time in five	4 = more than half the time
2 = less than half the time	5 = almost always

1. Over the past month, how often have you had a sensation of not emptying your bladder completely after you finished urinating?   Score_____
2. Over the past month, how often have you had to urinate again less than 2 hours after you finished urinating?   Score_____
3. Over the past month, how often have you found you stopped and started again several times when you urinated?   Score_____
4. Over the past month, how often have you found it difficult to postpone urination?   Score_____
5. Over the past month, how often have you had a weak urinary stream?   Score_____
6. Over the past month, how often have you had to push or strain to begin urination?   Score_____
7. Over the past month, how many times did you most typically get up to urinate from the time you went to bed at night until the time you got up in the morning?   Score_____

TOTAL SCORE _____

Symptoms of prostate enlargement are classified as **Mild** if your total score is 0 - 7; **Moderate** if your score is 8 -18; and, **Severe** if your score is 19 - 35.

A second way to obtain objective information about your prostate is to assess your ability to urinate as measured by the urinary-flow rate. The urinary-flow rate is the single best non-invasive test to quantify obstruction of the urinary outlet and is determined by electronically recording the velocity of the urine as it flows out. The AUA Symptom Index and the urinary-flow rate help the physician to decide upon treatment and then determine if that treatment is working.

WHAT IF YOU DON'T TREAT BPH? Prostatitis and urinary bleeding are frequent complications of BPH. The bladder muscle squeezes hard to force the urine through the narrowed urethra (tube connecting the bladder and penis). As the passage gets smaller and smaller, the urine is expelled by a bladder muscle that must become stronger and consequently thicker. The thickened and stronger bladder also becomes more sensitive and causes a stronger urge to urinate more frequently. Often the bladder cannot empty completely, or sometimes not at all, requiring a catheter to relieve the build up of urine. Other complications of long standing BPH include bladder stones and kidney failure. In the US, approximately 1 to 2 men per 100,000 die of BPH complications. A physician cannot predict who will develop these complications.

ESTABLISHING THE DIAGNOSIS OF BPH. A physcian will take a medical history, do a physical examination that includes a digital rectal exam, inspect the urine for infection or bleeding, and get a blood test to assess kidney function (serum creatinine). The PSA (Prostate Specific Antigen) does not need to be done routinely, but if it is, the value may be elevated above the normal range of 0 to 4 ng/ml. In fact, about 25 percent of men with BPH have elevated PSA levels between 4 and 10. And about 5 percent have levels above 10.1 ng/ml. An elevated PSA may necessitate an ultrasound study of the prostate in an attempt to rule out cancer.

Tests that are not generally helpful: Cystoscopy; IVP – study of the kidneys with a dye, ultrasound of the kidneys; and filling cystometry - records the rate of bladder filling.

TREATMENT OF BENIGN PROSTATIC HYPERPLASIA should be done only if its symptoms are severe, or if the anatomy of your urinary tract is affected. There are several options:

• NO TREATMENT - if your symptoms do not bother you (AUA Symptom score 0-7). To decrease your symptoms, decrease liquids just before going to bed, and do not take antihistamines or decongestants. BPH symptoms may get better, stay the same, or get worse with no treatment.

• MEDICAL DRUGS -

Terazosin, an alpha-blocker drug, relaxes the smooth muscle in the prostate gland and **improves urinary symptoms and urinary flow.**[2] Terazosin may cause dizziness, lightheadedness, headaches, fatigue, and possible low blood pressure.

Finasteride, a 5 alpha reductase inhibitor, can shrink the prostate by blocking the conversion of testosterone to dihydrotestosterone, but **does not relieve any symptoms.**[2] Finasteride decreases the serum Prostatic Specific Antigen (PSA) by 50%. Finasteride has side effects including impotence, decreased libido, and ejaculation problems. Finasteride's warning insert:

> "**Esposure to Women - Risk to Male Fetus**
> It is not known whether the amount of finasteride that could potentially be absorbed by a pregnant woman through either direct contact with PROSCAR [finasteride] tablets or from the semen of a patient taking PROSCAR can adversely affect a developing male fetus. .....Therefore, because of the potential risk to a male fetus, a woman who is pregnant or who may become pregnant should not handle crushed PROSCAR tablets; in addition, when the patient's sexual partner is or may become pregnant, the patient should either avoid exposure of his partner to semen or he should discontinue PROSCAR."

Dutasteride, another 5-alpha reductase inhibitor, shrinks the prostate by blocking the conversion of testosterone to dihydrotestosterone. It **increases maximum urinary flow rates** and reduces lower urinary tract symptoms.[3]

Saw Palmetto (*Serenoa repens*) comes from a small palm tree found along the southeastern coast of the US and the West Indies. In early winter, a blue-black fruit appears and an extract from this berry is the major component of most commercial products. Although its mechanism of action is not fully understood, it does not work by inhibiting 5 alpha reductase. A systematic review shows that saw palmetto **improves symptoms of BPH and flow measures** with few side effects.[4] Recommended dose: 160 mg twice a day.

Pygeum africanum is an evergreen found in the mountains of Africa. The bark is composed of lipid-soluble phytosterols and pentacyclic triterpenes that appear to act synergistically to **improve symptoms of BPH**. The phytosterols, especially beta-sitosterol,[5] compete with androgen precursors and decrease prostate inflammation by decreasing prostaglandin levels in the prostate. The triterpenes also decrease inflammation and swelling. Ferulic acid esters in pygeum reduce the levels of cholesterol in the prostate, limiting androgen synthesis.[6] *Pygeum africanum* does not work by inhibiting 5 alpha reductase. A review of the clinical literature that involved over 2,000 patients show significant improvement in symptoms when objectively measured.[7] Extracts of Pygeum africanum should contain 14% triterpenes and 0.5% n-docosanol. Recommended dose: 100 mg – 200 mg per day in tablet form.

Cernitin is a pollen extract that may be the best natural product to treat BPH. Multiple trials involving close to 3,000 patients, both open and blinded, all show **improvement in the signs and symptoms of BPH and chronic prostatitis,** no matter what criteria were used.[8] Cernitin decreases inflammation and edema of the prostate. Dose: 120 mg, three per day.

- **INVASIVE TREATMENTS used when AUA score is > 19**

Balloon dilation stretches the urethra where the prostate has narrowed it. At the location of the narrowing, the catheter tipped with a balloon is inflated. Some patients have been helped by this technique for only a short time. Side effects include bleeding, infection, and the inability to urinate for a period of time after the procedure.

Stents are flexible catheters that remain in the penis permanently. Stents are not often used in the US.

Transurethral Incision of the Prostate (TUIP) is often the procedure of choice for men with symptoms of BPH secondary to a smaller prostate gland (30 grams), or for those who want to preserve sexual function, or have medical conditions that preclude general anesthesia and extensive surgery. In four randomized trials, this procedure was as beneficial as the more invasive TURP procedure and had fewer complications and less recovery time.[9-11]

Transurethral Resection of the Prostate (TURP) is done by inserting a special instrument into the penile urethra, and reaming out the inside of the prostate, thus enlarging the obstructed area. Approximately 25% of men who have a TURP do not have long-term satisfactory results. Other side effects include: retrograde ejaculation of semen backwards into the bladder in 75% of men, impotence in 5 to 10%, incontinence in close to 5%, and blood transfusion required in 10%. About 15 to 20% of men need a second TURP within the first 10 years of the initial TURP.

Open prostatectomy is indicated for men with very large prostates and is performed by entering the abdomen to remove part of the prostate - major surgery with some complications.

Microwave therapy heats prostate tissue to destroy the obstructing area. Results are similar to medical drug treatment except that 35 percent of men are unable to pass urine for up to 10 days after the procedure.

Laser prostatectomy is one of the most promising treatments today. The physician can directly visualize the tissue to be destroyed, and can complete the procedure in less than 20 minutes with a minimal of bleeding. The maximum benefit is not appreciated by the patient for six to eight weeks because the treated tissue is gradually sloughed off.

TREATMENT OUTCOMES

Generally, your symptoms will improve the most with a treatment if you had a very high AUA Symptom Score. As the treatments become more invasive going from left to right in Table 1, so do the complications, risk of death within the first three months, incontinence (inability to control urination), impotence, and cost.

BPH INCREASES THE RISK FOR PROSTATE CANCER BY 400% TO 500%. Cells in BPH are constantly changing and have a higher chance of tranforming into a cancer particularly if you expose them to risk factors, like a high-fat, low-fiber diet, smoking, alcohol, etc. A study of 304 patients who underwent TURP for confirmed BPH, were followed for up to eight years. Close to 10 percent of this group developed prostate cancer.[12]

Table 1. Treatment Outcomes for Various Modalities					
Outcome	No Treat	Herbal	Finesteride	TURP	Open Surgery
Symptoms Improved	40%	60%	60%	80%	97%
Complication	None	5%	20%	85%	79%
Risk of Death	None	None	None	3%	1-5%
Incontinent	None	None	None	2%	1%
Impotent	None	3%	5%	20%	25%
Cost per year	None	$400	$1200	$9000	$14,000

GYNECOMASTIA is the condition in which the male breast enlarges. This male breast condition occurs when the influence of estrogen or estrogen-like chemicals is greater than the influence of testosterone. Gynecomastia generally affects the left breast more often than the right.[13] This condition may affect as much as one-third of the male population of all ages from puberty to old age and is seen in 57% of men over age 44.[14,15] Gynecomastia is associated with four causes:

1. Hormonal Changes
- Normal changes in the Neonatal period, Puberty, or Elderly
- Abnormal disease conditions:
  - Testicle fails to work
  - Puberty or Postpuberty abnormalities
  - Klinefelter's syndrome
- Testicle fails to work secondary to:
  - Radiation, or Trauma
  - Infection: orchitis, tuberculosis, leprosy
  - Cryptochidism
  - Hydrocele, or Varicocele, or Spermatocele
- Thyroid underactivity or overactivity
- Hormones produced from cancers of:

o Testicles – Seminoma, Teratoma, Embryonal cell carcinoma, Andro-
blastoma, Choriocarcinoma, Interstitial (Leydig) cell
o Adrenal – Hyperplasia, carcinoma
o Pituitary Gland – Adenoma
o Lung bronchogenic carcinoma
o Liver Hepatoma

2. Drugs

Amiloride	D-penicillamine	Marijuana	Reserpine
Amphetamines	Ergotamine tartrate	Methadone	Spironolactone
Anabolic steroids	Estramustine	Methyldopa	Sulindac
Busulfan	Estrogen	Metronidazole	Tamoxifen
Chlorpromazine	Fluphenazine	Neuroleptics	Theophylline
Cimetidine	Flutamide	Perphenazine	Thiazide
Clomiphene	Guanabenz	Phenothiazines	Thiethylperazine
Diazepam	Heroin	Procarbazine	Thioridazine
Diethylstilbestrol	Isoniazid	Prochlorperazine	Trifluoperazine
Digoxin	Ketoconizole	Propanolol	Tricyclics
Diphenylhydantoin	Leuprolide	Ranitidine	Vincristine

3. Systemic Disorders
Chronic disease of: liver, kidney, lung, brain
Malnutrition or starvation
Cancer of the colon, prostate, or lymphoma
Ulcerative colitis, Rheumatic fever

4. Idiopathic – Cause unknown

MALE REPRODUCTIVE HEALTH

About 25 percent of a couple's infertility can be attributed to
the male. A review of 61 studies from all over the world
demonstrate a decreasing concentration and quality of sperm
from 1938 to 1990.[16-18] The average sperm count declined
from 113 million per milliliter to 66 million/ml. During the
same period of time, there has been an increase in the number
and types of abnormalities in the male reproductive system
and an increase in the number of testicular cancers.

Estrogens or estrogen-like chemicals have been identified
as the culprits.[19,20] Men are subjected to higher concentrations
of estrogens while as a fetus *in utero* and as children and
adults. High concentrations of estrogens *in utero* seem to be
the trigger of these abnormalities. Then, as a child and adult,
the male is exposed to more estrogen compounds and environmental chemicals that possess estrogen-like activity. These

same environmental pollutants cause similar abnormalities in wildlife. It may take 20 to 40 years before effects from high estrogen exposure become evident.

The pesticides thought to be responsible for these abnormalities include organochlorine pesticides (DDT, aldrin, and dieldrin), polychlorinated biphenyls PCBs), dioxins and furans, and alkyphenol polyethoxylates. Phytoestrogens, estrogen compounds found naturally in plant foods, as well as phthalates, also contribute to these abnormalities.

The determination of the gender of a human occurs during the first 12 weeks of pregnancy. Therefore, any factors that influence this process can potentially influence the future of the fetus. DES (diethylstilbesterol), given to millions of women from the 1940s to the 1970s to prevent miscarriages, caused abnormalities in the reproductive systems of the fetuses. Women were also exposed to DES from eating livestock that were fed DES to increase muscle mass. Men exposed to DES *in utero* have a higher incidence of reproductive abnormalities and low sperm counts. Men are also exposed to DES when they eat livestock fed with DES.

Thousands of other man-made chemicals have estrogenic effects that are used in our homes, agriculture, or industry. Only a few have been studied, and then only by accident. Most pesticides will circulate in the environment for generations and get concentrated in our fat cells that act as reserviors and slowly release them into the bloodstream. Some are banned, like PCBs, but others are still used, like alkylphenol polyethoxylates (APEs). APEs are present in the water supply and water sediment because bacteria breakdown detergents and paints that contain them. Phytoestrogens are ingested from plants, and influence your body because they can be metabolized and excreted. We must take a stronger stand on chemical pollutants over which we have control.

ERECTILE DYSFUNCTION can be caused by disorders of various systems: endocrine, vascular, neurologic, and psychiatric. Erectile dysfunction is the failure to have an erection, ejaculation, or both. Men who are impotent usually complain about one or more of the following: loss of libido (no desire), unable to initiate or maintain an erection, premature ejaculation, no ejaculation at all, or inability to achieve orgasm.   A limited discussion of these symptoms and how the body's systems contribute to them are reviewed.

• **Loss of libido** (no desire) may be due to low blood testosterone levels, psychological issues, or drug abuse.

• **Failure to initiate or maintain an erection** is due to:

Endocrine. Low testosterone levels can be secondary to improper testicular function. Testosterone can be given to this patient. High blood levels of prolactin, another hormone, can cause impotence and a search for the cause usually reveals a pituitary tumor in the brain.

Drugs include:

> Anti-testosterones: H-2 blockers (eg. Tagamet), spironolactone (a diuretic), ketoconazole (an anti-fungal antibiotic).
> Antihypertensives: Clonidine, methyldopa, beta-blockers, thiazides
> Antidepressants: Tricyclics, Monoamine oxidase (MAO) inhibitors
> Antipsychotics.
> Sedatives like barbituates.
> Antianxiety drugs.
> Abused drugs: alcohol, heroin, methadone.

• **Penis diseases** like trauma, previous priapism (abnormal persistent erection of the penis), or Peyronie's disease (hard fibrous tissue in the penis impeding erection).

• **Neurologic diseases**. Disruption of nerves due to surgery for the removal of the prostate, urinary bladder, or rectosigmoid colon can lead to impotence. Diseases in certain areas of the brain (anterior temporal lobe), or spinal cord can result in impotence.   Impotence also develops in diabetics because their nerves gradually malfunction (diabetic neuropathy).

• **Vascular diseases**. Because erections develop as a result of blood rushing into elastic blood vessels of the penis, any disease that compromises the integrity of blood vessels will hinder potency. These include: atherosclerosis (hardening of the arteries), occlusions of arteries or aorta, venous leak from the penis after blood has flowed in, and enzyme degradation.

During sexual excitation a chemical called cyclic guanosine monophosphate (cGMP) is increased by nitric oxide and causes smooth muscle relaxation in the penis allowing blood to rush in to form an erection. Mother Nature provides an enzyme, Phosphodiesterase type 5 to degrade cGMP so that the erection is not permanent. The cGMP decreases with age causing softer erections. Several prescription drugs (sildenafil, tadalafil, vardenafil) inhibit Phosphodiesterase type 5 and thereby allow even small amounts of cGMP to work resulting in erections.

Premature Ejaculation is generally related to anxiety or other emotional disorders, but not always. **Failure to ejaculate** may be related to several causes: surgery of the bladder or prostate, diabetes, testosterone deficiency, and certain drugs (guanethidine, phenoxybenzamine, and phentolamine). **Inability to achieve orgasm** is usually related to a psychiatric disorder if libido and erectile function are normal. **There appears to be no link between developing prostate cancer and the frequency or infrequency of ejaculation as was commonly thought.**[21]

SIMONE TEN POINT PLAN FOR PROSTATE HEALTH
Point 1. Nutrition.
- Maintain an ideal weight – decrease calories.
- No four-legged animals, shellfish, or dairy products unless they are skim products, not whole, 1%, or 2%. Poultry cooked without the skin.
- Consume *soluble* and *insoluble* fiber (25-35 grams/day). Fruits, vegetables, cereals are mainly *insoluble* fibers. Pectins, gums, and mucilages have *soluble* fibers that can decrease cholesterol, trigylcerides, sugars, and carcinogens. Use a supplement of *soluble* fiber to insure a consistent amount each day.
- Supplement your diet with certain nutrients in the proper doses, form, and combination based on your lifestyle. Take high doses of all antioxidants (the carotenoids, vitamins C

and E, selenium, cysteine, bioflavonoids, copper, zinc), and the B vitamins with food. Calcium and its enhancing agents should be taken at bedtime.

- Eliminate salt, food additives, smoked and pickled foods. Limit barbecues.
- Take 325 mg aspirin every other day if you are able.

Point 2. Tobacco. Do not smoke, chew, snuff, or inhale other people's smoke.

Point 3. Alcohol and Caffeine. No alcohol or less than 2 drinks a week. Avoid caffeine (coffee, tea, chocolate).

Point 4. Radiation. X-rays only when needed. Use sunscreens, and wear sunglasses. Avoid electromagnetic fields.

Point 5. Environment. Keep air, water, workplace clean.

Point 6. Sexual-Social Factors, Hormones, Drugs. Avoid promiscuity, hormones, and any unnecessary drugs.

Point 7. Learn the Seven Early Warning Signs

- Lump in breast
- Nonhealing sore
- Change in wart/mole
- Unusual bleeding
- Persistent cough/hoarseness
- Change in bowel/bladder habits
- Indigestion/trouble swallowing

Point 8. Exercise

Point 9. Modify Stress, Spirituality, Sexuality

Point 10. Comprehensive Physical Exam Yearly. Correct diagnosis is important. Prevention is the key to wellness.

THE PROSTATE CANCER PREVENTION TRIAL involved close to 19,000 men (92% white, 4 % African American) to see whether the drug finasteride could prevent prostate cancer in men ages 55 and older. The study began in 1993 at 221 sites in the United States and was stopped in 2003 because finasteride reduced the risk of developing prostate cancer by only 6 percent and increased the risk of high-grade cancers for those who developed prostate cancer.[22] The trial was funded by the National Cancer Institute with $74 million and conducted by the Southwest Oncology Group.

Men taking finasteride had only 6 percent fewer prostate **cancers** compared to the placebo group, **but the cancers in**

the finasteride group were of a higher grade (37 percent vs. 22 percent of the cancers in the placebo group). **Men are more likely to die from a high-grade cancer** because the high-grade cancers are more aggressive and are more likely to spread outside the prostate. Finasteride may cause these high-grade aggressive tumors to develop either by preventing only low-grade tumors, or by making the prostate gland more favorable to high-grade tumors.

Any drug used in a prevention trial should be totally safe. As you have already read, finasteride is not safe for women and male fetuses. In the trial just done, men are more likely to die from a high-grade cancer that finasteride caused. Should men with a benign condition – benign prostatic hyperplasia – take finasteride as treatment knowing that finasteride could develop a high-grade prostate cancer?

It would make a lot more sense to modify an entire lifestyle over a lifetime to prevent prostate cancer or any other cancer. We must continue to identify men who are at high risk for developing prostate cancer by using the self-assessment test in Chapter 3 combined with any biopsy, ultrasound, examination, and blood reports to make an overall prostate cancer risk assessment. We can then intervene by using the Simone Ten-Point Plan to promote a healthy lifestyle. One must decrease fat, increase fiber foods, eliminate smoking and alcohol consumption, use certain antioxidants and other nutrients, exercise, reduce stress by way of a stress modification program, and thereby change your risk for developing prostate cancer before it ever starts. We don't have the quick fix that most Americans want, a single pill like finasteride to get rid of all their ills.

If you have an illness, then take medicine for it. If you don't have an illness but are at high risk for it, change your lifestyle. It is your responsibility to keep yourself healthy. No single pill is a green light for you to continue eating the wrong foods, smoking, drinking alcohol, etc.

3

An Overview of Risk Factors

Numerous risk factors are associated with cancer. Many of them are also risk factors for cardiovascular and other chronic diseases. Learn and modify these risk factors and your risk for all illnesses will be reduced.

DIET AND NUTRITIONAL RISK FACTORS

There is a strong correlation between nutritional factors and many cancers (Table 1). The National Academy of Sciences and others estimate that nutritional factors account for 60 percent of cancer cases in women and 40 percent in men.[1-3] Cancers of the prostate, breast, colon, rectum, uterus, and kidney are closely associated with consumption of total fat and protein, particularly meat and animal fat. Other cancers that are directly correlated with dietary factors are cancers of the stomach, small intestine, mouth, pharynx, esophagus, pancreas, liver, ovary, endometrium, thyroid, and bladder.[4-9] Aflatoxin, a fungus product that is found on certain edible plants (especially peanuts), is related to human liver cancer.[10] Obesity is also an independent risk factor for cancer, especially breast cancer.

Japanese men and women who leave Japan and settle in Hawaii or the continental United States have a lower risk of stomach cancer than those who remain in Japan. Stomach cancer in the United States has been steadily decreasing with the advent of refrigeration and the consequent removal of carcinogenic chemicals as food preservatives. Also, the Japanese gen-

Table 1. Risk Factors and Associated Cancers

Risk Factor	Associated Human Cancer
Nutritional Factors	
High-fat, low-fiber	Prostate, colon, rectum, breast, stomach, mouth, pharynx, esophagus, pancreas, liver, ovary, endometrium, thyroid, kidney, bladder
Iodine deficiency	Breast, thyroid
Aflatoxin (fungus)	Liver
Obesity	Prostate, breast, endometrium, colon,
Tobacco Smoking, Chewing, Snuffing	Prostate, breast, lung, larynx, mouth, pharynx, head and neck, esophagus, pancreas, bladder, kidney
Involuntary Inhalation	Breast, lung, cervix, mouth
Alcohol	Prostate, breast, mouth, pharynx, esophagus, liver, GI, pancreas, head and neck, larynx, bladder
Radiation	
X-rays, etc.(ionizing)	Prostate, breast, skin, myelogen. leukemia, thyroid
Sunlight (UV)	Skin. [Lack of sunlight (low vitamin D) – Prostate]
Hormonal Factors	
Late/never pregnant	Breast
Lumpy Breast disease	Breast
DES-diethylstilbestrol	Breast, vagina, cervix, endometrium, testicle
Conjugated Estrogen	Breast, liver
Androgen-17 methyl	Prostate, liver
Undescended Testicle	Testicle
Sexual-Social Factors	
Female promiscuity	Cervix
Male homosexual promiscuity	Kaposi's sarcoma, anus, tongue
Poor male hygiene	Penis
Sedentary Lifestyle	Prostate, breast, colon, other sites
Stress	Implicated in multiple sites
Immune Abnormality	Lymphomas, carcinomas
Age greater than 55	Multiple sites
High Blood Pressure	Breast, colon
Environment	Leukemia, lung, skin, other sites
Pesticides	Prostate, breast, lung, liver, skin, other sites
Hair dye	Lymphoma, multiple myeloma
Occupation or Workers in:	
Chemists	Brain, lymphoma, leukemia, pancreas
Flight personnel	Prostate, breast, skin, melanoma, leukemia
Furniture/Shoe/Textile	Nasal sinus
Painters	Leukemia

Table 1. (continued) Risk Factors and Associated Cancers	
Risk Factor	**Associated Human Cancer**
Petroleum, tar	Lung, skin, scrotum
Printers / Foundry	Lung, mouth, pharynx
Rubber workers	Lung, bladder, leukemia, pancreas
Infections – specific	Stomach, lymphoma, leukemia, brain, cervix, anus

erally have lower rates of prostate, breast and colon cancer, but when they immigrate to the United States, after only twenty years, they have the same rate of colon cancer as Americans. After only two generations, they have the same rate of breast cancer. Cancers and their relationship to diet and nutritional factors are discussed in depth in later chapters.

CHEMICAL RISK FACTORS

Chemical and environmental factors, including diet and lifestyle, may be responsible for causing 80 to 90 percent of all cancers. Most cancers could be prevented if the factors that cause them were first identified and then controlled or eliminated. People are exposed to many chemicals and some drugs in small amounts and in many combinations unique to their culture and environment. Many drugs and chemicals are now known to cause human cancer, and many more are suspected carcinogens.[11] The drugs include: calcium channel blockers,[12,13] chlorambucil, chloramphenicol, cyclophosphamide, dilantin, hair dyes,[14] melphalan, phenacetin, and thiotepa. The chemicals include: acrylonitrile, aminobiphenyl, aniline, arsenic, asbestos, auramine, benzene, benzidine, beryllium, cadmium chemicals, carbon tetrachloride, chlormethyl ether, chloroprene, chromate, isopropyl alcohol, mustard gas, nickel, radon, and vinyl chloride.

Due to differences in their genetic make-up, individuals exposed to a carcinogen (a chemical substance that causes cancer) will not all have the same probability of getting cancer. Enzymes can break down or activate the carcinogen at different speeds in different people to either render it harmless or promote it to cause cancer. Food sources that induce these enzymes are vegetables of the *Brassicaceae* family – Brussels sprouts, cabbage, broccoli.[15]

ENVIRONMENTAL RISK FACTORS

Environmental factors are just as important. Those living in cities encounter many sources of pollution. More people smoke cigarettes in cities than in rural areas. Air pollution is a risk factor for cancer, especially lung cancer. Carcinogens derived from car emissions, industrial activity, burning of solid wastes and fuels remain in the air from four to forty days and thereby travel long distances.[16] Asbestos, a potent carcinogen, can also be found airborne in cities.

Our drinking water contains a number of carcinogens, including asbestos, arsenic, metals, and synthetic organic compounds that are associated with gastrointestinal cancers, skin cancers, and urinary bladder cancers.[17,18]

With many carcinogens, the time between exposure to the carcinogen and actual development of cancer may be quite long. Hence, a cancer initiated by trace amounts of either airborne or waterborne carcinogens years before the cancer appears may be attributed to an unrelated or unknown cause at the time of diagnosis.

We are able to detect many carcinogens in our environment, but many others exist in low concentrations. These environmental carcinogens may themselves cause cancer in certain individuals, or they may interact with other risk factors to initiate or promote cancers. Therefore, we must avoid introducing harmful substances into the environment.

RADIATION RISK FACTORS

The more radiation to which a person is exposed, the higher is the risk of developing cancer, especially if the radiation exposure is to bone marrow, where the blood cells are made. Almost 85 percent of the radiation to which we are exposed in developed countries is from natural sources, but 15 percent is from human-made sources. Of these, about 97 percent is from diagnostic radiology – mainly CT scans.[19]

The lifetime risk of developing cancer attributable to diagnostic X-rays is 1-2%, except in Japan where it is 3.2%.[20]

Table 2. Number of Cancers per Year from Diagnostic X-rays

Australia	431	Germany	2049	Poland	291
Canada	784	Japan	7587	Sweden	162
Croatia	169	Kuwait	40	Switzerland	173
Czech Republic	172	Netherlands	208	United Kingdom	700
Finland	50	Norway	77	United States	5695

Women who received many chest X-rays to follow the progress of treatment for tuberculosis had an increased incidence of breast cancer with as little as 17 cGy total dose. A cGy, or centiGray, is a defined amount of energy absorbed by a certain amount of body tissue. One chest X-ray using modern equipment delivers about 0.14 cGy. Riding in an airplane at 35,000 feet for six hours exposes a person to 0.01 cGy.

People who received radiation to shrink enlarged tonsils or to treat acne have a higher risk of developing cancer of the thyroid and parathyroid glands located in the neck. Survivors of the bombings of Hiroshima and Nagasaki had an increased incidence of leukemia, lymphoma, Hodgkin's disease, multiple myeloma, and other cancers. Female radiology technologists may have only a small increased risk for developing breast cancer. People who painted radium on wrist-watch dials have a high incidence of osteogenic sarcoma, a bone cancer. Chronic exposure of fair-skinned, easily sunburned people to sunlight (ultraviolet light) will lead to a higher rate of skin cancer.

People who work in or live near nuclear power plants have a higher risk of cancer. A higher incidence of childhood leukemia has been reported in children living near several nuclear facilities, most notably a fuel reprocessing plant located at Sellafield in England.[21] The results of another study involving over 8,000 men who worked in the Oak Ridge National Laboratory in Tennessee between 1943 and 1972 show that they had a higher risk of developing cancers, especially leukemia.[22] Another study shows no such increase in cancer incidence.[23]

Female flight attendants have a two-fold increased risk of developing breast cancer because they have chronic disturbances in sleep-wake cycles (circadian rhythms) with a resultant deficiency of melatonin.[24] Male cockpit flight members flying 5000 hours or more in jets have a higher risk of acute myeloid leukemia and prostate cancer.[25,26]

Workers in many industries are chronically exposed to low-dose radiation and, hence, may be at risk for cancer and heart disease. We therefore have to reexamine standards for acceptable radiation levels in industry.

OCCUPATIONAL RISK FACTORS

About 10 percent of all cancers are related to exposure to carcinogens on the job. The relationship between a person's job and cancer was noted in the eighteenth century when it was observed that the incidence of cancer of the scrotum was very high in chimney sweeps. Occupations and their associated human cancers are listed in Table 1.[27]

AGE AS A RISK FACTOR

The older you are, the higher the risk of developing any cancer. The Biometry Section of the National Cancer Institute shows that with every five-year increase of age there is a doubling in the incidence of cancer[28] because of the amount of time you have been exposed to risk factors. The elderly often suffer from nutritional deficiencies, and they have an increased number of infections, autoimmune diseases, as well as cancer. Werner's syndrome, which prematurely ages very young children so that they die in early adolescence, is characterized by an impaired immune system. These facts suggest that the immune system in the elderly is working inefficiently, partly due to poor nutrition.[29] Because the gastrointestinal tract absorbs nutrients less efficiently with age, the elderly need more nutrients in their diets. The number of elderly aged 65 or older in the US for the year 2000 is about 35 million and in 2030 will be 66 million.

Prostate cancer is related to age. Between ages 40 and 59, one in 44 men will develop prostate cancer. Between ages 60 and 79, about one in seven men will develop prostate cancer.

The overall lifetime risk for a man to develop prostate cancer is one is six.

GENETIC RISK FACTORS

People with certain inherited diseases are more prone to getting cancer. There are over 200 genetic conditions that have an increased incidence of cancer,[30] including mongolism or trisomy 21 syndrome, the immunodeficiency syndromes, Gardner's syndrome, and many more. These genetic abnormalities, although important for the physician to recognize, make a minor contribution to the causation of cancer. *Inherited genetic factors account for only a small fraction of all human cancers – less than 7 percent.* [31,32]

ATHEROSCLEROSIS AND CANCER   Atherosclerosis is a major cause of death. Commonly called "hardening of the arteries," it is a disease that narrows the inside diameter of the artery and thereby restricts the blood flow and oxygen beyond the narrowed portion causing tissue death. Pain is a symptom of either very low oxygen or outright death of tissues. When a person has a "heart attack," pain occurs because some tissues die and others don't receive enough oxygen.

What does atherosclerosis have to do with cancer? Well, a cancer-like growth of cells may be responsible for the development of heart and vessel disease. The first step in the formation of a narrowed artery is the manufacture of cells (endothelial cells) that line the inside of the artery. Then cholesterol gets deposited in these cells after they have increased in number – called a plaque. There is good evidence that these cells come from a single cell, that is, they are cloned from one common cell. Cloning is a form of cancer [33] and can be initiated by carcinogens, like hydrocarbons. If we eat food contaminated with these hydrocarbons or are otherwise exposed to them so that they get into our bloodstream, atherosclerosis may begin to develop. Of course this is just one of many factors involved in the development of atherosclerosis.

There is a relationship between high blood pressure and cancers of the prostate, breast, colon, and others.[34-36] The higher

the blood pressure and the older the person, the more alterations of DNA occur in cells. The more abnormal the DNA, the
more often it will lose control and form a cancer.

HORMONAL RISK FACTORS

Hormones influence a cell's growth and development, so if
there is an excess or deficit of hormones in the body, cells will
not function properly and may grow abnormally or aberrantly
and become cancer cells.

The longer a woman's body is bathed with estrogen, the
higher is her risk for breast cancer. Women who start menstruating early (age 11), or stop menstruating late (after age 55), or
who have never been pregnant, or who have become pregnant
after the age of 35, all have a greater risk for developing breast
cancer. Women who become pregnant before age 20 have a
reduced risk. Women whose mothers or other close relatives
have breast cancer have three times the normal risk of getting
breast cancer. Women who do not menstruate during their lifetime have a three to four times higher risk of developing breast
cancer after the age of 55. A lower risk of breast cancer is seen
in women whose ovaries cease to function or are removed surgically before age 35. Women who use oral contraceptives before age 25 for four years or more, or women who use hormone
replacement therapy for 5 years or more have a two-fold higher
risk for developing breast cancer.

Daughters of women who received DES (diethylstilbestrol)
therapy during pregnancy have developed cancer of the cervix
and vagina.[37] Sons of women who took DES have a higher risk
of developing cancer of the testicles because DES causes urinary tract abnormalities including undescended testicles,
which, if not corrected surgically before age 6, can develop
into cancer of the testicles.[38] Furthermore, women exposed to
these same synthetic estrogens in adult life have a higher risk
of developing cancer of the cells that line the inside of the
uterus (endometrial cancer). Male hormones can predispose to
both benign and malignant liver tumors.

Benign lumpy breast disease, a disease that affects about 80
percent of all women sometime during their lives, probably

represents a hormone imbalance. If a woman has had the disease over many years, she is at an increased risk of developing breast cancer. We have shown that benign lumpy breast disease can respond to certain nutrients and dietary modification.

SEXUAL-SOCIAL RISK FACTORS

Cancer of the cervix is associated with having sexual intercourse at an early age and with having multiple male sex partners, especially uncircumcised male partners. The human papilloma virus is usually responsible.

Cancer of the penis is a very rare disease in the United States. The primary risk factor is poor hygiene, especially in the uncircumcised male. Secretion and different organisms retained under the foreskin produce irritation and infection that predispose to cancer's cellular changes.

Promiscuous male homosexuals have a higher risk of Kaposi's sarcoma, cancer of the anus, cancer of the tongue, AIDS, and an abnormal immune system.

INFECTIOUS DISEASES AS RISK FACTORS

The International Agency for Research on Cancer concludes that certain infectious diseases cause human cancer[39,40](Table 3).

Table 3. Infectious Disease Pathogen – Human Cancer Associations	
Helicobacter pylori	Stomach Cancer
	Mucosa-Associated Lymphoma Tissue
Schistosoma haematobium	Bladder Cancer
Chlamydia trachomatis	Cervix Cancer
T-cell Lymphoma/Leukemia Virus I	Adult T-cell Lymphoma/Leukemia
T-cell Lymphoma/Leukemia Virus II	Hairy Cell Leukemia
Hepatitis B and C virus	Liver Cancer
Human Herpes Virus 8	Kaposi's Sarcoma
Epstein Barr Virus	Lymphoproliferative disorders
	Nasopharyngeal cancer
	Burkitt's Lymphoma, Hodgkin's
Human Papilloma Virus	Cervix Cancer, Anal-Genital Cancer
Simian Virus 40 – from monkey	Lymphoma, Brain, Osteosarcoma,
	Mesothelioma
JC Virus – from animal	Medulloblastoma
BK Virus – from animal	Neuroblastoma

Some animal viruses cause cancer in animals, like feline leukemia virus that causes leukemia in cats. Some of these animal viruses can cross over to humans and cause human cancers.[41-44] Up to 80 percent of the adult population worldwide is positive for polyomavirus viruses – Simian Virus 40, JC and BK Virus. The major source of known human exposure to Simian Virus 40 is from contaminated poliovaccines as well as monkey laboratory animals.

Cats infected with feline leukemia virus should be kept away from pregnant women (developing human fetus), children, and immunosuppressed people.

RISK FACTOR ASSESSMENT

My Cancer Risk Factor Assessment test that follows has been designed to assess your own risk factors based upon diet, weight, age, lifestyle, and other variables covered in this chapter. Take the test to evaluate your risk. We define risk for potentially developing cancer based upon the following letter combination totals:

Risk Level	Number A's	Number B's	Number C's
High Risk	2+	Any	Any
	1	4 or more	Any
Moderate Risk	1	3 or less	Any
	0	4 or more	Any
	0	2 to 3	2 or more
Low Risk	0	0	0
	0	1	2 or less
	0	0	2 or less

A person in a high-risk category will not necessarily develop cancer, but simply he/she is more at risk than a person in another category. Following are a few examples of persons with various risk factors, their relative degrees of risk for developing cancer, and what they should do to modify those risks, thereby reducing their chance of developing cancer (and/or cardiovascular disease). After each risk factor, the score is indicated in parentheses.

Consider Linda, a 56-year-old (C) New Jersey (B) house-wife (0). She is 5 feet 5 inches tall, weighs 160 pounds (B), eats red meat daily, eats several eggs per week, drinks milk daily, consumes very little fiber-containing foods, and does not eat a balanced diet (A). She also smokes two packs of cigarettes a day, and has done so for over fifteen years (A). Linda drinks socially (0) and has never had cancer (0), but her mother had breast cancer (B). She started having sexual intercourse at age 20 (0), first got pregnant, at age 24 (0), has a history of lumpy breast disease (C), never had any radiation (0), and is usually calm (0).

Linda's total score is two A's, three B's, and two C's. She is in the high-risk group. What can she do to modify her risk factors? She directly controls the most serious ones. I would advise her to terminate cigarette smoking abruptly and completely. Then I would suggest that she permanently modify her diet in order to reduce two other serious risk factors: her high-animal fat, high cholesterol, low-fiber diet, and her overweight problem. This would serve also to counter any weight gain that may occur when she stops smoking. Linda has no control over her age, the state in which she has lived, or her history of fibrocystic breast disease; but these are minor risk factors. By modifying the risk factors that she directly controls, she will, over the course of time, lessen her overall risk category and reduce her risk of developing cancer or cardiovascular disease.

The second example is Dave, a 24-year-old sexually active male homosexual who has many male partners and uses a drug called amyl nitrite (C). He smoked two packs of cigarettes a day for eleven years but quit one year ago (A). Up until a few months ago, he ate red meat daily, ate cheese daily, ate very few fiber-containing foods, and took no vitamins (A). His weight is normal (0), and he has never had cancer (0) nor have any of his family members (0). Until Dave was 21 years old, he lived in Alaska (0), but he has since lived in New York City.

Dave's total score is two A's, zero B's and one C. He is in the high-risk group, but by continuing not to smoke and by modifying his diet, he can dramatically lessen his overall risk.

Next is Nancy, a 27-year-old woman who smoked two packs of cigarettes a day until she quit eight years ago (B). She eats a well-balanced diet consisting of red meat five times a week, low-fat dairy products, and an average intake of fiber (B), and she is twenty pounds overweight (C). As a lifelong resident of Vermont (C), Nancy has been working in the furniture industry for the past seven years (B). She is taking birth control pills (B) and has been doing so for the past ten years. She is fair-skinned, sunburns easily, and enjoys sunbathing and using a suntanning booth year-round (B).

On the surface of things it looks as though Nancy's overall risk is not so bad, but when you examine the whole picture, you find she is in the moderate-risk category. Her total score is five B's and two C's. However, she is on the right track. She should do the following to reduce her overall risk: continue not to smoke, lose twenty pounds, modify her nutritional status, seek another means of birth control, use sun screens when sunbathing, and avoid suntanning booths.

The last example is Bob, a 50-year-old (0) male chemist (B) who is twenty-five pounds overweight (B) and a meat-and-potatoes man all the way (A). He has smoked two packs of cigarettes a day for the past thirty years (A), drinks four ounces of whiskey every day (A), has lived in Illinois most of his life (B), and is easily angered (C). His father died of lung cancer (B).

You know that Bob is in the high-risk category: three A's, four B's, and one C. As you can see, he does have risk factors that he can directly control. He should: stop smoking, modify his diet and lose weight, stop drinking alcohol or less than 2 drinks per week, and learn how to relax. All these modifications will greatly reduce his overall risk.

What can *you* do to reduce *your* risk for cancer? You have now identified the problem areas that need modification. Simple preventive measures can be taken to help you reduce your chances of developing cancer or cardiovascular disease. This book will show you how you can make relatively minor adjustments in your lifestyle to lessen your risk. In the following chapters, I will review nutritional risk factors and other risk factors that can lead to the development of prostate cancer. I will also tell you how the risk factors can be modified. Maintaining a good weight, eating a healthful diet (one that is low in animal fat, low in cholesterol, and high in fiber), choosing not to smoke or drink alcoholic beverages, avoiding or limiting exposure to the sun – all of these are just a few of the ways you can protect yourself from cancer. You must strive to maintain good health. Good health is no accident!

SELF-TEST

What is your risk of developing cancer? Take my **Cancer Risk Factor Assessment Test** to determine your risk for developing cancer according to your lifestyle factors. You will be able to determine which factors pose a risk, and then how to modify them according to my recommendations. Repeat the test in the future to see if your risk has been reduced.

Choose the statement that most applies to you and mark the score accordingly. After completely the questionnaire, add up your scores. The zero scores won't count in the total.

Cancer Risk Factor Assessment Test

Risk Factor	Score

1. Nutrition
- If during 50% or more of your life two or more apply to you:
  - (1) one serving of red meat daily (including luncheon meat)
  - (2) 6 eggs per week
  - (3) butter, milk, or cheese daily
  - (4) little or no fiber foods (3 gm or less daily)
  - (5) frequent barbecued meats
  - (6) below average intake of vitamins and minerals   Score A__
- If during 50% or more of your life two or more apply to you:
  - (1) red meat 4-5 times a week (including luncheon meat)
  - (2) 3-5 eggs per week
  - (3) margarine, low-fat dairy products, some cheese
  - (4) 4-15 gm fiber daily
  - (5) frequent barbecued meats
  - (6) average intake of vitamins and minerals   Score B__
- If during 50% or more of your life two or more apply to you:
  - (1) red meat and one egg once a week or none at all

    (2) poultry or fish daily or very frequently
    (3) margarine, skim milk, or skim milk products
    (4) 15-20 gm fiber daily
    (5) above average intake of vitamins and minerals   Score C__

2. Weight

Ideal weight for men is 110 lbs + 5 lbs per inch over 5 feet.
Ideal weight for women is 100 lbs + 5 lbs per inch over 5 feet.

- If you are 25 pounds overweight   Score B __
- If you are 10-24 pounds overweight   Score C __
- If you are less than 10 pounds overweight   Score 0 __

3. Tobacco

- Smoke 2 packs or more per day for 10 years or more   Score A __
- Smoke 1-2 packs for 10 yrs or more, or quit less than 1 yr Score A __
- Smoke less than 1 pack for 10 yrs or more, or pipe/cigar Score B __
- Smoked 1-2 pks/d, pipe or cigar, but stopped 7-14 yr ago Score B __
- Chew or snuff tobacco   Score B __
- Inhaled others' smoke for 1 or more hrs/day up to age 25 Score B __
- Inhaled others' smoke for 1 or more hrs/day from age 25 Score C __
- Never smoked, quit 15 years ago, never inhaled others'   Score 0 __

4. Alcohol

- If you drink 4 oz whiskey, and/or 8 oz wine, and/or
  24 oz beer daily or more   Score A __
- If you drink 2-4 drinks per week   Score B __
- If you drink less than that indicated above   Score 0 __
- If you drink 4 oz whiskey, 8 oz wine, 24 oz beer daily, and also
  Smoke less than 1 pack /day, or chew or snuff tobacco Score B __
  Smoke 1-2 packs per day, pipe or cigar   Score A __
  Smoke 2 or more packs per day   Score A __
- If you do not drink at all   Score 0 __

5. Hormonal

- If you started menstruating between ages 8 and 12   Score C __
- If you stopped menstruating at age 50 or older   Score C __
- If you never had menses at all   Score C __
- If your mother took DES, or you took DES or estrogens Score C __
- If you took oral contraceptives for 4 years + before
  age 25, or 10 or more during your lifetime   Score B __
- If had miscarriage/abortion in 1st trimester, 1st pregnancy Score C __
- If 1st pregnant after age 35, or never were pregnant   Score C __
- If you have/had lumpy painful breasts premenstrually   Score C __
- If your bra cup size is D or greater   Score C __

6. Prostate Biopsy Report

- If your biopsy showed high-grade PIN (Prostatic
  Intraepithelial Neoplasia)   Score B __

7. Radiation Exposure
- If you received multiple X-rays or radiation treatments, or if you were exposed to radioactive isotopes, radioactive weaponsScore C __
- If you are fair-skinned and sunburn easily   Score B __
- If neither applies   Score 0 __

8. Occupation
- If you are a radiologist, chemist, painter, luminous dial painter, or worker in: leather, foundry, flight, dye, printing, rubber, petroleum, furniture, textile, nuclear, slaughterhouse, plutonium/uranium   Score A __
- Never was one of the above workers   Score 0 __

9. Chemicals
- If you worked with: acrylonitrile, aminobiphenyl, aniline, arsenic, asbestos, auramine, benzene, benzidine, beryllium, cadmium chemicals, carbon tetrachloride, chlormethyl ether, chloroprene, chromate, isopropyl alcohol, mustard gas, nickel, radon, and vinyl chloride   Score A __
- If you worked indirectly with one of the above   Score C __
- Never worked with one of the above   Score 0 __

10. Sexual-Social History
- If you are a female who started having intercourse before age 16 with multiple male partners, particularly uncircumcisedScore C __
- If you are a promiscuous male homosexual   Score C __
- If neither applies   Score 0 __

11. Immunity, Drugs, Hormones
- If your doctor said you have an immune deficiency   Score A __
- If you had an organ transplant   Score A __
- If you've taken for prolonged time: calcium channel blockers, chlorambucil, chloramphenicol, cyclophosphamide, dilantin, hair dyes, melphalan, steroids   Score A __
- If you've taken for prolonged time: phenacetin, thiotepa Score A __
- If none of the above applies   Score 0 __

12. Geography
- If during most of your life you've live in the Northeast   Score A __
- If during most of your life you've lived in the Midwest   Score C __
- If during most of your life you've lived elsewhere in US   Score 0 __

13. Age
- If your age is 70 or more   Score B __
- If your age is 55 to 60   Score C __
- If your age is 54 or less   Score 0 __

14. Personal History
- If you had cancer   Score B __
- If you never had cancer   Score 0 __

15. Family History
- If your parents or grandparents had cancer   Score B __
- No family history of cancer   Score 0 __

16. Exercise
- If you exercise very little or not at all   Score C __
- If you exercise 3 or more times per week and get your
  heart rate 50% higher than normal for 20 minutes   Score 0 __

17. Stress
- If easily frustrated or angered, or can't control stress   Score C __
- If comfortable while waiting, and can control stress   Score 0 __

TOTAL SCORE: ____A's; ____B's; ____C's

PART TWO

The Body's Defenses

4
Nutrition, Immunity, and Cancer

Nutrition affects immunity [1,2] and also affects the development of cancer [3,4] either directly or indirectly via the immune system. The immune system is a complex interaction of blood cells, proteins, and processes that protect you from infections, foreign substances, and cancer cells that spontaneously develop.

White blood cells and antibodies are two major armies of the immune system. A lymphocyte is a type of white cell involved in cellular immunity. Lymphocytes are divided into two groups, T cells and B cells. T lymphocytes, or T cells, are derived from or are under the influence of the *thymus*, an organ in the neck and front part of the chest that is functionally active in early childhood. T cells fight cancer, fungi, certain bacteria (intracellular), some viruses, transplant rejections, and delayed skin reactions (tuberculosis skin test). T cells can be divided into helper T cells and suppressor T cells, those that either help or hinder normal immune cellular function. B cell lymphocytes produce proteins called antibodies or immunoglobulins. B cells originate in the *bone* marrow, from which they derive their designation. Antibodies are formed by the B cells in response to a foreign substance introduced into the body.

In 1980, I showed how a white blood cell and complement proteins kill abnormal cells. They do so by making holes in the abnormal cell's membrane, thereby allowing water to rush in

and explode the cell. White blood cell extends feet-like processes that kill the targets. [5]

Phagocytes are another group of white cells that reside in
the blood and body tissues to recognize and dispose of abnormal cancer cells and other foreign substances. Phagocytes can
perform this task alone or can recruit antibodies and complement proteins to aid in the disposal.

IMMUNOLOGY AND CANCER

The immune system is extremely intricate and finely tuned.
If any one aspect of the system malfunctions because of poor
nutrition, or if it is destroyed, you may become susceptible to
cancer and foreign microbial invaders. The white blood cell
army and the antibody army must be functioning perfectly to
destroy any cancer cell or foreign invader and prevent either
one from gaining a foothold in your body.

The major histocompatibility complex is part of your genetic make-up and is another component of the immune system, acting as a commander of the white blood cell and antibody armies. This complex allows the immune system to recognize the parts of your body so that it does not destroy them
as it would destroy foreign substances. At the same time, it can
recognize a substance or tissue (histo-) that does not belong to
its body and subsequently take the necessary steps to destroy it.

Killer cells of the immune system watch, or keep a surveillance on, all cells in the body and immediately destroy any
cells that start to have a malignant or cancerous potential.[6] The
most convincing evidence for this comes from observations of
patients with suppressed immune systems caused by drugs or
radiation or an inherited disorder. Patients with inherited im-
munodeficiencies, whose immune systems do not function
normally from birth, or patients whose immune systems ac-
quire a malfunction later in life have 100 times more deaths
due to cancer than the expected cancer death rate in the normal
population.[7,8] Kidney transplant patients, who receive drugs to
suppress the immune system's ability to reject the new kidney,
also have a higher rate of cancer than expected.[9,10] The cancers

most frequently seen in these cases are the lymphomas and epithelial cancers; however, all other types of cancers have been reported.

The immune system is relatively immature in infancy, and then becomes weak with advancing age. These two times of life have the highest incidence of lymphocytic leukemia. Other immune-deficiency states that can lead to cancer are seen with malaria, acute viral infections, and malnutrition.

NUTRITION AND THE IMMUNE SYSTEM

Nutritional deficiencies decrease a person's capacity to resist infection, and decrease the capability of the immune system.[11] In old age, the immune system is impaired mainly because of nutritional deficiencies.[12] Poor nutrition adversely affects all components of the immune system, including T cell function, other cellular-related killing, the ability of B cells to make antibodies, the functioning of the complement proteins, and phagocytic function. When several of these functions or processes are impaired, the ability of the entire immune system to keep a watchful eye for cancer cells, abnormal cells, or foreign substances and to dispose of them is also markedly impaired. Table 1 summarizes the factors that affect the functioning of the immune system.

Table 1. Factors That Influence the Immune System

Enhance	Suppress
Nutrition	Nutrition
Low-fat, high-fiber diet	High-fat diet
Antioxidants	High sugar level
Carotene, vitamins E & C,	Obesity
Selenium, cysteine, copper	Soy and Corn oil
flavonoids, zinc	Tobacco
B vitamins, pantothenic acid	Alcohol
Calcium	Radiation
Exercise	Lead, cadmium, mercury
Stress Modified; Loving	Certain Drugs
Clean air and pure water	Environmental pollutants
	Ozone depletion [13,14]
	Stress
	Sedentary Lifestyle
	Exhaustive Exercise [15,16]

Protein deficiency impairs the ability of phagocytes and T cells to kill.[17,18] Antibody production is reduced as is the speed with which it attaches to an "enemy."[19] Complement proteins also are impaired.

Sugar levels – high or low – adversely affects the immune system. The function of phagocytes, and T and B cells are impaired if the sugar is too high (diabetes) or too low (hypoglycemia).[20-22] The degree of impairment correlates well with the fasting blood sugar level and improves as the sugar level becomes normal.

Lipids have a significant effect on the functioning of the immune system. Cholesterol and fats inhibits antibody production[23] and the functioning of T cells and phagocytes.[24,25]

The Epstein-Barr virus may manifest itself by causing entirely different diseases in different people as a result of varying degrees of impairment of the immune system. The extent to which the immune system is weakened or damaged is partly determined by the nutritional status of the individual prior to infection. Epstein-Barr virus is implicated in many diseases: a relatively benign disease, infectious mononucleosis; a slow-growing cancer, nasopharyngeal cancer; and a rapidly growing, usually fatal cancer, Burkitt's lymphoma; as well as other diseases. Why does one person's immune system permit infectious mononucleosis to develop and another person's immune system permit a fatal cancer to develop? The answer is very complex and not well defined at all, but nutritional status is a factor.

Your nutritional status is determined by how well your diet and supplementation program is meeting your nutritional needs. The better your nutritional status, the better your immune system, and the better off you will be.

5

Antioxidants and Other Cancer-Fighting Nutrients

Living cells contain proteins, nucleic acids, carbohydrates, lipids, and certain organic substances that function in very small amounts, called vitamins. Vitamins are essential to life and the immune system, and play a crucial role as helper enzymes in important chemical functions of the body. Vitamins interact with each other, and some can be stored for long periods of time, while others have to be supplied on a daily basis. Certain drugs and hormones can produce a gradual vitamin deficiency.

A person who is grossly deficient in vitamins demonstrates specific symptoms and complaints. But a person with only marginal deficiencies demonstrates no such signs or symptoms and does not appear to be ill.

Do you consider your diet to be well balanced? Do you think it is meeting your nutritional needs? Although you may believe it is fulfilling your requirements, you will most likely find that your diet is deficient in at least one nutrient. Consider the following sections.

MARGINAL DEFICIENCIES

Marginal deficiency is a gradual vitamin depletion in which there is evidence of personal lack of well-being associated with impairment of certain biochemical reactions.[1,2] The person may complain of non-specific symptoms such as fatigue, decreased mental acuity, loss of appetite, irritability, inability to sleep, and decreased resistance to disease, infection, as well as poor wound healing. Comprehensive studies confirm marginal deficiencies by measuring blood levels or assessing dietary ingestion.[3-6] **About 50 percent of all people examined and surveyed, whether rich or poor, educated or not, had at least one, and usually two or three marginal nutrient deficiencies.**

LIFESTYLE AND EATING PATTERNS

Lifestyle and eating patterns can lead to nutrient deficiencies. There is an increased demand for convenience foods and fast-food. Eating patterns have changed. About 25% of Americans skip breakfast, 25% skip lunch, almost 50% snack, and most eat one meal a day away from home. In 1965 affluent whites ate less healthy compared to poor African-Americans; by 1991, the diets of both were similar.[7]

In the federally sponsored HANES II study, people were asked to choose a food that they liked and considered "balanced." For a "balanced" vegetable, the majority chose French fries over broccoli; for meat/legume, hot dogs over split peas; and for grain, white bread over whole wheat. In the same study, favorite foods included coffee, doughnuts, soft drinks, and hamburgers. The percentage of calories in the American diet derived from fat is 42; from sugar, 24.

When caloric intakes fall below 1,600 calories, most nutritional guidelines cannot be met.[8] And below 1,800 per day, which about 50 percent of the population consumes at times, trained nutritionists have trouble designing meals to provide the minimum RDIs.[9] The Nationwide Food Consumption Survey[10] found that over 50 percent of people who thought they ate the "well-balanced" diet had deficiencies in vitamins A, C, B1, B2, B6, B12, calcium, magnesium, and iron. Women of all economic levels had low intakes of vitamins A, C, B6, calcium, iron, and zinc.[11]

Outright vitamin deficiencies occur in two groups of people. In the first group, people are unable to buy the right kinds of food either because of the expense or because they are not knowledgeable about the proper foods. The second group consists of people whose nutrient deficiency occurs as the result of a specific disease or a drug or other treatment therapy.

Americans unknowingly eat foods that are sprayed with chemicals, refined, processed, over-cooked, frozen, canned, stored, and trucked around the country. Many of our meats contain the hormones and chemicals that have been fed to animals. All of these foods have been depleted of nutrients to varying degrees. Some methods of cooking can totally destroy nutrients or decrease their concentration, and some nutrients are not stable in heat or boiling water. As a result, Americans do not or cannot eat a healthful balanced diet.

We get about one-third of our calories from sources of little or no nutrient value. The average American consumes about 60 pounds of sugar each year and four to five times the amount of salt necessary, favors carbonated drinks to others when not consuming 2.6 gallons of alcoholic beverages each year (if of drinking age). In short, it is very difficult to find an individual who consistently, on a daily basis, eats a "well-balanced diet" – that is, one containing foods that are freshly prepared, varied, and nutritionally adequate.

GROUPS AT RISK FOR NUTRIENT DEFICIENCIES

There are multiple groups of our population that may not be "healthy" and that may be considered to be "at risk" for inadequate nutrient intake. The RDIs do not take into account the special needs of these people. The greater requirements of the groups listed in Table 1 need to be recognized and addressed.

ANTIOXIDANTS REDUCE CANCER RISK

Since the 1950s a huge volume of evidence has demonstrated that antioxidants reduce the risk of cancer. The evidence is so overwhelming that I will cite only the main references and review articles.

Oxidation causes cancer, and inflammation causes cancer because of free radical production.[92-104] Antioxidants reduce the risk of cancer because they neutralize free radicals (Chapter 6) and the oxidative reaction that is caused by free radicals, thus interfering with the initiation and promotion phases of cancer.

Table 1. Candidates for Nutrient Supplementation		
Risk Group	**Million**	**Nutrient Deficiencies**
Alcohol drinker (3+ drinks/week)	90	Carotene, vitamins A, B6, D, folate, thiamine [12-22]
People with Alleriges or Food Intolerance	80	Any or all
Cigarette Smokers	50	Carotene, vitamins C, E, B6, Folate [23-32]
Dieters	45	Any or all [33-37]
Hospitalized Patients	36	Any or all [38]
Osteoporosis Patients	34	Calcium, vitamin D, others
People with Chronic Diseases	31	Any or all [39-44]
Elderly Patients	25	Folate, vitamins C and D [45-51]
Surgical Patients	24	Any or all
Oral Contraceptive Users	18	Carotene, folate, B6 [52-57]
Teenagers	17	Vitamin A, folate [58,59]
Diabetics	11	Vitamins C, D, B6, Magnesium [60,61]
Pregnant Women	7	All [62]
People with Infections	5	Any or all
Strict Vegetarians	1	Vitamins B12 and D
Stressed People	*	B vitamins, any and all
Athletes, Exercisers	*	B vitamins, any and all
Consumers of High-Fat Foods	*	Any and all
Low income people	*	Vitamin A and C, B vitamins, iron [63]
Premature Infants/Toddlers	*	Vitamins A,C,E, iron [64-68]
Children with low IQs	*	Any and all [69-83]
Psychiatric Patients	*	Any and all [84]
People with Aggressive / Criminal Behavior	*	Any and all [85-90]
Drug Addicts	*	Antioxidants, any and all [91]

*Unknown Millions

formation.[105,106] Antioxidant nutrients include beta-carotene, vitamin C, vitamin E, selenium, alpha-lipoic acid, copper, zinc, bioflavonoids, and cysteine.

CELLULAR AND ANIMAL STUDIES [107-115]
Hundreds of studies demonstrate that antioxidants protect normal cells from transforming to cancer and animals from developing cancer. Antioxidants like the carotenes, vitamins E and

C as well as selenium protect the cell membrane from carcinogens by allowing it to communicate efficiently and by preventing uncontrolled growth characteristic of cancer. Antioxidants can even reverse the transformation process.

HUMAN EVIDENCE
Epidemiological and Cohort Studies

An **extensive review** of the evidence **shows that vitamin E and C reduce the risk for cancer,** and neither antioxidant cause any harm.[116,117] Multiple observational studies, including the Iowa Women's Health Study, demonstrate protection against colorectal cancer with vitamin E, some protection with vitamin A, but none with vitamin C. [118,119]

A cohort study is one that investigates a specific group of people prospectively. **A review of 24 cohort studies demonstrate that supplemental vitamins C, E, A, carotene, selenium, multivitamins, or any combination of these confer protection against cancer or had no effect, but none report harm.** [118] This is a massive amount of data. Below are some additional studies.

- *Breast Cancer* [119-125] Antioxidants, including beta-carotene, vitamins C and E, or vitamin A, other nutrients, and/or fiber alone or in combination decrease the risk for breast cancer by as much as 20 percent. In one of these studies, vitamin E was shown to reduce the risk for cardiovascular disease.
- *Endometrial Cancer* [126] occurs mainly in older women who are obese and eat a high-fat diet. Antioxidants help protect against it. The antioxidant enzymes glutathione S-transferase and superoxide dismutase were significantly lower in patients who had cancer of the endometrium compared to patients undergoing hysterectomy without cancer.
- *Cervical Cancer* [127] Patients who had cervical cancer or cervical dysplasia had significantly lower levels of beta-carotene than women who had normal cervices.
- *Oral And Pharyngeal Cancer* [128-130] People who took supplements containing vitamins A, C, E, and B complex had a much lower risk for oral and pharyngeal cancer after control-

ling for the effects of tobacco, alcohol, and other risk factors. This was confirmed by a US National Cancer Institute study. Another study showed people with high levels of carotenoids including beta-carotene, alpha-carotene, cryptoxanthin, leutin, and lyocopene – but particularly beta-carotene – had a much lower rate of getting oral cancer than the control population. High blood levels of vitamin E and beta-carotene together provided the most protection against oral cancer.

- *California Study* [131] investigated over 11,600 people during 8 years. Women with higher dietary intakes of vitamin C, vegetables and fruits or fruits alone, had a lower risk for developing cancer at all sites, especially colon cancer. Taking supplements of beta-carotene, vitamin A as well as vitamin C and E were associated with a lower risk of getting lung cancer, colon cancer, and bladder cancer.
- *Hawaiian Study* [132] Beta-carotene, alpha-carotene, and lutein all conferred protection against lung cancer. Lycopene and beta-cryptoxanthin showed no such protective effects. It was found that beta-carotene conferred the most protection.
- *Finland Study* [133] Over 4,500 men entered a 20 year study. The nonsmokers who had low intakes of carotenes, vitamin E, and vitamin C had high risk of developing lung cancer. Those who had the least intake of these antioxidant nutrients were twice as likely to develop lung cancer.
- *Switzerland Study* [134] Serum levels of vitamins A, C, and E as well as beta-carotene were measured in almost 3,000 men. Men with low levels of beta-carotene and vitamin C had a higher risk of dying from lung and stomach cancer. Men who had low levels of both vitamin A and beta-carotene had an increased risk of all cancers.

Case Control Studies

Over 45 case control studies have been done and several reviews of them have been written.[118,135] **The overwhelming conclusions are that antioxidants reduce the risk of cancer and no harm is caused by them.** Additional studies below:

- *Pediatric Brain Cancer Study* [136] The risk of a child developing brain cancer decreased by 30% if the mother took antioxidants for 2 trimesters of the pregnancy.
- *Basel Study* [137] showed that high plasma levels of vitamins C, E, retinol, and carotene reduced the risk of death overall and reduced the risk for lung cancer and prostate cancer.
- *Physicians' Health* Study [138,139] found that higher levels of lycopene and vitamin C reduced the risk for prostate cancer.

Intervention Studies involve a specific treatment, like nutrients, over a course of time to determine an outcome. The best known are: Linxian study, ATBC study, Physician's Health study, Carotene and Retinol Efficacy Trial (CARET), Clark's study of selenium. The authors who reviewed all of these state: **"Overall there is evidence for protective effects of nutrients from supplements against several cancers."**[118]

- *Linxian, China Study* [140-142] In north central China in the county of Linxian, Henan Province, are people who have the world's highest rates of esophageal cancer and a high rate of stomach cancer. The people of Linxian also have a very high rate of marginal nutritional deficiencies. In Linxian, esophageal cancer deaths are one hundred times higher than the rate for Caucasian Americans and ten times higher than the rate for China in general. Since poor nutrition is linked to these two cancers and since marginal deficiencies are very common in the people of Linxian, an intervention trial was conducted.

  Researchers from the Cancer Institute of the Chinese Academy of Medical Sciences and the US National Cancer Institute studied almost 30,000 adults, randomizing them over five years. The findings were spectacular.
  - Three antioxidant nutrients taken together daily – beta-carotene (15 mg), vitamin E (60 IU), and selenium (50 mcg organic) – significantly reduced total mortality (9 percent) especially from all cancers (13 percent) and particularly stomach cancer (21 percent).
  - These antioxidants also reduced the risk of cancer.

- o These antioxidants substantially reduced the prevalence of cataracts in the oldest patients (aged 65-74 years).
- o These antioxidants reduced the mortality from stroke.

The doses used in the study are relatively low; I recommend much higher doses. Five years is a short time; imagine what the results would be in a population taking these antioxidants as well as other nutrients in higher doses for a lifetime.

- *Small Cell Lung Cancer Study* [143] Patients who received conventional therapy and also antioxidants lived longer than those who just received conventional treatment. The patients receiving the antioxidants were able to tolerate chemotherapy and radiation therapy better. And when antioxidant treatment was started earlier, survival was longer.

ANTIOXIDANTS AND PRE-CANCER CONDITIONS

- *Esophageal Dysplasia Intervention Study* in Linxian, China [144] More than 3,300 patients with esophageal dysplasia, a precursor to esophageal cancer, were studied by the same team of researchers from China and the United States as above. One group received a placebo. The other group received a multiple vitamin-mineral supplement daily for six years that contained doses two to three times higher than the U.S. Recommended Dietary Intake: beta carotene 15 mg, vitamin A 10,000 IU, vitamin E 60 IU, vitamin C 180 mg, folic acid 800 mcg, thiamin 5 mg, riboflavin 5.2 mg, niacinamide 40 mg, vitamin B6 6 mg, vitamin B12 18 mcg, vitamin D 800 IU, biotin 90 mcg, pantothenic acid 20 mg, calcium 324 mg, phosphorus 250 mg, iodine 300 mcg, iron 54 mg, magnesium 200 mg, copper 6 mg, manganese 15 mg, potassium 15.4 mg, chloride 14 mg, chromium 30 mcg, molybdenum 30 mcg, selenium 50 mcg, and zinc 45 mg. The group that took the supplement:
  - o 8% lower mortality from esophageal, stomach cancers.
  - o 7% lower overall mortality.
  - o 4% lower rate of death from cancer in any site.
  - o 38% lower risk of dying from stroke.

Here again the results are spectacular despite the short duration of time and the low doses. Other trials with positive results used 30 to 90 mg of beta-carotene[145,146] and 800 IU of vitamin E to treat precancerous oral lesions.[147,148]

● *Colorectal Polyp Adenomas*
Most colon cancers arise from adenomas. Patients with colorectal adenomas[149] were given vitamins A, C, and E for six months after complete polypectomy. After thorough analysis, those who received the vitamins were less likely to develop future adenomas compared to the placebo group.

ANTIOXIDANTS AND OTHER DISEASES
Free radicals are now considered to be the cause of many chronic illnesses (Free Radical Chapter). It is therefore crucial that we be aware of the protection offered by antioxidants. Only the major studies or reviews will be cited in Table 2.

Table 2. Antioxidant Supplementation

Decreases Risk for	Enhances
Aggressive Behavior [85-90]	I.Q. [69-83]
Angina [150]	Memory [219]
Arthritis and Inflammation [151]	
Cardiovascular Disease [152-182]	
Cataracts [140-142, 182-200]	
Drug Addiction [91]	
Hepatitis C [201]	
Hypertension [202]	
Macular Degeneration [203-207]	
Neurological Diseases	
Alzheimer's [208, 209]	
Dementia [210]	
Epilepsy [211]	
Lou Gehrig's Disease [212]	
Parkinson's Disease [213-215]	
Tardive Dyskinesia [216-218]	

INDIVIDUAL ANTIOXIDANTS
You should be aware of the beneficial effects, recommended doses, and the possible toxicity of:

Beta-carotene
- Most potent antioxidant of free radicals and singlet oxygen.
- Cancer and Cardiovascular Disease risk – reduced. [220-222]
- Immune System – enhanced. [223]
- Cataracts and other eye disease risk – reduced. [224]
- Toxicity: None in any amount. [225]

The ATBC and CARET studies erroneously suggested that beta-carotene increased the risk of lung cancer in heavy smokers who drank alcohol and had asbestos exposure. Multiple reasons cast doubt that carotene increases cancer risk: [226,227]

1. Cancers start between 10 and 20 years before symptoms occur or our technology can detect them. These heavy smokers and drinkers already had developed their cancers that were simply not detected with the methodology used.
2. The smokers who had high carotene serum levels at the start of the study had the lowest incidence of lung cancer.
3. Most of the study participants were alcoholics, and all ate a high fat diet – both risk factors independently increase cancer risk. Other risk factors were not indicated.
4. Beta-carotene did not increase the risk of lung cancer for those who smoked less than 20 cigarettes a day and drank little or no alcohol.
5. Beta-carotene works most efficiently at the early stages of carcinogenesis, not at the later stages when a cancer is already formed.
6. Over 200 studies have demonstrated that beta-carotene is safe and can lower the risk of cancer and cardiovascular disease, or has no effect, including harm.
7. All intervention studies show that beta-carotene and other nutrients can decrease cancer rates and cancer progression.
8. A total of 22 epidemiological studies that included 400,000 smokers and nonsmokers have shown those who

had a high blood level of beta-carotene had a lower incidence and mortality of lung cancer.

9. None of these studies reported any association with an increased incidence of lung cancer, including the Physician's Health Study which was the longest and largest trial of beta-carotene in which 11% of the physicians remained smokers. In fact, the reduction in risk was more pronounced in smokers than in nonsmokers.

It is important to rely on the synergism of all the antioxidants, including the carotenoids, vitamins C and E, selenium, and also the B's, etc., as well as lifestyle changes to decrease one's risk of cancer and heart disease. It is foolish to expect that a single nutrient can give the "green light" to continue lifestyle behavior that will cause disease.

- Simone recommended dose: 30-40 mg per day.

Vitamin E

One vitamin E molecule fits snugly between polyunsaturated fat molecules. This location and closeness to the polyunsaturated fats is extremely important because vitamin E competes with the polyunsaturated fat for free radicals that are formed when polyunsaturated fats react with oxygen. This means that if there are more vitamin E molecules than polyunsaturated fat molecules, the radicals will be taken out of the system and neutralized by vitamin E. The more polyunsaturated fats you eat, the more vitamin E you require.

- Potent antioxidant.
- Cancer risk – reduced, [228-258] especially bladder, breast, cervix, colon polyps, colon, lung, oral cavity, prostate, skin, stomach – as shown in intervention, prospective, retrospective studies.
- Cardiovascular Disease risk – reduced and reduces progression of coronary artery blockages. [259-263]
- Smog – protects you from free radicals of smog. [264]
- Lumpy Breast Disease (fibrocystic) – reduced. 85% of women who took 600 IU of vitamin E daily for eight weeks

had relief of their breast pain pre-menstrually, and some had demonstrable regression of disease. [265]

- Diabetes complications – reduced when taking 600 to 1200 IU of vitamin E daily. [266]
- Allergy Reactions – reduced. [267]
- Toxicity: There is no case on record of vitamin E toxicity or any indication of vitamin E toxicity. A daily intake of 800 IU of vitamin E per 2.2 pounds of body weight for five months has not been toxic. This equals 56,000 IU for an average man weighing 140 pounds, or about 5,600 times the RDI.

As ridiculous as it may sound, some people, including some physicians, "believe" that vitamin E causes cancer. They reason that since the molecule of vitamin E looks similar to estrogen, it can cause breast cancer. This is absolutely absurd! There are hundreds of molecules in the body that are formed from the same basic cholesterol ring structure. The body is able to discriminate one molecule from another even if there is only a slight difference between their structures. For instance, what differentiates men from women is a mere methyl group, CH_3, on a cholesterol-steroid chemical compound. Obviously, Mother Nature has this under control.

- Toxicity – None. Vitamin E has never been shown to cause cancer or changes in the DNA or RNA, nor has it ever been shown to cause changes in fetal development – even at very high doses of 3,200 IU per day. [268-270]
- Simone recommended dose: 400-1600 IU per day.

Vitamin C
Vitamin C is a major factor in controlling and potentiating multiple aspects of human resistance to many diseases including cancer. Unlike most animals, humans do not manufacture their own vitamin C.

- Potent antioxidant. Deficiency of vitamin C leads to deficiency of other antioxidants. [271]
- Cancer risk – reduced [229, 238, 272-308] especially bladder, breast, cervix, colon, colon polyp, lung, upper digestive tract, pancreas, prostate, stomach – as shown in intervention, prospec-

tive and retrospective studies. It also inhibits the spread of cancer by neutralizing an enzyme (hyaluronidase) made by cancer cells.[309,310]

- Hypertension – decreased. [311]
- Bone density – increased. [312]
- Gall Stones – reduces formation. [313]
- Immune System – enhanced. [314]
- Viral infection – reduced.
- Smoking reduces vitamin C in blood.
- Ultraviolet light harm – reduced.
- Toxicity: Doses of 3 to 30 grams of vitamin C in more than 1,000 patients since 1953 has not caused one miscarriage, kidney-stone formation, or any other serious side effect. [315] Klenner has given patients 10 grams of vitamin C daily for over thirty years without any serious toxic side effects. [316]
- Simone recommended dose: 350-6,000 mg per day or more, depending upon circumstances.

Bioflavonoids
- An antioxidant.
- Cancer and Cardiovascular Disease risk – reduced. [317,318]
- Helps vitamin C to work efficiently.
- Toxicity: None reported.
- Simone recommended dose: 10-20 mg per day.

Selenium [319]
- A powerful antioxidant.
- Cancer and Cardiovascular Disease risk – reduced.
- Immune System – enhanced.
- HIV progression to AIDS – inhibited.
- Arthritis inflammation – reduced.
- Brain function and mood – enhanced.
- Miscarriage risk – reduced.
- Thyroid function – enhanced.
- Neutralizes toxic metals (mercury, cadmium, arsenic).
- Vision – enhanced.

- Toxicity: Occurs after prolonged ingestion of 2,400 to 3,000 micrograms of selenium per day.[320] Approximately 500 micrograms of selenium per day is safely tolerated by people in Japan.[321] Supplemental "organic" selenium from yeast is less toxic than inorganic selenium; it also resists chemical changes, and is stable during food processing.
- Simone recommended dose: 200-300 mcg per day.

Zinc
- An antioxidant.
- Cancer risk – reduced. [322]
- Immune System – enhanced. [323]
- Toxicity: 80-150 mg/day or more.
- Simone recommended dose: 15-20 mg per day.

Copper
- An antioxidant.
- Cancer and Cardiovascular Disease risk – reduced.
- Immune system – enhanced.
- Cholesterol and Glucose levels – helps to control.
- Toxicity: 10 mg/day for prolonged periods.
- Simone recommended dose: 3-5 mg per day.

alpha-Lipoic Acid
- Powerful antioxidant.
- Recycles vitamins C and E, regenerates glutathione, removes heavy metals, generates energy.
- Liver damage is repaired.
- Diabetes – improved. [324-328] Makes cells more sensitive to insulin. Improves peripheral neuropathy (painful feet/hands).
- Cataracts – decreases formation. [329]
- Glaucoma – improves pressures (150 mg per day). [330]
- Ischemia-Reperfusion Injury. A stroke or heart attack deprives that area of the body of blood for a while. When blood gains access to the deprived tissue, a burst occurs of free radicals that can be neutralized by alpha-Lipoic acid. [331]

- Other uses: Prevents HIV replication in animals, protects against radiation injury, prevents neurological disorders.
- Toxicity: None reported for doses between 2,000-3,000 mg per day. Some people have reported allergic skin reactions.
- Simone Recommended Dose: 300-600 mg per day

Cysteine (an amino acid)
- An antioxidant.
- Cardiac toxicity of adriamycin – reduced
- Immune System – enhanced.
- Toxicity: None.
- Simone recommended dose: 20-500 mg per day.

OTHER NUTRIENTS also protects against cancer.

Vitamin A
- Cancer risk – reduced. [332-336]
- Immune System – enhanced. [337]
- Cataract risk – reduced. [338]
- Hearing – enhanced. [339]
- Toxicity: Daily doses of 100,000 IU (30 milligrams of retinol) have been given to adults for many months without serious side effects. [340] Children who ingest 50,000 to 500,000 IU (15 to 150 milligrams of retinol) per day do exhibit toxicity. [341] The safety of vitamin A is extensively reviewed. [342]
- Simone recommended dose: 5,000-7,500 IU per day.

Vitamin D
- Cancer risk – reduced, especially breast, colon cancer. [343-345]
- Oncogene c-myc - inhibited. [346]
- Immune System – enhanced [347]
- Osteoporosis risk – reduced.
- Toxicity: A daily dose of 100,000 to 150,000 IU of vitamin D (250 to 375 micrograms of cholecalciferol) for many months can be tolerated by a healthy adult.[338]
- Simone recommended dose: 400-600 IU per day.

Vitamin K
- Cancer risk – reduced. [348]
- Immune System – enhanced.
- Toxicity: Not toxic in large doses.
- No supplement is needed.

Thiamine (B1)
- Cancer and Cardiovascular Disease risk – reduced. [349]
- Immune System – enhanced.
- Toxicity: None recorded.
- Simone recommended dose: 10-15 mg per day.

Riboflavin (B2)
- Immune System – enhanced.
- Toxicity: None.
- Simone recommended dose: 10-15 mg per day.

Niacin
- Cancer and Cardiovascular Disease risk – reduced. [350]
- Cholesterol and Triglycerides – reduced. [351]
- Toxicity: Timed-release niacin can damage your liver. Use only immediate-release form and do not exceed 1,500 milligrams per day. Take it with food to decrease the red flush to skin. Niacin may aggravate gout, and stomach problems.
- Simone recommended dose: 40-80 mg per day; 1000-1500 mg per day to lower cholesterol and triglycerides.

Pantothenic Acid
- Energy - boosted.
- Diabetes – controls sugar.
- Toxicity: None.
- Simone recommended dose: 20-30 mg per day.

Pyridoxine (B6)
- Cancer risk – reduced. [352]
- Immune System – enhanced.
- Toxicity: Taking 500 mg/d for months will damage nerves.
- Simone recommended dose: 10-15 mg per day.

Vitamin B12
- Immune system – enhanced.
- Toxicity: None.
- Simone recommended dose: 18-30 mcg per day.

Folic Acid
- Cancer risk – reduced, breast, colon, and colon polyps. [353,354]
- Immune system – enhanced; Neural tube defects – reduced.
- Toxicity: None.
- Simone recommended dose: 400-800 mcg per day.

Biotin
- Its deficiency results in depression, anemia, sleepiness, muscle pain, hair loss, and increased cholesterol levels.
- Immune system – enhanced.
- Toxicity: None.
- Simone recommended dose: 150-250 mcg/day.

Calcium
The average daily calcium intake for Americans is 450-500 mg, an amount well below even the US RDI of 1000 mg per day for those under age 50 or menstruating, and 1500 mg per day for those over 50 or menopausal.
- Cancer risk – reduced, especially breast, colon, and pre-colon cancer (adenomas). [355-359]
- Cardiovascular Disease risk – reduced.
- Osteoporosis risk – reduced. Adolescent girls have evidence of osteoporosis. [360,361] Even eight year old girls and women of all ages benefit from calcium supplemention. [362,363] Based on 3 studies, $2.6 billion could be saved from hip fractures if people over age 50 took 1200-1500 mg/day of calcium. [364]

The following increase the risk of osteoporosis:
- Smoking and Caffeine – 2 to 3 cups of coffee/day [365-370]
- Sedentary Lifestyle, Aging
- High Sodium, High Protein diet, and High Blood Acid
- Soft drinks (high phosphates).
- Steroid treatment of arthritis, asthma, inflammatory bowel disease;[371] and excessive thyroid hormones.

- Anti-depression medications: fluoxetine, fluvoxamine, paroxetine, sertraline, nortriptyline, protriptyline, desipramine, amitriptyline, desipramine, clomipramine, doxepin, imipramine, and trimipramine. [372]
- Cadmium – a toxic metal found in tobacco smoke and also dolomite, a common calcium tablet. [373]

- Hypertension – reduced. [374]
- Alzheimer's disease risk – reduced. [375]
- Asthma flares – reduced.
- Some male infertility problems – reduced.
- Kidney stone risk – reduced. [376,377]
- Calcium carbonate is the most bioavailable form of calcium. Take at bedtime or between meals with a little orange or tomato juice. [378-380] Calcium should be taken with several other nutrients that aid calcium absorption and metabolism. Some of these nutrients, like vitamin D and vitamin C, should be taken only with food, while others, like magnesium, potassium bicarbonate, boron, silicon, threonine, and lysine, should be taken with calcium at night or between meals. [381]
- Simone recommended dose: 1500 mg per day for age 50 or older or post menopause, otherwise 1000 mg per day.

Magnesium
- Cardiovascular Disease risk and death – reduced. [382,383]
- Hypertension – reduced. [384]
- Asthma – improved. [385]
- Low magnesium causes low levels of calcium and potassium.
- Simone recommended dose: 420 mg per day for age 50 or older, otherwise, 280 mg per day.

Iron
- Iron should not be taken unless you have an iron deficiency anemia because iron causes free radicals and excess stores of iron increase the risk of cancer in men and women. [386,387]
- Cancer risk –increased especially breast and colon. [388]
- Toxicity: Acute effects occur above 75 mg daily for adults.

- Simone recommended dose: None unless you have iron deficiency anemia, and then only in therapeutic doses for 30 days with a doctor's supervision. Avoid routine supplementation.

Amino Acids

Amino acids are the building blocks for all proteins and are necessary for brain function. We can make some in our bodies, others we cannot. The ones that cannot be made by us are called essential amino acids. All are important for our health.

Amino acid deficiencies or abnormalities can be found in:

- Athletes, Body builders, people with muscle wasting or connective tissue disorders.
- Depression, hyperactivity, attention deficit disorder.
- Substance abuse.
- Immune System disorders, Viral Infections (herpes, Epstein Barr syndrome), Allergies.
- Eating disorders.
- Surgery, Sepsis, Trauma.
- Simone recommendations include the following groups of amino acids: Essential, Branched Chain (BCAA), Neurotransmitters, Glycogenics, Urea Cycle, Connective Tissue.

Dietary Fiber

- Cancer risk – reduced. On the basis of hundreds of clinical studies, a global review of 4500 research studies, studies and statements by the US National Cancer Institute, international governmental agencies, and seven international Consensus Statements, there is little doubt that fiber lowers the risk of colorectal cancer, and other cancers. [389-392]
- Cardiovascular Disease, Diabetes, Obesity, Diverticulosis risk – reduced.

Soluble fiber gets into the bloodstream and binds to and thereby decreases bile acids, cholesterol, triglycerides, sugars, poisons, and carcinogens. *Insoluble* and *soluble* fibers increase the weight and amount of stool, which dilutes and excretes carcinogens, and keeps the intestinal flora healthy.

You need about 25 to 35 grams of fiber daily for this protection: 6-11 servings of grains (cereal, rice, past, bread), 2-4 servings of fruits, 3-5 servings of vegetables, and legumes once or twice a week. However, Americans consume only about 10 grams of fiber per day. Therefore a dietary fiber supplement must be used to attain the protective effect.
- Toxicity: None. Dietary fiber is safe.
- Simone recommended dose: 25-35 grams per day.

Essential Fatty Acids
- Cancer risk and Cardiovascular risk – reduced.[393,394]
- Toxicity: None known.
- Simone recommendations: Linolenic Acid – 2 to 8 grams per day; Linoleic Acid – 3 to 9 grams per day.

NATURAL PROTECTORS IN FOODS
Researchers, prompted by epidemiological evidence have studied foods that can protect your health – Table 3.

Table 3. Natural Food Protectors		
Protector	**Food**	**Protective Action**
Carotene	Carrots, sweet potatoes,	Neutralizes singlet oxygen
Lycopene	Yams, Pumpkins, broccoli,	and free radicals
Lutein	Kale, cantaloupe, tomato	Cancer risk – reduced
Indoles	Cabbage Family: cabbage, broccoli, cauliflower, mustard greens, etc.	Destroys estrogen that causes cancer.
Lignans	Flaxseed, walnuts, fatty fish	Inhibits estrogens, & certain protaglandins that promote cancer
Polyacetylene	Parsley	Inhibits certain protaglandins Destroys some carcinogens
Quinones	Rosemary	Inhibits carcinogens
Sterols	Cucumbers	Decreases cholesterol
Sulfur	Garlic	Inhibits carcinogens Lowers cholesterol
Terpenes	Citrus Fruit	Destroys carcinogens Lowers cholesterol
Triterpenoids	Licorice	Inhibits estrogens & some prostaglandins, Slows down rapidly dividing cells.

Lycopene content varies with different food sources (content in micrograms/100gram wet food): Tomato raw – 3100, tomato juice – 8600; tomato sauce – 6300; watermelon – 4100; guava pink – 5200; and pink grapefruit – 350. [395]

PROSTATE CANCER PREVENTION[396]

- **ANTIOXIDANTS.** Evidence suggests that prostate cancer is caused by free radicals.[397]
  - **Lycopene**, part of the carotene family, protects against prostate cancer.[398,399]
  - **Vitamin E**, when given to men in the Alpha Tocopherol Beta-Carotene Cancer Prevention Study, decreased the incidence of prostate cancer.[400] Another large study involving 47,700 men showed that those who recently quit smoking had a reduced risk of prostate cancer with vitamin E supplementation.[401]
  - **Selenium** supplementation prevents prostate cancer.[402,403]
- **VITAMIN D** can inhibit the growth of prostate cancer cells and therefore has been added to some prostate cancer prevention trials.

REDUCE YOUR RISK OF CANCER

Cancer takes decades to develop. Cancers begin and grow early in life at a time when people do not receive enough antioxidants because they are simply not eating enough of the recommended 9 servings of fruits and vegetables that might provide some of these antioxidants in modest amounts. We now have enough positive scientific data to conclude that antioxidants reduce the risk for cancer because they protect against the initiation and promotion of a cancer. **So we must begin taking antioxidants consistently early in life for long periods of time because they are protective, but they should not be used as a sole weapon to kill cancer.**

Almost 40 percent of people take vitamins, but the vitamins they take are not necessarily the ones they need.[404,405] A proper formulation should consist of four factors: the **correct nutrient**, the **correct dose**, the **correct chemical form** of that nutrient, and the **correct ratio of one to another**. Often, a person will hear or read about a specific nutrient and run to the store to buy that nutrient without knowing the correct dose, chemical form, and ratio of it to another.

President Reagan's Administration said, "This new strategy [vitamin use] holds promise for reducing the incidence of cancer more successfully than an attempt to remove from the environment all substances which may initiate the cancer process." (*Medical Tribune*, June 30, 1982). And in 1995, US National Cancer Institute researchers stated: The field of chemoprevention...is now considered to be an extremely promising approach to the prevention of invasive cancer." [406]

YOUR IDEAL SUPPLEMENT PROGRAM

I recommend taking the following combinations of antioxidants, vitamins, minerals, amino acids, fibers, and other nutrients as supplementation shown below. These nutrients can be taken daily unless otherwise specified by your physician. Pregnant or lactating women should not follow this program unless approved by their physician.

Simone Antioxidant – Nutrient Supplementation

Carotene	30 mg	**Selenium**	200 mcg
Lutein	20 mcg	**Copper**	3 mg
Lycopene	20 mcg	**Zinc**	30 mg
Vitamin A	5500 IU	Iodine	150 mcg
Vitamin D	400 IU	Potassium	30 mg
Vitamin E	400 IU	Chromium	125 mcg
Vitamin C	350 mg	Manganese	2.5 mg
Folic Acid	400 mcg	Molybdenum	50 mg
Vitamin B1	10 mg	Inositol	10 mg
Vitamin B2	10 mg	PABA	10 mg
Niacinamide	40 mg	**Bioflavonoids**	10 mg
Vitamin B6	10 mg	Choline	10 mg
Vitamin B12	18 mcg	**L-Cysteine**	20 mg
Biotin	150 mcg	**L-Arginine**	5 mg
Pantothenic acid	20 mg		

*Antioxidants are bolded

Simone Calcium Formula	
Calcium carbonate	1000 mg
Magnesium	280 mg
Potassium bicarbonate	200 mg
Boron	4 mg
L-Lysine	4 mg
Silicon	4 mg
Threonine	4 mg

Simone Fiber Formula	
Soluble Fiber	800 mg
Pectin, Gums (Guar, oat)	
Mucilages (kelp, psyllium)	
Insoluble Fiber	200 mg

Simone Essential Fatty Acids
Linolenic Acid 2 to 8 grams
Linoleic Acid 3 to 9 grams

I am advocating simple common sense. Modify your risk factors and thereby reduce your risk of cancer, cardiovascular, and other chronic diseases. This includes following our Ten Point Plan and taking the correct nutrients, the correct doses, the correct chemical forms, and the correct ratio of one to another according to your individual lifestyle needs.

6

Nutritional and Lifestyle Modification Augments Oncology Care

Charles B Simone, II, Nicole Simone, M.D., Victoria Simone, RN, Charles B. Simone, M.D.

The successes in cancer treatment plateaued in the 1970s, and no real advances have been made since then. Chemotherapy and radiation therapy, however, continue to have a large role in cancer treatment but produce great morbidity. Two prescription medicines, Amifostine and Dexrazoxane, both antioxidants, reduce cancer therapy side effects without interfering with tumor killing. Amifostine (WR-2721) is an antioxidant analog of cysteamine discovered by the Armed Forces at Walter Reed Army Hospital that reduces side effects and increases response rates without interfering with cancer therapy [1-9] (29 studies). Dexrazoxane (ICRF-187) protects the heart from adriamycin toxicity without interfering with the antitumor effect [10-13] (21 studies) by chelating iron that would otherwise form free radicals. [14-17]

Despite the common use of Amifostine and Dexrazoxane, and in direct opposition to clear scientific findings since the 1970s, many patients have been told not to use food supplement antioxidants and other nutrients during chemotherapy and/or radiation therapy because there is an erroneous but seemingly logical belief that antioxidants interfere with radiation and some chemotherapies because those modalities kill by generating free radicals that are neutralized by antioxidants, and also, that folic acid interferes with methotrexate. [18-23]

Front page Sunday <u>New York Times</u> article on October 26, 1997: "Research at [Memorial Sloan Kettering] showed that large doses of vitamin C could blunt the beneficial effects of chemotherapy for breast cancer...It is also known that folic acid can negate the effects of methotrexate, a drug used to treat cancer."[18]

The research referred to was finally published almost two years later demonstrating only the mechanism by which cancer cells obtain vitamin C and that more vitamin C was found in mice cancer cells compared to normal mice cells.[20] However, the senior author of that paper stated in a news release on the day of publication (September 15, 1999), "It's possible that taking large amounts of vitamin C could interfere with the effects of chemotherapy or even radiation therapy."[21]

A single front page interview in the Sunday <u>New York Times</u> in 1997 based on no published scientific work, and a single mouse paper and comments in 1999, led to the erroneous notion that vitamin C interferes with chemotherapy and radiation in humans. This notion soon applied to all antioxidants as physicians, patients, the media, the American Cancer Society[22,23] and scores of web sites took the same position without reviewing the scientific evidence.

NUTRIENTS AUGMENT CHEMOTHERAPY AND RADIATION THERAPY

Since the 1970s, 280 peer-reviewed *in vitro* and *in vivo* studies, including 50 human studies involving 8,521 patients, 5,081 of whom were given nutrients, have consistently shown that non-prescription antioxidants and other nutrients do not interfere with cancer therapeutic modalities, and can enhance their killing capabilities, decrease their side effects, protect normal tissues, and in 15 human studies, 3,738 patients actually had prolonged survival. **For each section below, only representative references will be cited, however.**

CHEMOTHERAPY AND RADIATION THERAPY DECREASE SERUM NUTRIENT LEVELS OF ANTIOXIDANTS due to lipid peroxidation and thereby exhibit a higher level of oxidative stress.[24-30] Iron could be the possible intermediate cause of this oxidative stress,[14-17] and therefore supplemental iron should be given only if the cancer patient has an iron deficiency anemia.

In Vitro **Cellular Studies** [31-39](close to 100 studies) **and Animal Studies**[40-52] (over 100) using nutrients that include vitamins C, A, K, E, D, B6, B12, beta-carotene, selenium, or cysteine as single agents or in combination given concomitantly with chemotherapy, or tamoxifen, or interferon alpha-2b, or radiation, or combinations of these modalities show the same effect: No interference, increased protection of normal tissues, increased tumor killing, and, in some studies, increased animal survival.

Human Studies [53-102]
Fifty human studies, involving 8,521 patients, 5,081 of whom were given food supplement nutrients, have consistently shown that non-prescription **antioxidants and other nutrients**:

- **Do not interfere with cancer therapeutic modalities**
- **Can enhance cancer therapy killing capabilities**
- **Decrease cancer therapy side effects**
- **Protect normal tissues from cancer therapy, and**
- **Prolong lifespan in 15 studies for 3,738 patients**

Table 1 lists the effects of nutrients on patients receiving systemic or radiation treatment in randomized and observational studies. Observational studies provide valid information, do not overestimate the effects of treatment, and provide virtually identical results compared to randomized studies. [103-105]

Folic Acid does not interfere with methotrexate[106-108]
The effects of methotrexate, a chemotherapy, can be reversed with folinic acid, which is an analog of the vitamin folic acid. Folic acid itself does not reverse methotrexate's effects. In order to reverse the effects of methotrexate, folinic acid has to be given in high doses. Folinic acid cannot be obtained over the counter, it must be prescribed.

Table 1. Effects of nutrients with systemic or radiation treatment

Author Type Study (ref #)	# Patients	Nutr ient	Systemic Treatment	Local Treatment	Higher Response Rate	Decrease Side Effects	Increased Survival
Israel R* (53)	100 Breast	A	Chemo (site appropriate)	None	Yes	Yes	Yes
Komiyam O* (54)	275 Neck	A	5FU	RT	Yes	Yes	Not addressed
Meysken R* (55)	153 CML	A	Busulfan	None	Yes	Yes	Yes
Recchia O* (56)	40 Lung	A	Cisplatin, vindesine, 5FU, interferon	None	Yes	Yes	Yes
Recchia O* (57)	23 Oral	A	5FU, cisplatin	None	Yes	Yes	Yes
Recchi O* (58)	36 Breast	A	Chemo (site appropriate),steroid, interferon, tamoxifen	None	Yes	Yes	Yes
Recchia O* (59)	22 Pancreas	A	Epirubicin, mitomycin C, interferon,5FU	None	No Difference	No Difference	No Difference
Recchia O* (60)	49 Breast	A	Tamoxifn Interferon	None	Yes	Yes	Yes
Mills R* (61)	20 Oral	Carot ene	Vincristine,MTX Bleomyin	RT	No Difference	Yes	No Difference
Santamari O* (62)	15 Various	Carot ene	Chemo (site appropriate)	RT	Yes	Yes	Yes
Besa O* (63)	66 Myeldy splasia	E	13-cis-retinoic acid	None	Yes	Yes	Yes
Dimery O* (64)	39 Neck Lung	E	13-cis-retinoic acid	None	Not Addressed	Yes	Not Addressed
Ganser O* (65)	17 Myeldy splasia	E	Trans-retinoic erythropoietin	None	Yes	Yes	Not Addressed
Gottlobe O* (66)	1 Benign	E	None	RT	Yes	Yes	Not Applicable
Legha O* (67)	21 Breast	E	CAF	None	No Difference	No Difference	Not Addressed

Author Type Study (ref #)	# Patients	Nutrient	Systemic Treatment	Local Treatment	Higher Response Rate	Decrease Side Effects	Increased Survival
Lenzhofer R* (68)	12 Breast	E	Doxorubicin	None	Yes	Yes	Not Addressed
Lopez R* (69)	20 Leukemia	E	for AML, transplant	None	Yes	Yes	Not Addressed
Wadleigh R* (70)	18 Various	E	Chemo (site appropriate)	None	Not Addressed	Yes	Not Addressed
Weitzman R* (71)	16 Various	E	Adria regimen	None	No Difference	No Difference	Not Addressed
Wood O* (72)	16 Various	E	Adriamycin	None	Not Addressed	Yes	Not Addressed
Copeland O* (73)	58 Various	Antioxidants	Chemo (site appropriate)	None	Yes	Yes	Not Addressed
Filler O* (74)	41 Various	Antioxidants	Chemo (site appropriate)	Surgery	Yes	Yes	Not Addressed
Jaakkola O* (75)	18 lung small cell	Antioxidants	CTX Adria VCR	RT	Yes	Yes	Yes
Lockwood O* (76)	32 Breast	C, E, Carotene Selenium	Chemo (site appropriate)	RT	Yes	Yes	Yes
Osaki O* (77)	63 Oral	C, E, Glutathion	5FU Peplomycin	RT	Yes	Yes	Not Addressed
Pyrhone R* (78)	41 Gastric	A, E	FEMTX	None	Not Addressed	Yes	Yes
Rougerea O* (79)	17 Esophageal	Antioxidants	None	RT	Yes	Yes	Yes
Sakamoto O* (80)	20 Various	A, C, E	Chemo (site appropriate)	None	Yes	Yes	Not Addressed
Thiruvengadam O* (81)	10 Various	A, E, C Selenium	Chemo (site appropriate)	None	Not Addressed	Yes	Not Addressed
Wagdi R* (82)	24 Various	E, C Cysteine	Chemo (site appropriate)	RT	Yes	Yes	Not Addressed
Kim R* (83)	25 Neck Melano	Nicotinamide	None	RT Hyperthermia	Yes	Yes	Not Addressed
Ladner R* (84)	6300 Gyn, Breast	Pyridoxine	Chemo (site appropriate)	RT	Yes	Yes	Yes

Type of Study: R* = Randomized; O* = Observational

Author Type Study (ref #)	# Patients	Nutrient	Systemic Treatment	Local Treatment	Higher Response Rate	Decrease Side Effects	Increased Survival
Wiernik R* (85)	248 Ovarian	Pyridoxine	Cisplatin, hexamethyl-amine	None	Not Addressed	Yes	Not Addressed
DeRosa O* (86)	44 Myelodysplasia	Retinoic acid, D₃	Ara C	None	Yes	Yes	Yes
Margolin O* (87)	51 Various	K₃	Mitomycin C	None	Yes	Yes	Not Addressed
Nagoumey O* (88)	14 Various	K₃	Chemo site appropriate	None	Yes	Yes	Not Addressed
Bohm O* (147)	50 Ovarian	Glutathione	Cisplatin, Carboplatin	Surgical Debalk	Yes	Yes	Yes
Bohm, O* (90)	35 Ovarian	Glutathione	Cisplatin, CTX	None	Yes	Yes	Not Addressed
Cascinu R* (91)	50 Gastric	Glutathione	Cisplatin	None	Yes	Yes	Not Addressed
Cozzaglio O* (92)	11 Colon	Glutathione	5FU, Cisplatin	None	Not Addressed	Yes	Not Addressed
Di Re O* (93)	79 Ovarian	Glutathione	Cisplatin, CTX	RT	Yes	Yes	Yes
Di Re O* (94)	40 Ovarian	Glutathione	Cisplatin, CTX	None	Yes	Yes	Not Addressed
Fontanelli O* (95)	27 Cervix	Glutathione	Cisplatin, Bleomycin	Surgery	Yes	Yes	Not Addressed
Leone O* (96)	12 Lung	Glutathione	Cisplatin	None	Yes	Yes	Not Addressed
Locatelli O* (97)	20 Ovarian	Glutathione	Cisplatin	None	Yes	Yes	Not Addressed
Nobile O* (98)	13 Various	Glutathione	CTX	None	Not Addressed	Yes	Not Addressed
Oriana O* (99)	16 Ovarian	Glutathione	Cisplatin, CTX	None	Not Addressed	Yes	Not Addressed
Parnis R* (100)	36 Ovarian	Glutathione	Cisplatin	None	Not Addressed	Yes	Not Addressed
Plaxe O* (101)	16 Various	Glutathione	Cisplatin	None	Not Addressed	Yes	Not Addressed
Smyth O* (102)	151 Ovarian	Glutathione	Cisplatin	None	Yes	Yes	Not Addressed

Type of Study: R* = Randomized; O* = Observational

SUMMARY. Since the 1970s, 280 peer-reviewed *in vitro* and *in vivo* studies, including 50 human studies involving 8,521 patients, 5,081 of whom were given nutrients, have consistently shown that non-prescription antioxidants and other nutrients do not interfere with cancer therapeutic modalities, and can enhance their killing capabilities, decrease their side effects, protect normal tissues, and in 15 human studies, 3,738 patients actually had prolonged survival.

LIFESTYLE MODIFICATION AUGMENTS ONCOLOGY CARE

BREAST CANCER – QUALITY OF LIFE IS IMPROVED WITH LIFESTYLE MODIFICATION AND NUTRIENTS. Using Quality of Life Scales, 50 patients with early staged breast cancer evaluated treatment side effects of radiation and/or chemotherapy while taking therapeutic doses of nutrients.[109,110] The patient decided if the nutrients used during treatment had improved, worsened, or made no change in her life during the treatment period. The qualities of life tested were physical symptoms, performance, general well being, cognitive abilities, sexual dysfunction, and life satisfaction.

All 50 patients had lumpectomy, axillary node dissection, and radiation therapy (4500 cGy to whole breast + 1500 cGy to tumor bed); but for 25 patients with positive nodes, 6 cycles of chemotherapy were given – cytoxan, 5-FU, and then methotrexate was added after radiation was completed. Each patient followed the Ten Point Plan as described in Chapter 26 and took nutrients as outlined on page 60 in Chapter 4.

Patients in both groups generally indicated improvement in their quality of life, a few indicated no change, and none indicated worsening. Those who followed the Ten Point Plan and took certain nutrients in the correct doses, correct chemical form, and correct ratio of one to another, had a better quality of life while receiving chemotherapy or radiation therapy.

JAPANESE EXPERIENCE – HEALTHY LIFESTYLE INCREASES LIFESPAN. Elderly Japanese women rarely get breast cancer, but when they do, they live longer than American women stage for stage[111-118] because (1) they are less obese, (2) they eat a low-fat, high-fiber diet with vitamins and minerals, (3) they don't smoke, or drink, (4) they exercise and mentally relax. Younger Japanese women have now adopted a more Western culture and diet[102] and have a higher rate of breast cancer.

Obese breast cancer patients have a greater chance of early recurrence and a shorter life span compared to non-obese patients.[119-123] And breast cancer patients who have a high-fat intake and a high serum cholesterol also have a shorter life span than patients with normal or low-fat intake and low serum cholesterol.[124] Fat can initiate and also promote a cancer, especially a dietary cancer like breast cancer. If cholesterol intake is dramatically limited, cancer cell growth is severely inhibited.[125]

U.S. NATIONAL CANCER INSTITUTE EFFORT. Armed with this information, the US National Cancer Institute, National Institutes of Health in Bethesda, Maryland conducted a research protocol in the mid 1980s to see if a low-fat diet would increase the life span of breast cancer patients. However, in January 1988, after only a brief time and an expenditure of about $90 million, it was decided to end the proposed ten year study because: (1) Physicians did not "believe" that there was a relationship between breast cancer and fat or other nutritional factors and, subsequently, did not refer patients to the study; and (2) Once a woman was enrolled in the protocol, she subsequently "failed out" because she did not want to give up pizza, ice cream, and other high-fat foods.

HOFFER-PAULING STUDY. Professors Hoffer and Pauling asked whether therapeutic nutrition could help 129 cancer patients.[126] All ate a low-fat diet supplemented with therapeutic doses of vitamins C, E, A, niacin, and a multiple vitamin/mineral supplement, in addition to following the advice and treatment of traditional oncology care. Those who did not follow nutritional modification (31 patients) lived an average of 6 months less. The other 98 patients fell into three categories: 32 patients with breast, ovarian, cervix, and uterus cancer had an average life span of over 10 years; 47 patients who had leukemia, lung, liver, and pancreas cancer had an average life span of over 6 years; and 19 patients with end-stage terminal cancer lived an average of 10 months.

OTHER CLINICAL STUDIES

Other clinical studies show similar findings: Patients who undergo conventional oncology therapy generally live longer and/or have a lower recurrence rate if they modify their lifestyle, which includes diet changes, nutrient supplementation, and other lifestyle changes.[127-131]

The effect of vegetable consumption was examined over a period of 6 years in 675 patients with lung cancer. Those who lived longer ate more vegetables.[127] In another study, 200 patients who made significant dietary changes, experienced regression of their cancers without conventional treatment: 87 percent changed their diet dramatically to mainly vegetables, fruits, and whole grains; 65 percent consumed nutrient supplements; and 55 percent used a detoxification method.[128]

The effect of eating a macrobiotic diet on survival was studied in 1490 patients with pancreas cancer and 18 patients with prostate cancer.[129] Twenty-three matched patients with pancreas cancer changed to a macrobiotic diet and 12 (52%) were alive after one year; 1467 continued their high-fat, low-fiber diet and of these, 146 (10%) were alive after one year. Similarly, nine patients with prostate cancer who ate a macrobiotic diet were matched to nine patients with prostate cancer who ate their "normal" high-fat diet. Those eating the macrobiotic diet lived longer (median survival 228 months) than those who did not (median survival 45 months).

Tumor recurrence rate was decreased by 50 percent in patients with transitional cell bladder cancer who took higher than Recommended Dietary Intake (RDI) doses of certain vitamins compared to matched controls taking RDI doses.[131]

RECURRENCE RISK IS DECREASED[132]

Low intake of fat and calories decreases the risk of recurrence and increases lifespan for breast cancer patients.

LIFESPAN IS INCREASED

• **Nutrients + Chemotherapy and/or Radiation therapy increase lifespan** in eight studies for patients who received vitamin A or antioxidants concomitantly with chemotherapy and radiation therapy compared to patients who did not receive the nutrients. This finding is observed for patients with cancers of the breast, lung, stomach, mouth, nasopharynx, and myelodysplastic syndromes.

• **Lifestyle Modification (including nutrients) + Chemotherapy and/or Radiation Therapy increase lifespan** as demonstrated in twenty studies with more than 2700 patients. The patients in these studies had the following cancers: breast, ovarian, cervix, uterus, head and neck, lung, pancreas, prostate, and bladder.

CONCLUSION

Many of the nutrients used in the above studies are antioxidants. Antioxidants neutralize free radicals. Most cancer modalities exert their cancer killing effects by generating free radicals. Therefore it would seem inconsistent that these nutrients can help the cancer patient. However, hundreds and hundreds of *in vitro* and *in vivo* studies, including scores of clinical studies have repeatedly shown that certain vitamins and minerals can enhance the killing of cancer therapeutic modalities while at the same time protect normal tissues and decrease side effects from these modalities.

How is this possible? Because cancer cells accumulate excessive amounts of antioxidants[133] due to a loss of the homeostasis control mechanism for the uptake of these nutrients. Normal cells do not have this membrane defect and do not accumulate large amounts of antioxidants. Accumulation of excessive antioxidants in cancer cells can:

- Shut down oxidative reactions necessary for making energy
- Inhibit protein kinase C activity[134] which normally increases cell division and increases cell proliferation
- Inhibit oncogene expression[135,136]
- Increase the amount of growth inhibitory growth factors[137]

With higher levels of cancer intracellular accumulation of nutrients, more of these cellular alterations occur. These changes can lead to a higher rate of cancer cell death, and a reduction in the rate of cell proliferation and induction of differentiation. These acquired changes of cancer cells due to high doses of nutrients actually override any protective action that antioxidants have against free radical damage on cancer cells.

Cancer patients should modify their lifestyles (Ten Point Plan), that includes modifying nutritional factors and taking certain vitamins and minerals in the correct doses, especially if they receive chemotherapy and/or radiation. No one should take "a multiple vitamin/mineral formula" that simply has the correct words on the label. The studies indicate that it is important to take the correct nutrients, in the correct dosages, in the correct chemical form, and in the correct ratio of one to the other.

PART THREE

The Risks

7
Free Radicals

Free radicals are made in our bodies all the time and, if not destroyed, can lead to the development of cancer and other diseases. You already are familiar with free radicals – they cause oxidation – rusty metal, rancid butter, the greenish hue on outdoor copper statues. Antioxidants, like beta-carotene, vitamins C and E, selenium, and others, can neutralize the harmful free radicals and thereby prevent disease and protect us.

By definition, free radicals are chemical substances that contain an odd number of electrons. Every atom has a nucleus and a certain number of electrons that orbit around the nucleus. This setup is very much like our solar system, with the sun in the middle and all the planets orbiting around the sun. The nucleus has a positive charge, and the electrons have a negative charge. The negative charges of electrons balance out the positive charge of the nucleus to give an overall charge of zero. Hence, the energy of a single atom is very stable at zero.

When high energy in any form (from light, radiation, smog, tobacco, alcohol, polyunsaturated fats, etc.) hits an atom, an electron is kicked out of orbit. All of the energy that forced the electron out of orbit is transferred directly to the electron, making it highly energetic and unstable. Because it is so unstable, this electron quickly seeks *another* atom to reside in. This excited high-energy electron transfers very high energy to the new atom, which then becomes extremely unstable because of the newly acquired high energy. The process is depicted below.

FREE RADICAL FORMATION CAUSING CELL DAMAGE

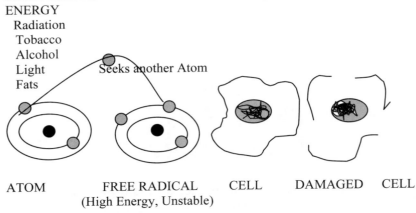

ENERGY
  Radiation
  Tobacco
  Alcohol
  Light   Seeks another Atom
  Fats

ATOM   FREE RADICAL   CELL   DAMAGED   CELL
              (High Energy, Unstable)

This excited high-energy atom with its extra electron is called a free radical. A free radical is unstable and must get rid of all the extra energy for the atom to become stable once again; hence the radical transfers its energy to nearby substances. All these reactions take place in a fraction of a second. When free radicals are made, the high energy is transferred to body tissues, particularly to the polyunsaturated fats found in the cell membranes, thereby causing cell damage. The more fats you eat, the more of them will be absorbed by cell membranes and the higher the risk will be for membrane disruption by free radicals. If the free radicals are not neutralized, this process can lead to cancer in the tissue affected by the radical.

FORMATION OF RADICALS

The following produce free radicals and can lead to the development of cancer:

• **Oxygen** can be activated or split with high energy into very potent damaging radicals (superoxide) or a high-energy, unstable nonradical called singlet oxygen. Singlet oxygen has extremely high energy and is very unstable, and thus is very destructive to normal body tissues and cells.

- **Polyunsaturated Fats** react with oxygen or enzymes to release their energy and thereby form a free radical. This free radical reacts with another polyunsaturated fat to produce a hydroperoxide. The more unsaturated the fat is, the more hydroperoxides are made that produce more radicals, damage cell membranes, and can lead to the development of cancer.
- **Metals** accumulate in the body and can also initiate free radical formation by activating oxygen. Iron is one example.
- **Radiation** produces free radicals and electrons that react to yield many different kinds of free radicals. At high levels of radiation, hydroperoxides are produced in addition to all the other free radicals.
- **Sunlight (Photolysis)** produces free radicals in skin cells, which can damage the skin and lead to skin cancer, the most common of all human cancers. The three kinds of skin cancers are basal cell, squamous cell and melanoma. Chronic sun exposure in Caucasians directly damages the skin and results in wrinkling, the formation of tiny networks of blood vessels, and the appearance of discrete small raised bumps on the skin called actinic keratosis (which are precancerous). And ultraviolet light harms the immune system. Use sunscreens, sunglasses, protective clothing and don't use suntanning booths.
- **Smog** causes more tissue damage than background radiation. Ozone and other compounds of smog react with almost every type of molecule in the body to form free radicals that damage cells. Ozone in normal amounts in the air can even form radicals with polyunsaturated fatty acids.
- **Alcohol and Chloride-Containing Compounds.** Vinyl chloride, chloroprene, and carbon tetrachloride react with some liver enzymes (microsomal mixed function oxidase) to produce free radicals that damage liver cells and potentiate liver cancer.

FREE RADICALS CAUSE DISEASE
Free radicals are the main cause of many human diseases – Table 1.[1,2] Free radicals cause cancer by damaging the membrane and the nucleus of the cell and subsequently the DNA. When certain segments of the DNA are affected, a malignant change

occurs, altering the genetic code and leading to cancer.[3-5] Antioxidants neutralize free radicals and protect against cancer.

Table 1. Conditions Associated with Free Radicals	
Cancers: all types	**Central Nervous System Diseases**
	Senile dementia
Cardiovascular Disease	Parkinson's disease
Alcohol heart condition	Hypertensive stroke
Selenium heart condition	Encephalomyelitis
(Keshan disease)	Aluminum overload
Atherosclerosis	Ataxia-telangiectasia
Adriamycin toxicity	
Heart Attack	**Iron Overload**
Lung Disease	**Radiation Injury**
Emphysema	
Pneumoconiosis	**Kidney Diseases**
Respiratory distress syndrome	
Bleomycin toxicity	**Gastrointestinal Diseases**
Air pollutant toxicity	Free-fatty acid pancreatitis
	Nonsteroidal anti-inflam-
Alcohol-related diseases	matory drug lesions
	Liver injury from toxins
Immune System Diseases	Carbon tetrachloride injury
Glomerulonephritis	
Vasculitis	**Skin Diseases**
Autoimmune diseases	Solar radiation damage
Rheumatoid Arthritis	Contact dermatitis
Eye Diseases	**Red Blood Cell Diseases**
Cataracts	
Retinal Damage	**Aging**

Free radicals cause cardiovascular disease by damaging the cells that line the inside of all blood vessels.[6] Due to this initial injury, fats and fibrin (blood-clotting protein) and other elements of the blood ultimately form clots and block the arteries.[7] Once a person sustains a heart attack, the injury that occurs within the first twelve to twenty-four hours is secondary to free radical damage.[8,9] Therefore, antioxidants have an important role not only in the prevention of cardiovascular disease but also at the time of an ongoing heart attack. The process of aging is due to oxidation – related to free radicals.

OUR BODY'S DEFENSES AGAINST RADICALS

We know that all life requires oxygen, but sometimes oxygen can produce radicals and high-energy (singlet) oxygen. Because of this, Mother Nature has given us three major lines of defense against free radical formation to preserve our very existence and to lessen the chance of abnormal cell (cancer) development.

The first is the *protective protein coat* that lines the surface of the cell membrane and prevents oxygen from reacting directly with lipids in the membrane, a reaction that would produce many free radicals. A second defensive mechanism involves the *protective enzymes* that float around in all cell membranes and act as antioxidants. They include *superoxide dismutase, catalase,* and selenium-containing *glutathione peroxidase.* Vitamin E is also an antioxidant and is the third mechanism that inhibits formation of free radicals in the cell membrane.

Mother Nature did not realize just how abusive we would be to our bodies. And although these three lines of defense are important, they are simply not enough given all that we now do to generate free radicals. That's why we should take antioxidant supplements.

8
Nutritional Factors

Jason's History
Jason loves steak, hot dogs, pizza, and ice cream. Who doesn't? He has been eating these foods for all his 53 years. His new PSA shows an abnormality that was not seen on his prior three PSAs.

The National Academy of Sciences estimates that 60 percent of all women's cancers and 40 percent of all men's cancers are related to nutritional factors alone.[1-3] Overall, it has been estimated that 75 to 90 percent of all cancers are related to life-style: nutritional factors, smoking, alcohol consumption, occupational factors, chemicals, environmental factors, etc.

Nutritional factors are most closely associated with cancers of breast, prostate, colon/rectum, and endometrium. The number of new cancers continues to rise each year, especially diet related cancers. You can readily understand the enormous impact that proper nutrition can have in lowering the overall incidence of cancer in the United States and the world.

NUTRITIONAL EVOLUTION
The human race has existed for about two million years, and our prehuman ancestors existed for at least four million years. Today, we are confronted with diet-related health problems that were previously of minor importance or totally nonexistent. Dietary habits adopted by Western society over the past hundred years have greatly contributed to the development of coronary heart disease, hypertension, diabetes, and cancer. These illnesses have dominated the past century and are virtu-

ally unknown among the few surviving hunter-gatherer populations, like the Bantu tribesmen in Africa, whose way of life and eating habits today resemble those of people before agricultural development. Members of primitive cultures today who survive to the age of sixty or more are relatively free of these illnesses unlike their Western "civilized" counterparts.[4,5]

With the development of agriculture over 10,000 years ago, we began eating less meat and more vegetables. With less protein in our diets, our height declined by six inches. After the Industrial Revolution, the pendulum started to swing back, and we started to increase the protein content of our diets. Height increased and we are now nearly the same height as were the first biologically modern people. But our diet is still very different from theirs. We are affluently malnourished.

Animals that live in the wild have less fat than domesticated ones because they are more active and have a less steady food supply. Domesticated animals and farm-raised fish are fed high fat foods to produce tender meat. Wild game has fewer calories and more protein per unit of weight. Even modern plant foods have more fat than non-commercially grown vegetables and fruits. Table 1 lists the various nutrients consumed by primitive people compared with those eaten by Americans today.[6] Primitive people consumed more dietary vitamins, more protein, less harmful fats, and much more essential fatty acids.

Table 1. Diet Comparison of Primitive and Modern Person

Nutrient	Primitive Person	Modern American	Simone Recommendations
Percentage of Total Calories			
Protein	34%	12%	35%
Carbohydrates	45%	46%	45%
Fats	21%	42%	20%
Daily Consumption			
Cholesterol	591 mg	600 mg	250 mg
Fiber	45.7 g	12 g	30-45 g
Sodium	690 mg	5000 mg	1000 mg
Calcium	1580 mg	500 mg	1500 mg
Vitamin C	392 mg	80 mg	400 mg

We have created a food supply very different from that of our ancestors with the development of food technology and the chemicals used for its growth and production. This "advancement" is costly to the human race.

> The vitamin and mineral content continues to decrease in our food supply because of pesticides, herbicides, processing techniques, freezing, thawing, transporting around the country, etc.

EPIDEMIOLOGICAL PATTERNS

Epidemiological studies demonstrate that a high-risk diet for cancers of the breast, colon, rectum, prostate, endometrium, as well as cardiovascular disease and other chronic illnesses is one that has high-fat, high-cholesterol, low-fiber, low intake of vitamins and minerals, more refined sugar, salt-cured, pickled, charred, smoked, or burned foods.[7-15] The more industrialized a country is, the higher is the rate of diet-related cancers.

Epidemiological studies assess cancer trends. They show a sixfold variation in breast cancer incidence in different parts of the world. High-incidence countries such as the United States are characterized by diets rich in cholesterol and animal fat. In high-incidence countries, there is a constant increase in the rate of breast cancer development with age, but in low-incidence countries the rate decreases after menopause.

- **Migration studies** show that if people emigrate from a country with a low incidence rate of a dietary cancer to a country with a high rate, they incur the higher rate fairly quickly.
  - **Japanese immigrants** to the United States, particularly the young, have the same colon cancer rate after only twenty years of consuming the American diet and have the same incidence of prostate and breast cancer after only two generations. Older Japanese are less apt to adopt American dietary customs and therefore have less risk for these cancers. Only 20% of the daily calories in Japan is derived from fat compared to 40% in America. But now, as the diet in Japan has become more Westernized, especially among the young, the rates of prostate, colon, and breast cancer have risen.[16]

○ **Southern Italian women immigrants** to Australia adopt a higher fat diet and incur a higher breast cancer rate as well.[17]

• **Bantu** people of Africa eat a low fat, high fiber diet and have an extremely low incidence of cancer compared to people in industrialized nations.

• **Seventh-Day Adventists and Mormons** in the United States have a very low incidence of cancer and heart disease because they consume a high fiber, low fat diet.[18-20]

• **American-born Jews of European descent** are at high risk for developing colon and rectal cancer. A twenty-year prospective study conducted in Israel showed that a high-fiber, low-fat, high vitamin C diet substantially reduced the number of colon and rectal cancer cases in that group.[21]

• **Finns** have a high fat intake, mainly from dairy. They have a high incidence of heart attacks but a low incidence of colon cancer because they consume a large amount of fiber from rye that suppresses fecapentaene, a cancer-causing chemical. Fecapentaenes are found in stools of people on fiber-depleted diets. These people have a higher incidence of colon cancer. This chemical, produced by bacteria in the large bowel and then released by them when they die, is not present in fiber-eating populations who are free from colon cancer.[22,23] When fiber is added to the diet, the bacteria stay healthy, they don't die and they don't release fecapentaenes.

• **Chinese**, compared to Americans, consume 20% more calories, three times the amount of fiber (33 to 77 grams), one-third the amount of fat, less protein from animal sources, have a lower cholesterol, eat twice the amount of starch, half as much calcium (all from vegetables) as Americans yet do not have osteoporosis, and are less obese. Because of a lower fat diet, Chinese women start menstruating three to six years later than American women and have less breast cancer. Chinese men have much less prostate cancer[Nutrition, Environment, Health Project, Chinese Academy of Preventive Medicine, Cornell].

Chinese people are a genetically similar population, but there are differences in dietary habits, environmental exposures, and disease rates in China from region to region. For instance, the cancer rate varies by a factor of several hundred from one region to another. The genetic contribution to cancer in China is minimal. Chinese who do eat more protein and fats have more heart disease, cancer, and diabetes. Any differences in cancer rates and other chronic illnesses, like heart disease, are attributed to dietary and other environmental exposures.

• **Diet Recall Studies** ask people what they ate every day for the last number of months or years. Can you to remember what you ate two nights ago for dinner? Most people tend to under-estimate their consumption of fat and/or other unhealthy foods particularly when they know that a high-fat diet is not healthy. Despite this, most diet recall studies suggest that a high fat intake increases the risk for breast cancer.[24-31] However, the Nurses Health Study,[32] widely publicized, suggested otherwise. Many scientist-physicians agree that the study is flawed for several reasons: (1) The patients consumed a high-fat diet of 32% compared to a low-fat diet of 20% that protects against breast cancer – in fact, other investigators[33] showed that the percentage of fat was even higher than 32% - and the authors of the Nurses Health Study freely admit that a 20% or less fat diet does decrease the risk of breast cancer;[34] (2) The study involved middle-aged women and totally ignored diet earlier in life, a time critical to breast cancer development; (3) This was an eight-year study, most cancers take decades to develop.

High-fat diets are correlated with a higher risk of cancers like colon, prostate, breast, endometrium, etc. I recommend a 20% or less fat diet.

• **Breast fluid** also influences the development of breast cancer. Breast fluid secretion occurs in most women, but in varying amounts. For example, Oriental women have much less breast fluid secretion than white women. Breast fluid bathes the ductal cells of the breast gland where most cancers originate. A high blood cholesterol level increases the breast fluid level of a carcinogen called cholesterol epoxide.[35] Nicotine and its close relative cotinine appear in breast fluid within five minutes after smoking or inhalation of other people's smoke.

Carcinogens get into breast fluid, bathe breast tissue for long periods of time, and increase the risk of cancer.

PHYTOESTROGENS

The belief that soy, a bean containing phytoestrogens, protects against breast cancer originates in the fact that older Japanese women have a lower incidence of breast cancer than older American women. However, this lower incidence of breast cancer is not because of soy, but because of their better overall lifestyle: a low-fat diet that includes soy but little or no red meat or dairy foods, less obesity, little or no smoking and alcohol, exercise, stress modification and other healthy habits.[36]

Soy has two phytoestrogens – genistein and daidzem. They were initially thought to be weak estrogens because they bound weakly to the alpha Estrogen Receptor. Now, however, it is known that they have strong estrogen capability because they bind strongly to the beta Estrogen Receptor.[37] Animal studies have demonstrated that soy can stimulate the growth of estrogen receptor positive breast cancer cells implanted into nude mice[38] and increase DNA synthesis which represents a marker for increased cancer risk.[39]

In animal experiments, ovaries were removed from rats so that a minimal amount of estrogen was made. Phytoestrogens were then given to them for 30 days. A decreased blood level of luteinizing hormone (LH) was found indicating high circulating levels of estrogens were present. Since the rats had no ovaries and could not produce their own estrogen, the drop in LH could only have resulted from the phytoestrogens given to the rats. Additionally, the uterus of each rat got larger from the phytoestrogens as it would to any estrogens.

A growing body of evidence suggests that phytoestrogens are not safe.[40-65] Soy, extracts of vitex, dong quai, American ginseng, and cohosh – all phytoestrogens – bind estrogen receptors in exactly the same way as estrogens made by the body. Phytoestrogens have the same effect as estrogens produced by the body. DON'T CONSUME PHYTOESTROGENS UNLESS YOU HAVE PROSTATE CANCER.

FATS

In 1942 Dr Tannenbaum first showed that dietary fat significantly favored the development and growth of both spontaneous and induced breast cancer in animals.[66] Dietary animal fat is found in all four-legged animals (red meat), luncheon meats, and all dairy products, including milk, cheese, and eggs.

- **Animal fat promotes and initiates cancer**[67-87] because:
  - o Fats increase sterol chemicals and bile acids that bacteria convert to carcinogens and carcinogenic estrogen.[88,89]
  - o Overweight women have fatty breasts that accumulate carcinogenic estrogens and are attacked by free radicals.
  - o Fats increase prolactin, a carcinogenic hormone.[90]
  - o Fats inhibit the immune system.
- **Fats decrease lifespan, increase prostate cancer aggressiveness, and increase death rate in prostate cancer patients.**[91-99]
  - o Men who eat the most meat and dairy products are the most likely to die from prostate cancer, and those who eat plenty of grains and nuts are least likely to die from the disease.
  - o Being overweight and having high cholesterol decreases both disease-free survival and lifespan.
  - o In Japan, older prostate cancer patients live longer with fewer disease events than men in America with similar prostate cancer because of a lower fat diet. Extent of disease and histology did not account for this difference.

FIBER

Dietary fiber is safe. Hundreds of studies involving tens of thousands of subjects demonstrate that 25 to 35 grams of dietary fiber daily will reduce the risk of cancer.[100] The most compelling and the most comprehensive review and evaluation of the link between diet and the development of cancer concludes that 3 to 4 million cases of cancer per year could be prevented by appropriate diet and lifestyle changes. A panel of over 150 scientists who reviewed and evaluated 4,500 research studies published their findings in a 670 page report, <u>Food, Nutrition and the Prevention of Cancer: A Global Perspective</u>.

Decreased cancer risk is most convincingly linked to fiber from vegetables, followed by fibers from non-soluble polysaccharides, starches, and fiber foods with carotenoids. Most Consensus Statements indicate that 25-35 grams of fiber each day is needed to protect against colon cancer. Unless a person has the time or the inclination to become a grazing animal, it would be difficult to attain the protective level of fiber each day without taking a supplement because Americans typically consume an average of only 8 to 15 grams of fiber per day. Food Guide Pyramid suggests daily: 6 to 11 servings of grains (cereal, rice, pasta, bread), 2 to 4 servings of fruits and 3 to 5 servings of vegetables daily, and legumes at least once or twice a week. Not very many of us can consume this amount without a supplement.

Prostate cancer patients should increase dietary fiber because fiber increases the fecal excretion of estrogen and decreases the plasma concentration of estrogen.[101] In fact, it might be wise to extend this modified diet to other diet-sensitive cancers – colon and rectal, breast, endometrium – in an attempt to increase lifespan and disease-free survival.

PROTEIN AND CARBOHYDRATES

High protein consumption is linked to a higher risk of breast cancer,[102] colon and rectal cancer,[103,104] prostate, and other cancers. A high sugar intake increases the risk for prostate and other cancers.[105,106] Excessive carbohydrate ingestion contributes to obesity, that, in turn, increases prostate cancer risk.

NATURALLY OCCURRING CARCINOGENS AND MUTAGENS

Some foods have naturally occurring carcinogens or mutagens. Plants have certain molecules to protect them against microorganisms and insects, and some of these are carcinogenic or mutagenic in humans.

For instance, certain foods contain nicotine. Eggplant has the highest amount of nicotine per gram of vegetable (0.1 mcg) followed by potato (0.007 mcg), then tomato (0.004 mcg).[107-]

[110] Although there is no cotinine (breakdown product of nicotine) in these foods, it may show up in the bloodstream of people eating these foods.

Some other foods and the carcinogens they contain are: black pepper (piperine and safrole), bruised celery (psoralen), herbal teas (pyrrolizidine, phorbol esters), mushrooms (hydrazines), and all foods containing mold (aflatoxin) or certain bacteria (nitrosamines).[111] Many of these are occasional contaminants, whereas others are normal components of relatively common foods.

Mutagens are chemicals that cause DNA changes. Mutagens are found in charred foods, coffee (quinones), and horseradish (allyl isothiocyanate). Mutagens pose a minimal risk for cancer development.

DIETARY TRENDS FOR FAT AND CHOLESTEROL

It has been estimated that if Americans reduce their fat content from 40% to just 30% (still higher than the protective 20%), about 42,000 of the 2.3 million annual deaths in the United States could be deferred.[112]

Studies indicate that patients fail to follow sound dietary advice.[113-117] This indicates that unless there is a strong motivating factor, and it is hard to imagine that a person's life is not such a motivating factor, people simply will not change habits even though they are told it will benefit them medically.

People who are aware of the health benefits of a low-fat, high-fiber diet supplemented with certain nutrients chose, instead, to eat high-fat snacks, and gained an average of two to four pounds a year. This "pleasure revenge," as The New York Times labels it, is seen most often among the affluent and well-educated people who previously led the health and fitness frenzy. People now are giving themselves permission to be unhealthy – not worrying about weight or smoking cessation. Consider the facts.

- Sales of high calorie foods rose: butter, beef, soda, sugar, cheese, super premium ice cream, cookies, fast-foods.

- Sales of low-calorie foods declined: margarine, diet-soda, sugar substitute, yogurt, fruit, and popcorn.
- Many diabetics eat what they want because "their medicines will take care of them."
- Fast-food chains stopped offering lean foods because people don't buy them.
- Massage is more popular than exercise.

People know what is good for their health, but many people indulge themselves and do what they want, when they want. This unhealthy trend is happening at a time when the cost for health-care is rising. Who do you think is going to pay for all this indulgence? And why should people who are striving to be healthy pay for others who indulge themselves?

Jason's PSA abnormality proved to be a cancer. Unlike many who don't follow sound dietary advice, Jason did decrease his fat intake and increased his fiber. He is also modifying the rest of his lifestyle. These efforts will increase his lifespan.

9
Obesity

John's History

John was overweight all his life. He was allowed to eat whatever and whenever at an early age. By age 41, he developed arthritis, then heart disease, and prostate cancer by age 52.

Obesity affects about 65% of US adults and 13% of children. Close to 1 million teenagers already have evidence of diabetes and cardiovascular disease. Being obese carries with it a social stigma as well as a general health risk. There are about 900 million pounds of excess fat on American men and 1,500 million pounds of excess fat on American women, for a total of 2.4 billion pounds. The US medical costs attributed to obesity is $75 billion. The US taxpayer, via Medicare and Medicaid, pays $175 a year for obesity-related illnesses: cancer, cardiovascular diseases, diabetes, gallbladder disease, and many more.[1] More obesity occurs in middle-aged people and in people with low socioeconomic status. The percentage of African-American men who are obese is greater than the percentage of white men. Adopted children become obese if adoptive family members are obese.

The fat cell *size* is increased in all types of obesity. An increased *number* of fat cells is found in children and adults who were obese before the age of two. If children are obese before the age of two, they will likely be obese in adulthood because they already have an increased number of fat cells. Only 1 percent of obesity is caused by a disease or medical problem; 99 percent of all obesity is directly related to overeating.

Because obese individuals tend to develop a variety of diseases, some of which are life threatening, obese adults have a higher than normal death rate for their age group. The risk of death correlates almost directly with how much a person is overweight. Even if you are only a little overweight, you still have an increased risk of death compared to a person who is not overweight.

OBESITY INCREASES RISK FOR PROSTATE CANCER

• Overwhelming evidence from around the world involving millions of men demonstrate that obesity increases the risk of prostate cancer independently of other risk factors.[2-5] This fact is especially true for African-Americans.

OBESITY INCREASES PROSTATE CANCER AGGRESSIVENESS AND DEATH RATE[3-6]

OBESITY INCREASES RISK FOR ALL CANCERS[2]

• Colon, Rectal, Esophagus, Stomach, Liver, Pancreas
• Gall Bladder and Biliary Passages
• Breast
  o Obesity increases the risk of breast cancer.[7-11]
  o Weight gain from puberty to adulthood, especially between 20 and 30, increases the risk of breast cancer.[12]
  o A birth weight of more than 9 pounds increases the risk.[13]
  o Obese postmenopausal women, especially those with a waist size larger than their hip size, have a higher rate of breast cancer.[14-20] Obese women have more estrogens because they have more fat cells, the main site of estrogen production.[21-24] Fat cells convert adrostenedione to estrone, a more carcinogenic estrogen.[25] Obese women with a large waist who lose more than 10 pounds can lower their increased risk of breast cancer by 45 percent.[26]
  o After age 35, there is fat in breasts regardless of weight. Breast fat then serves as a local source of breast tissue estrone production that can be up to forty times the levels found in serum of menstruating, nonlactating women.[27,28]

o Estrogen and estrone levels can be lowered by 30 percent in three to six months when you reduce dietary fat from 35 percent to 20 percent, or by 15 percent when you reduce dietary fat modestly and add 35 grams of fiber per day.[29-32] Therefore women should reduce their weight and add fiber. **These concepts are similar for men**.

- Lung, Melanoma
- Bladder, Kidney, Brain
- Cervix, Endometrium, Ovary
- Leukemia, Lymphoma, Multiple Myeloma
- All Others

OBESITY INCREASES RISK FOR OTHER DISEASES

- Impaired Immunity – more infections and higher death rate from infections; lower resistance to tuberculosis, malaria, and pneumonia, and decreased antibody production.
- Diabetes - a two or three times higher risk.
- Impaired breathing
- Cardiovascular disease – heart attack, stroke, hypertension, high cholesterol, high triglycerides
- Gall bladder disease
- Higher risk of death

OBESITY DECREASES LONGEVITY [33]

ATTAINING YOUR IDEAL WEIGHT

How much should a person weigh? There is no one answer, but here is a good rule of thumb. Men who are 5 feet tall should weigh 110 pounds. For every inch over 5 feet, add another 5 pounds. Thus, if a man is 5 feet 11 inches tall, his ideal weight is about 165 pounds. Women who are 5 feet tall should weigh about 100 pounds. For every inch over 5 feet, add 5 pounds. Therefore, if a woman is 5 feet 6 inches tall, her ideal weight is about 130 pounds.

Attaining your ideal weight is not always easy. Lose weight gradually. Losing one or two pounds a week is safe, and that loss will probably be maintained. Do not lose more weight than called for by the formula. Successful weight loss and maintenance of that loss will be achieved only if you totally modify your eating habits. Many people are put on high-protein liquid diets consisting of 800 calories a day and lose a great deal of weight within the first few weeks. But over time, these pounds come right back on because the person did not learn new eating habits. Eating less than 800 calories per day is dangerous and not recommended.

A person whose body weight fluctuates often or greatly has a much higher risk of developing coronary heart disease and dying than does a person who has a relatively stable body weight. Those aged thirty to forty-four were shown to suffer the most detrimental effects of weight fluctuation. These harmful effects of weight fluctuation were independent of degree of obesity or existing cardiovascular risk factors.

> # To lose weight, you must eat less
> # and
> # increase your physical activity.

Every pound of fat you have contains about 3,500 calories. Therefore, to lose one pound, you have to burn off 3,500 calories more than you eat. You will lose a pound a week if you burn off 500 calories per day more than you consume. So, if you eat a diet containing 1,200 calories per day and burn off 1,700 calories per day, you will lose one pound a week.

Before you start a physical exercise program, let a physician examine you. An exercise program should start out gradually, with new goals set every week. Walking is very good exercise. Table 1 shows the approximate number of calories burned by a 150-pound person performing various activities.

If you lose weight suddenly or without a good reason, see a physician. Unexplained weight loss can be a sign of cancer or another serious medical problem. Even though it is difficult to lose weight, you must try. Obesity has no benefits, and its risks are very great.

Table 1. Activities and the Calories They Burn

Activities	Calories Used/Hour	Activities	Calories Used/Hour
Answering Telephone	50	Bowling	250
Bathing	100	Calisthenics	500
Bed making	300	Card Playing	25
Brushing teeth or hair	100	Cycling slowly (5.5 mph)	300
Chopping Wood	400	Cycling strenuously (13 mph)	660
Dishwashing	75	Dancing, slow step	350
Dressing, undressing	50	Dancing, fast step	600
Driving Automobile	120	Fishing	150
Dusting Furniture	150	Football	600
Eating	50	Golfing	250
Filing (office)	200	Handball	660
Gardening	250	Hiking	400
Housework	180	Horseback riding	250
Ironing	100	Jogging	600
Mopping Floors	200	Kissing vigorously	6-12
Mowing Lawn	250	Lovemaking	125-300
Preparing Food	100	Painting	150
Reading	25	Piano playing	75
Sawing	500	Running, fast pace	900
Sewing	50	Singing	50
Shoveling	500	Skating leisurely	400
Sitting	100	Skating rapidly	600
Sleeping	80	Skiing (10 mph)	600
Standing	140	Soccer	650
Typing	50	Swimming leisurely (1/4 mph)	400
Walking up and down stairs	800	Swimming rapidly	800
Recreation		Tennis, singles	450
Badminton	400	Tennis, doubles	350
Baseball	350	Volleyball	350
Basketball	550	Walking leisurely (2.5 mph)	200
Boating, rowing	400	Walking quickly (3.75 mph)	300
Boating, motor	150	Watching television	25

Source: Dr. Robert Johnson, Depart of Agriculture, University Illinois 1980.

John decided to lose weight to improve his well-being and lifespan.

10
Food Additives, Contaminants, and Pesticides

Bob's History
Bob thoroughly washes all fruits and vegetables but is concerned that the imported ones have extra contamination and pesticides. Is his risk higher for developing prostate cancer?

The "Delaney clause" of the Federal Food, Drug, and Cosmetic Act, written because of food additives, prohibits the addition of any known carcinogens to food. Currently there are about 3,000 intentional food additives. There are over 12,000 occasionally detected unintentional additives from packaging, food processing, and other phases of the food industry.

FOOD ADDITIVES AND CONTAMINANTS
Chemical food additives and food contaminants have been extensively studied because they come into contact with our bodies. Chemicals are used to prevent contamination and spoilage of food that has to be produced in great quantities, stored, and transported. Chemicals are also used for flavoring and appearance. Chemical contaminants may develop as a result of food processing procedures such as irradiation, cooking, pickling, or smoking. The trouble with the use of chemicals in food is that we are exposed to them constantly, repeatedly, and at low doses. Therefore, laboratory investigations rather than

large population studies must be done to determine whether the chemicals are potentially hazardous.

Intentional food additives are chemicals that are purposely added to food. Cyclamate, for example, has not been shown to cause cancer in humans, but it does produce testicular atrophy (shrinking) in rats. Saccharin produces bladder cancer in rats when comprising 5 percent or more in the diet,[1] but so far, there is no clear connection to human cancer.[2] Xylitol, a sweetener, causes bladder cancer in mice and adrenal cancer in rats. [3] Nitrites are used as preservatives in meats. They also add color to bacon and hot dogs. Nitrites can react with other compounds to form potent carcinogens called nitrosamines.[4] When bacon is cooked, nitrosamines form. There is a low level of nitrites in our saliva and in some vegetables, but there is no information on whether these nitrites can be activated to form nitrosamines. Vitamin C, also found in vegetables, can inhibit the formation of nitrosamines and is usually added to meat cures. Nitrites might be carcinogenic.[5]

Unintentional food additives are those chemicals used to prepare or store the food product; small amounts of these chemicals subsequently, unintentionally, become part of the food. Paraffin wax that lines many food containers, pesticides, and DES are unintentional food additives. Pesticides get into our bodies and are stored in fat cells, since they are fat-soluble. These pesticide-laden fat cells can then act as reservoirs to slowly, but constantly release the pesticide into the bloodstream. DES (diethylstilbestrol) is used to fatten cattle and has been found in trace amounts in dairy products and beef. DES causes cancer of the vagina in young women and cancer of the testicles in men whose mothers had taken DES. Keep in mind that a large amount of DES is needed to cause cancer, and only a small amount is in our food. But small amounts accumulate and do affect us.

Aflatoxin is a food contaminant that causes human liver cancer. Aflatoxin is a product of a fungus, *Aspergillus flavus*, that grows mainly on peanut plants. Other fungal products have been implicated in human cancers. *Gyromita esculenta*, a common mushroom used in cooking, contains a compound called N-methyl-N-formylhydrazine, a potent animal carcinogen.[6]

Certain food processing techniques, such as smoking and charcoal broiling, produce carcinogens.[7] Smoked food increases the risk of gastric cancer. The carcinogens that result from charcoal broiling appear to come from the fat that drips from the meat and is burned, forming the carcinogen, which then rises with the smoke back up into the meat.[8]

As yet, there are no definite proven cases of human cancers directly related to food additives, but many authorities agree that additives and contaminants do account for a small percentage of human cancers. Those chemicals implicated in animal cancers were removed from the market. However, nitrites are bothersome sources of carcinogens and should be avoided. The reduced incidence of gastric cancer in the United States is directly related to less food additives with the advent of refrigeration. Also naturally occurring food components like aflatoxins do cause human cancer and should be eliminated.

PESTICIDES

Pesticides are now in widespread use throughout the world. They control or kill pests or affect plant or animal life. There are about 1,200 pesticide chemical compounds, combined in 30,000 different formulations. Pesticides have made an important contribution to both food production and disease control. Some estimate that at least one-third of the crops in Third World countries are lost to pests.[8]

Pesticides have aided in the control of malaria, schistosomiasis, and filariasis in tropical countries, but there are still hundreds of millions of cases of these diseases each year. There is no way of knowing and no way of calculating how many lives will be saved or improved by the use of pesticides to control diseases and increase our food production. Likewise, there is no way to calculate how many lives will be lost from pesticide use. Some dangerous pesticides that are banned or restricted in

North America and Europe have been unloaded on Third World countries.

Pesticides enter your body by inhalation, absorption through the skin, or ingestion. And unlike industrial chemicals, which are used in a very controlled manner, pesticides are sprayed, powdered, or dropped as pellets or granules in and around places where the general public may walk or play. In fact, pesticide residues are commonly found in human tissue in almost everyone in the United States, averaging six parts per million in fatty tissue.[9] Pesticides are found in cow milk, human breast milk, and can even cross the placenta to the human fetus.[10]

The 1994 General Agreement on Tariffs and Trade (GATT) allows for substantially higher levels of pesticide residues on U.S. import produce. Specifically, 5000 percent higher levels of DDT than current U.S. standards are permitted on imported peaches, bananas, grapes, strawberries, broccoli, and carrots.

The health of Americans is apparently subordinate to political pressure.

Certain pesticides, such as DDT (an insecticide), are animal carcinogens that get into fatty tissue and are slowly released.

Some pesticides have estrogen-like activity in the human: endosulfan, dieldrin, toxaphene and chlordane. When they are together in various combinations, they have a 150- to 1600-fold greater estrogenic affect than each alone.[11]

The implications of this are enormous. People are commonly exposed to more than one pesticide and this synergistic action of estrogen activity increases the risk for prostate, breast and other cancers. The link of pesticides to cancer is not direct, but these findings are enough to dictate the reduction in pesticides.

PESTICIDES INCREASE PROSTATE CANCER RISK[12-14]

PESTICIDES INCREASE RISK FOR MANY CANCERS

Table 1 lists pesticides and their roles as human carcinogens.[15-18] Pesticides are associated with, but not necessarily the direct cause of, the following human cancers:[9,19-30]

- Breast
- Brain
- Esophagus
- Leukemia
- Liver

- Lung
- Lymphoma
- Melanoma
- Multiple Myeloma
- Nasal

- Ovarian
- Prostate
- Sarcoma
- Skin
- Stomach

PESTICIDES INCREASE RISK FOR:

- Parkinson's disease[31,32]
- Cardiovascular disease
- Allergies
- Skin diseases

- Hypertension
- Abnormal blood cholesterol
- Liver disease
- Fertility problems

Dioxin, also known as Agent Orange, and one of its associated contaminants, TCDD, was used during the Vietnam War. Hundreds of thousands of people were exposed to these agents, and Vietnam veterans and others raised serious allegations that Agent Orange and TCDD caused malignant tumors,[19-30] sterility, spontaneous abortions, birth defects, disfiguring skin diseases, and other illnesses. Most of these studies involved a short period of time between exposure and disease. It now appears that the longer the time from exposure to TCDD, the higher the risk for the development of cancer and the higher the incidence of cancer.[33-35]

MINIMIZING PESTICIDE USE

Nature provides us with biological controls, that is, natural predators that can control insects. For example, ladybugs can fight off aphid predators. Beetles controlled weeds in the western United States in the 1950s, and parasites controlled the citrus fly in Barbados in the 1960s. Wasps have been controlled

Table 1. Pesticides as Human Carcinogens [11-14]

Pesticide	Definite	Probable	Possible
Aldrin and dieldrin			•
Amitrole		•	
Arsenicals	•		
Atrazine		•	
Benzal chloride			•
Benzotrichloride		•	
Benzoyl chloride			•
Benzyl chloride			•
Carbon tetrachloride	•		
Chlordane			•
Chlorophenols		•	
p-Dichlorobenzene		•	
DDT		•	
Ethylene dibromide		•	
Ethylene oxide		•	
Formaldehyde		•	
Heptachlor			•
Lindane			•
4-chloro-2-methyl acetic			•
Methyl parathion			•
Pentachlorophenol			•
Phenoxy acids			•
Dioxin		•	
2,4,5-Trichlorophenol			•
2,4,6- Trichlorophenol			•
2,4,5-Trichlorophenoxy acetic			•
Vinyl chloride		•	

by parasites in greenhouses more effectively than with chemicals. The bacterium, *Bacillus thuringiensis,* is a good alternative to several toxic insecticides. Silicon and soap can be used in gardens as a nontoxic insecticide rather than the other commonly used pesticides for the garden. Minimize the pests by providing food and habitat for the pest's natural enemies.

Certain farming practices may be employed as well. Crop residues may be removed by plowing or flooding. Pest deterrents, crop rotation, proper drainage methods, and physical controls like traps or blocking of insects and/or other pests can be used.

WHAT CAN BE DONE

The number of tons of pesticides has increased thirty-three times since 1940, and their toxicity has grown tenfold. However, crop losses to microorganisms, insects, and weeds have gone up 35 percent. There are a number of reasons for this. As new pesticides are developed, insects develop resistance to them. But even more importantly, the government supports prices of various crops, which encourages farmers to produce only a single crop instead of rotating crops to inhibit the pests. By using crop rotation and biological pest control, pesticide use could be cut in half. Food prices would rise by one percent – about $1 billion a year – but the benefits would be enormous. The United States would save billion of dollars per year as a result of decreased cancers and other medical diseases, decreased damage to fish and water supplies, decreased costs of regulating pesticides, and decreased health-care costs for the 20,000 people poisoned each year from pesticides.

Pesticides certainly benefit people by increasing food production and decreasing certain diseases, but we should use the least toxic to us and the environment, and only when we must.

You should learn as much as you can about any pesticides you do use. Use alternatives to the current pesticides. Exposure to pesticides can be controlled. This is yet another risk factor for disease over which you have control.

Bob is correct to avoid imported fruits and vegetables because foreign countries can use harmful/carcinogenic pesticides that have been banned in the US.

11

Smoking

Nicole L. Simone, M.D.

Sean's History
As a young child Sean inhaled his parents' smoke and then began to smoke 1-2 packs of cigarettes each day starting at age 17. He tried quitting several times but still is smoking at age 39. Is he at risk for cancer and other medical diseases?

Smoking is a major health hazard. In 1995 the Brown and Williamson documents revealed that the tobacco industry knew of the harm brought on by its products.[1] About 10% of the world's deaths are related to tobacco use.[2]

The World Health Organization indicates that the annual number of premature deaths caused by tobacco will rise to 10 million by the year 2025. Over half a billion people today, including 200 million currently under the age of 20, will die from tobacco-induced disease, and half of these will be in middle age.[3] Worldwide, 1.1 billion people smoke and 330 million of them live in China. [4,5]

The WHO Conference said that the tobacco companies have targeted expansion in Third World countries, and women and girls, and young boys in the US. Smoking among children has increased dramatically. Since 1968, the number of girls between the ages of 12 and 14 who smoke has increased eightfold. Six million children between 13 and 19 are regular smokers, and over 140,000 children under 13 are regular smokers. Smoking among blacks exceeds that among whites.

More deaths and physical suffering are related to cigarette smoking than to any other single cause: over 228,700 deaths (and rising) each year from cancer, over 325,000 deaths from cardiovascular disease, and more than 50,000 deaths from chronic lung diseases. Compare these figures with the number of Americans who died in the following wars – Table 1. Over a ten-year period (1964-1974), research by the cigarette industry confirmed the fatal dangers of smoking cigarettes. [6]

Table 1. US Deaths: Wars vs. Smoking

World War I	116,708
World War II	407,316
Korean War	54,246
Vietnam War	58,151
Smoking Annually	603,700
Involuntary inhalation of smoke annually	55,000

The cost of smoking-related diseases is staggering. Over $100 billion dollars a year are spent on tobacco related diseases and disability. Over $900 million are spent on prescription smoking cessation products, and close to $800 million are spent on over-the-counter smoking cessation products.[7] A great deal of this cost is paid by nonsmokers as well as smokers through ever-increasing health insurance premiums, disability payments, and other programs. Nonsmokers should not have to pay one penny for self-induced smokers' diseases.

The longer a person smokes, the greater the risk of dying. A person who smokes two packs a day has a death rate two times higher than a nonsmoker. If a smoker stops smoking, the mortality rate decreases progressively as the number of nonsmoking years increases. Those who have stopped for fifteen years have mortality rates similar to those who never smoked, with the exception of smokers who stopped after the age of 65. Cigar and pipe smokers also have an increased risk of death.

SMOKING INCREASES LUNG CANCER RISK
- **Cigarette smoking.** The risk is increased by the amount of smoking, duration of smoking, age at which smoking starts,

and content of tar and nicotine. Deaths are rising from lung cancer making it the leading cause of women's cancer deaths.

- **Marijuana smoking** also increases risk (National Academy of Sciences, "Marijuana and Health"). Marijuana smoke has 50% more carcinogenic hydrocarbons than cigarette smoke.
- **Breast Radiation Therapy + Smoking ⇒ Lung Cancer**. After about 10 years, women with breast cancer who smoked at the time they received breast radiation therapy have a 75% higher risk for developing lung cancer on the same side as the breast that was treated.[8] The overall risk for developing lung cancer in a woman who smokes and gets radiation therapy is about thirty times that of a woman with breast cancer who doesn't smoke, and over seventy-five times for the same side lung as the treated breast. If this high-risk woman is not willing to stop smoking, then maybe she should have a mastectomy instead of radiation.

SMOKING INCREASES PROSTATE CANCER RISK [9-11]

- Smoking two packs a day for 20 years doubles a man's risk for prostate cancer and his chances that he will have cancer that has spread outside the prostate.

SMOKING INCREASES PROSTATE CANCER AGGRESSIVENESS AND DEATH [12,13]

- Smoking increases the aggressiveness of the prostate cancer and increases the death rate from it.

SMOKING INCREASES BREAST CANCER RISK [14-22]

- Women smokers have higher risk for breast cancer.

TOBACCO-RELATED CANCERS AND PRE-CANCERS

- Cervix [23]
- Cervix dysplasia, a pre-cancer [24]
- Colon polyp (adenomatous, precancer) – 2.7 higher risk [25-29]
- Esophagus
- Larynx
- Kidney
- Mouth
- Nasopharynx
- Pancreas
- Urinary Bladder

Alcohol and asbestos intensify the harmful effects of to-bacco smoking. Chewing tobacco or snuff dipping in non-smokers causes a fourfold increase of oral cancers and a sixfold increase in those who smoked tobacco and drink alcohol heavily.[30] Furthermore, countries such as India, Ceylon, China, and the Soviet Union have the highest rates of death from oral cancer because the people there combine snuff and/or chewing tobacco with other ingredients such as betel nut. A chemical in the betel nut (N'nitrosonornicotine) initiates tumors in animals.

CARCINOGENS IN TOBACCO SMOKE

There are over 2,000 chemical compounds generated by tobacco smoke. The gas phase contains carbon monoxide, carbon dioxide, ammonia, nitrosamines, nitrogen oxides, hydrogen cyanide, sulfurs, nitriles, ketones, alcohols, and acrolein. The tars contain extremely carcinogenic hydrocarbons, which include nitrosamines, benzo(a)pyrenes, anthracenes, acridines, quinolines, benzenes, naphthols, naphthalenes, cresols, and insecticides (DDT), as well as some radioactive compounds like potassium-40 and radium-226. Tobacco smoke, through its many carcinogens, produces harmful free radicals.

OTHER SMOKING-RELATED ILLNESSES

- Cardiovascular illnesses[31-35]
- Osteoporosis[36]
- Emphysema and other lung diseases
- Female infertility, higher risk of miscarriage or spontaneous abortion, more genetic mutations[37-40]

SMOKING IMPAIRS THE IMMUNE SYSTEM

- SMOKING IMPAIRS IMMUNE SYSTEM ANATOMY by destroying hair-like structures that line the respiratory tract. These hairs normally beat upward to remove mucous and microorganisms. Without them, bacteria and viruses can grow.

Smoking also causes an increase in macrophages, cells that defend the lung against invading organisms. Macrophages secrete enzymes against the invaders, which also causes emphysema by breaking down of the walls of the respiratory tree.

• **SMOKING IMPAIRS IMMUNE CELLS** - The function of T cells, natural killer cells, macrophages, and antibody levels.[41-43]

INVOLUNTARY INHALATION OF SMOKE causes the death of approximately 53,000 people each year. A nonsmoker who is exposed to tobacco smoke has many adverse reactions and is unjustly and unnecessarily subjected to risk factors detrimental to his or her health.[44] The smoke that comes from the lighted end of a cigarette contains more hazardous chemicals than does the smoke that is inhaled by the smoker. It is virtually impossible to avoid tobacco smoke because it is so prevalent in homes, work places, and public areas.

On March 19, 1984, R.J. Reynolds Tobacco Company asserted in the *Wall Street Journal* entitled Smoking in Public: Let's Separate Fact From Fiction, that: "But, in fact, there is little evidence and certainly nothing which proves scientifically that cigarette smoke causes disease in nonsmokers." Then came the Surgeon General's report in 1986 proclaiming for the first time that involuntary inhalation of cigarette smoke by nonsmokers causes disease, most notably lung cancer.[45,46] The National Academy of Sciences reported similar findings.[47]

A movement to stop all smoking in public areas began with the ban of smoking on all domestic flights in the United States since early 1990. Forty-two states have legislated smoking restrictions in public transportation, hospitals, elevators, indoor areas, cultural or recreational facilities, schools, and libraries.

• **BREAST CANCER RISK IS INCREASED.** Involuntary inhaled smoke increases breast cancer risk.[48-56]

• **LUNG CANCER RISK IS INCREASED.**[57,58] Nonsmokers married to smokers have a 1.34 times greater risk for lung cancer than do those married to nonsmokers. This is one hundred times higher than the person exposed to asbestos for twenty years.

About 17 percent of lung cancers in nonsmokers are a result of exposure to tobacco smoke during childhood and adolescence.[54-58] Innocent children are at tremendous risk for lung cancer because they inhale their parent's smoke.

Smoking during pregnancy increases by 50 percent the fetus's risk of developing cancer later in childhood.[59] Infants exposed to smoke through breast milk have a higher risk of sudden infant death syndrome [SIDS].[60]

- **CERVICAL CANCER RISK IS INCREASED BY THREE-FOLD** for those who inhale smoke involuntarily for three or more hours daily.[61]

- **BLADDER CANCER RISK IS INCREASED** for nonsmokers who inhale other people's smoke.[62]

STOP SMOKING. More than 95 percent of former smokers quit on their own, usually at the recommendation of their physician. Seek help to quit smoking.

- Smoking cessation for 10 years lowers the risk of heart disease, and for 15 years lowers the risk of cancer to the same rates as a nonsmoker of that age.
- Smokers who have existing heart disease can reduce their risk of future heart attacks and death if they quit smoking, even if they are 65 or older.[63,64]
- Weight gain may occur for only a small percentage of those who stop smoking.[65] To guard against possible weight gain, follow the Ten-Point Plan.

CURRENT PUBLIC POLICIES

Federally sponsored programs support tobacco prices, benefiting allotment holders (a unique monopoly situation) and tobacco growers. In addition, other federally sponsored programs benefit the tobacco industry. On the other hand, federal funds are spent to discourage smoking, to research the health effects of smoking, and to provide a great portion of the cost of medical care for people who are suffering from and dying of smoking-related diseases. Patients with *self-induced* smoking-related diseases and their families receive Social Security benefits.

The American Medical Association's official policy since 1986 has stated that it: (1) Opposes any efforts by the government or its agencies to actively encourage, persuade, or compel any country to import tobacco products; and (2) Favors legislation that would prevent the government from actively supporting, promoting, or assisting such activities. However, the AMA's Political Action Committee has been giving money to United States representatives who actively oppose the AMA's official policy and who are responsible for getting tobacco into foreign markets.[66]

TIME FOR NEW PUBLIC POLICIES

Tobacco smoke is a threat to all of our lives. It is time now to prohibit smoking in all public areas and work places.

Nonsmokers incur higher risk from involuntarily inhaling others' smoke but also have to pay higher health insurance premiums for diseases related to smoking (cancer, cardiovascular diseases, lung diseases, etc.). Moreover, nonsmokers subsidize the tobacco industry through their tax dollars. We should pressure our senators and congressmen to force the American government to stop subsidizing the tobacco industry.

The United States has adopted uncompromisingly restrictive measures concerning food additives, but only a verbal statement of caution is required on every package of cigarettes. The Delaney Clause legislation prohibits the sale of any product to the American people that has been shown to be carcinogenic to humans and animals, and thus applies to situations in which the human hazard may be minimal. Tobacco is a major risk factor for cancer, cardiovascular diseases, lung diseases, and others.

CONCLUSION

If you smoke, stop. If you have not started, don't! Seek professional help if you must, but stop smoking!

Sean stopped smoking after we reviewed the scientific data. He knows he can lower his risk for diseases by following our Ten Point Plan. He's won his battle.

12
Alcohol and Caffeine

Bob's History
Bob drinks a glass of wine every night for dinner – sometimes two on the weekend. He likes how it tastes and how it relaxes him. However, his recent PSA is abnormal.

About 100 million Americans drink alcohol, and over 28 million – 1 of every 8 Americans – are children of alcoholics. Alcohol-related costs are about $120 billion every year. Many more billions of dollars are added to this figure when you consider that alcohol is involved in 50 percent of all traffic fatalities, 30 percent of small-aircraft accidents, and 66 percent of all violent crimes. The totals are higher still when you consider the losses due to diseases aggravated by alcohol use, and losses due to alcohol-induced poor decision-making in government, industry, education, law, the military, and medicine. About 68 percent of adult Americans abuse alcohol. Alcohol-related hospitalizations among the elderly are common. All of society pays for this. Employers lose productivity, taxpayers pay the bill for programs and services, and consumers pay higher insurance premiums.

Alcohol is a risk factor for cancers of the prostate, breast, mouth, pharynx, larynx, esophagus, pancreas, liver, and head and neck. Alcohol acts synergistically with tobacco smoking in the development of other gastrointestinal cancers and urinary bladder cancer. Alcohol causes cirrhosis of the liver, the seventh leading cause of death in the US. Fifty percent of alcoholics die from cardiovascular diseases and 20 percent from accidents, suicides, and homicides.

ALCOHOL CAUSES NUTRITIONAL DEFICIENCIES

Alcoholics will consume about 20 percent of their total calories as alcohol and therefore vitamin deficiencies are common in alcoholics. Thiamine (vitamin B1) deficiency causes a severe brain disease called Wernicke-Korsakoff syndrome that can be rapidly reversed by the administration of thiamine. Folic acid and vitamin B12 deficiencies cause anemias. Pyridoxine (B6) deficiency causes peripheral nerve problems. Alcoholics have a deficiency of vitamin C because of their liver disease. Mineral deficiencies include calcium, zinc, magnesium, and iron. Some alcoholics develop the Plummer-Vinson syndrome that is characterized by a cluster of symptoms including difficulty swallowing; a red, smooth tongue; and iron deficiency anemia. People with this syndrome have a high rate of cancer of the mouth.

ALCOHOL SUPPRESSES IMMUNITY

- Decreases the number and function of neutrophils, lymphocytes, monocytes, and natural killer cells.
- Decreases the rate of antibody production.
- Decreases the complement protein defense system.
- Increases risk for cancer, tuberculosis, viral infections.

ALCOHOL INCREASES PROSTATE CANCER RISK BY 150%-250%.[1-3] Men who consume between three to seven drinks a week, have a higher risk for developing prostate cancer independently of other prostate cancer risk factors. Twelve ounces of beer equals four ounces of wine, which equals one and a half ounces of whiskey in alcohol content. Drinking this amount will increase your risk because alcohol is immunosuppressive, carcinogenic, and, can alter hormone levels, and increase your testosterone levels that stimulate prostate cells to grow. Other studies that are less well controlled show no relation between alcohol and prostate cancer risk.

ALCOHOL INCREASES SPREAD OF CANCER. Alcohol may actually speed up an existing cancer.[4] Animals were injected with a cancer that always spreads to the lungs. At the time of injection, the animals were allowed to get drunk. Those with a blood alcohol content of 0.15 percent, which represents about four to five drinks an hour, later developed more than twice the number of new lung metastases compared to the animals that did not drink alcohol. Those with a blood level of 0.25 percent had eight times more tumors in their lungs.

These same levels of alcohol are seen in humans who drink excessively in one hour. Men with prostate cancer who drink this amount are probably at an increased risk for developing metastatic disease.

ALCOHOL INCREASES RISK FOR OTHER CANCERS, AND OTHER DISEASES

- Mouth, pharynx, and esophagus cancers – alcohol is a topical carcinogen. People who use mouthwash that contains alcohol have a high rate of oral cancer. Alcohol and tobacco account for 75 percent of all oral cancers in the United States.
- Alcoholic liver cirrhosis increases the risk for liver cancer, varicose veins in the esophagus, ascites (fluid in the abdomen); muscle wasting; kidney failure, pancreas and heart abnormalities, and stroke.[5,6]
- Breast, and colon-rectal cancers.
- Premature testicle and ovary shrinkage.
- Peptic ulcers.
- Adult brain shrinkage that may normalize after abstinence.[7]
- "Fetal alcohol syndrome" – defects in the brain, in intellectual development, physical growth, and in the facial features of infants born of alcoholic mothers.

CAFFEINE

Caffeine is the most popular drug in North America and in many other parts of the world. It is found in coffee, tea, cola beverages, and chocolate. Caffeine is linked to:
- Breast Cancer [8,9]

- Urinary Bladder cancer[10] – more than three cups per day.
- Miscarriage and Infant Prematurity – one cup per day[11-13]
- Low Infant Birth Rate.
- DNA damage – increases cancer, fetal malformations[14,15]
- Heart Disease risk – more than 5 cups per day [16]
- Osteoporosis [17]

Caffeine Concentrations in Milligrams			
COFFEE (12 oz)		**SOFT DRINKS (12 oz)**	
Brewed (drip method)	275	Cherry Cola	36-46
Brewed (percolator)	190	Diet Cherry Cola	36-45
Instant	155	Cola (all), Dr Pepper	30-46
Brewed, Decaffeinated	7	Diet Colas & Dr Pepper	38-45
Instant, Decaffeinated	5	Lemon-lime, Orange	0
TEA (12 oz)		Root Beer and diet	0
Brewed (imported)	145	Ginger Ale & diet, Tonic	0
Brewed (domestic)	95		
Iced Tea	70	**OVER-THE-COUNTER MEDS**	
CHOCOLATE		Vivarin	200
Baker's chocolate (1.5 oz)	39	No-Doz	100
Dark or semisweet (1.5 oz)	30	Excedrin	65
Hot cocoa (12 oz)	10	Vanquish	33
Milk chocolate (1.5 oz)	9	Midol	32
Chocolate Milk (12 oz)	7		

CONCLUSION

Alcohol and caffeine are two important risk factors for cancer. The decision to consume them is *yours*. You can again decide about the status of your health!

Bob's PSA abnormality was found to be a cancer. He stopped drinking and modified his lifestyle according to the Ten Point Plan. He knows his life will be extended.

13

Hormonal and Sexual-Social Factors

Carl's History
Carl is 51. He had been a body-builder for years and used steroids in the process. What's his risk?

Hormonal factors and sexual-social behavior are directly related to the development of cancer. The risk for certain cancers is increased because more hormones are used and there is a relaxation of sexual mores that increases promiscuity.

SEX HORMONES AND IMMUNE SYSTEM REGULATE EACH OTHER

CRITICAL TIMES OF HORMONE INFLUENCE
The prostate grows in spurts – during puberty and during ages 40 to 50 – as a result of hormonal changes, especially the conversion of testosterone to dihydrotestosterone (DHT) via the enzyme 5 alpha-reductase. DHT stimulates cellular growth within the prostate. Also, estrogen begins to rise as men age and further enhances DHT.

NATURAL HORMONAL INFLUENCE FOR CANCER
■ **TESTOSTERONE AND ESTROGEN.** High levels of circulating testosterone and low levels of estrogen increase the risk for developing prostate cancer.[1] If, however, testosterone is high but in the normal range, there seems to be no increased risk.[2]

■ **BENIGN BREAST DISEASE.** About 60% of men over the age of 40 develop breasts because their testosterone levels begin to fall allowing estrogen levels to influence the growth of breast tissue. This has been reviewed in ***The Truth About Breast Health – Breast Cancer***. A low-fat, high fiber diet with certain vitamins and minerals, together with the avoidance of caffeine and nicotine inhalation can decrease breast tenderness and swelling after six months and breast swelling and nodularity are reduced in 60% of the patients.

Since 1979, I have treated patients with benign breast disorders, specifically lumpy breast disease. All the patients followed my Ten-Point Plan. Almost 90 percent of the patients had decreased breast pain, and about half of the patients experienced a decrease in the size of their cysts. In most cases the size of the breast diminished somewhat.

ADMINISTERED HORMONES INCREASE RISK

■ **TESTOSTERONE INCREASES RISK FOR CANCER AND HEART DISEASE.** Athletes use testosterone to increase muscle bulk and performance. Testosterone causes cardiovascular illnesses, prostate cancer, liver cancer, and osteosarcoma, as well as benign liver disease.

Because testosterone levels fall with aging, more men in their 50s and 60s are being treated with some form of testosterone. Transdermal testosterone gels represent an effective alternative to injectable testosterone preparations. However, elevated PSA and biopsy-proven prostate cancer has been reported in about 2% of men who used transdermal gels.[3]

Also, a case of prostate cancer has been reported in a patient with Klinefelter syndrome who had undergone long-term testosterone replacement therapy since childhood for chronically depressed levels of testosterone.[4]

Testosterone is undoubtedly involved in the growth of benign prostatic nodules, the initiation of prostate cancer and in the promotion of the growth of active prostate cancer.[5]

■**DES INCREASES RISK FOR CANCERS OF THE BREAST, VAGINA, CERVIX, AND TESTICLE.**[6-9] DES (diethylstilbestrol) was used to avert miscarriages in the 1940s and 1950s.

- Sons of DES-exposed mothers have reproductive and urinary tract abnormalities. One of these is undescended testicles, that may lead to cancer of the testes if uncorrected before the age of 6.

- Increases risk for vaginal and cervical cancer and dysplasia in women who were exposed to DES as fetuses.

- Increases risk for breast cancer for women who took it.

- Breast enlargement in children who ate meat that had DES.[56]

For women who were exposed to DES:
  1. Tell your daughter or son.
  2. Try to obtain the details of your DES dosage and duration.
  3. Have Pap smear, breast exam by a physician, mammogram.
  4. Practice breast self-exam and report anything.
  5. Report any unusual bleeding or discharge from the vagina.
  6. Avoid oral contraceptives, hormone replacement, etc.

For daughters of DES-exposed mothers:
  1. Report unusual bleeding or discharge from the vagina.
  2. Annual Pap smear at age 14 or when you begin menses.

For sons of DES-exposed mothers:
  1. Have physician check reproductive and urinary systems to make certain there are no abnormalities.

■**ESTROGENS ADMINISTERED IN LARGE AMOUNTS INCREASED THE RATE OF BREAST CANCER** in male transsexuals[10] as well as in male heart and ulcer patients.

■**PHYTOESTROGENS** can decrease the risk of prostate cancer[11] for men who consume phytoestrogens from soy, etc, and have high serum concentration of phytoestrogens. This case-control study in Japan (Japan Collaborative Cohort (JACC) Study) showed that a low risk for prostate cancer was associated with high serum levels of genistein, daidzein, and equol.

SEXUAL-SOCIAL FACTORS

■ PENIS CANCER is not common in the continental United States, it occurs more frequently in many parts of the world where circumcision is not performed routinely. Penile cancer has been studied extensively in Puerto Rico. The epidemiological evidence there suggests that uncircumcised males with poor hygiene techniques, that is, those who do not routinely clean beneath the foreskin, have a very high incidence of cancer of the penis. Routine circumcision almost completely eliminates the risk for this cancer.

■ AIDS is one of the most feared diseases in the world affecting hundreds of millions of people. AIDS patients develop several cancers. The prevalence of AIDS in the homosexual population received much media attention; however, today over 60 percent of the cases of HIV infection worldwide have been acquired heterosexually. Intravenous drug users, their sexual partners, and their children represent the next largest portion of all cases.

■ **Mode of Spread.** In June 1987 Dr. F. Noireau reported from the Congo that the isolation of a retrovirus from monkeys was closely related to the human immunodeficiency virus (HIV) and strongly suggested a simian origin of this virus. HIV is widely thought to have originated in central East Africa where the virus may have existed in an endemic state for a while. The indirect transmission of the virus from the monkey to man may have occurred through bites, through the cutting up and consumption of monkey meat, or from insects. In a book on the sexual practices of people in the Great Lakes area of Africa, Kasharmura writes the following: "To stimulate a man or woman and induce them to intense sexual activity, monkey blood (for a man) or she-monkey blood (for a woman) was directly inoculated in the pubic area and also the thighs and backs." These magic practices could be responsible for the emergence of AIDS in humanity.

■ AIDS has been reportedly transmitted by:
    Breastfeeding[12]

Oral-genital transmission[13,14]
Mother to child transmission via the placenta[15]
Heterosexual transmission[15]
Blood transfusions of unscreened blood.
Blood transfusions of screened or unscreened blood[16]
Female to female transmission[17]
Transmission by human bite[18]
Insect-borne transmission[19]
Acupuncture[20]
Faulty condoms[21]
Transmission between two siblings[22]

In addition, HIV has been isolated from dead infected patients up to eleven days after death[23]

The risk of developing AIDS increases each year after infection by the virus. Evidence from San Francisco's Health Department and the Centers for Disease Control has shown that only 4 percent of those infected with the virus will develop the disease within three years. But after five years of exposure that figure climbs to 14 percent, and after seven years it jumps to 36 percent. Hence the longer you are infected, the higher your chances for developing AIDS.

■ AIDS INCREASES RISK FOR CANCERS OF THE ANUS, TONGUE, KAPOSI'S SARCOMA, AND LYMPHOMA

CONCLUSION

All the studies reviewed suggest a consistent theme: If you tamper with Mother Nature's hormonal milieu by taking hormone pills, or by disrupting reproduction, you have a higher risk of developing certain cancers, including prostate cancer.

Carl knows his risk for developing cancer is very high based on his hormonal and sexual-social factors alone. He is now modifying his lifestyle to decrease his risks.

14
Air and Water

Henry's History
Henry is 41 with four children. They use special filters on their vents. The children are fed well, the house is clean, and all chemicals locked up. They drink distilled water.

Mounting evidence suggests that our environment contains many carcinogens. The air we breathe, the water we drink, the radiation to which we are exposed, and the power lines that supply us with energy pose threats to our health. As with many carcinogens, the time between exposure to environmental carcinogens and actual development of cancer may be quite long. Therefore, the cause of a cancer initiated by trace amounts of either airborne or waterborne carcinogens years before may be attributed to an unrelated or unknown factor at the time of diagnosis. This is why we must constantly clean our environment of carcinogens.

OUTDOOR AIR POLLUTION costs $50 billion a year.
- Cancer rate is increased in cities due to: (1) more cigarette smoking; (2) more involuntary inhalation of tobacco smoke (3) occupational exposures.[1-3]
- Workers exposed to air pollutants have an increased risk for lung cancer – gas production workers (coal carbonization); steel workers at coke ovens; and roofers exposed to hot pitch
- City air pollution has more than 100 particulate carcinogens that come from the burning of any material containing carbon and hydrogen, including petroleum, gasoline, and diesel

fuel.[4] Many studies indicated that tiny particulate air pollution in cities is linked to higher mortality rates.[5-7]

- Gas phase of the air also has carcinogens: benzene, carbon tetrachloride, chloroform, and vinyl chloride, among others.[8] These carcinogens are derived from car emissions, industrial activity, burning of solid waste, forest fires, and evaporation of solvents.[9]

- Asbestos is a potent carcinogen for lung cancer and is found in roofing and flooring, car brakes and clutches, dry walls, home heating and plumbing. Family members of persons who work with asbestos or asbestos products are exposed to very high levels of asbestos also. Cigarette smoking acts synergistically with asbestos to greatly enhance the risk of lung cancer. It is *extremely* rare for lung cancer to develop in an asbestos worker in the absence of exposure to tobacco smoke.

- Diesel exhaust increases risk of lung cancer for workers exposed to diesel engine emissions.[10]

ACID RAIN is made when sulfur dioxide and nitrogen oxide are released into the atmosphere and converted into sulfuric acid and nitric acid from fossil fuel combustion and power plant emissions.

- Affects soil: releases toxic metals – aluminum, mercury, lead, nickel, cadmium, and manganese that get into the water supply adversely affecting aquatic life in 10% of Eastern lakes and streams. Reduces selenium content in soil.

- Decreases the number of red spruce at high elevations, and contributes to the corrosion of buildings and materials.

- To control acid rain – use fossil fuel with low sulfur content.

DEPLETION OF NATURAL UPPER ATMOSPHERIC OZONE INCREASES RISK FOR SKIN CANCER

The naturally occurring ozone layer in the upper atmosphere is crucial to the protection of living organisms because it absorbs harmful ultraviolet radiation. About 3 percent of the sun's electromagnetic output is emitted as ultraviolet radiation, but only a fraction of this reaches the surface of the Earth.

• Ultraviolet exposure is associated with melanoma, basal cell, and squamous cell cancer of the skin. People with fair skin, blond hair, and blue eyes who also sunburn easily are at highest risk for the development of these skin cancers. The US Environmental Protection Agency calculates that a 1 percent decrease in the ozone concentration will increase the incidence of most skin cancers by 3-5 percent.

• Ultraviolet exposure causes skin damage and skin aging

• Phytoplankton, zooplankton, and the larval stages of fish, are very sensitive to small increases in ultraviolet exposure. The resultant decrease in the food chain and in the oxygen output from the oceans' plants will have serious and dramatic repercussions on all human life.

Addressing the Problem

Chlorofluorocarbons, commonly known as CFCs, are chemical compounds that cause holes in the protective ozone layer. CFCs are in aerosols, foam blowers for items such as hamburger cartons and drinking cups, refrigerants and cooling systems, and solvents for computer circuits. In most instances, nonchlorinated substitutes are available or can be developed. Some CFCs remain in the air for over a century. For every 2.5 percent increase per year of chlorofluorocarbon, an additional million skin cancers and 20,000 deaths will occur over the lifetime of the existing United States population.

If pentane is used instead of chlorofluorocarbons as the blowing agent to produce foam products, *ozone is produced* both in the stratosphere and at the ground level. These products are less costly than paper products. A paper cup costs more to make: raw materials (wood, bark, petroleum fractions), finished weight, wholesale price, utilities needed to produce it (steam, power, cooling water), waste products produced, and air emissions (chlorine, chlorine dioxide, reduced sulfides).[11] The polystyrene cup is easier to recycle and ultimately to dispose. Here again, we have the proper technology to solve this problem.

OZONE AT GROUND LEVEL CAUSES DISEASES

• Ozone at ground level is harmful to us whereas the naturally occurring protective ozone layer in the upper atmosphere shields us from harmful ultraviolet rays. Ozone at ground level is the most widespread air pollutant in any industrialized country and is formed when car exhaust and other industrial emissions react with sunlight.

• Smog is derived predominantly from ozone as well as from carbon monoxides, nitrogen oxides, sulfur oxides, particulates, and volatile organic compounds. These compounds are derived from bakeries during fermentation; dry cleaning chemicals; paints; wood-burning stoves and starter fluid used to ignite charcoal; industries and motor vehicles using fossil fuels.

• Cities with the highest ozone: Los Angeles, New York, Philadelphia, Trenton, Baltimore, Hartford, Chicago, and Houston. Some national parks like Acadia, Shenandoah, and Sequoia national parks have higher ozone levels than some cities because of their proximity to the major cities with smog and/or the air currents around them.

• Ozone at ground level has been linked to cancer, lung and heart disease, impaired immunity, and other illnesses.

• Ozone impairs oxygen absorption.

• Ozone causes lung damage similar to that seen from smoking

• When ozone levels are high, asthmatics, cardiac patients, and older people who have respiratory illnesses do poorly.

ULTRAVIOLET SUNLIGHT has two forms: ultraviolet A (UVA) and ultraviolet B (UVB). The UVB is the more harmful causing sunburn and skin cancer. It has wavelengths between 290 and 320 nanometers. UVA causes skin cancer, skin damage, and premature aging of the skin. UVA has wavelengths between 320 and 400 nanometers, which is where the visible light spectrum begins.

Sunglasses should be used to protect your eyes from the harmful ultraviolet rays of the sun. Regardless of cost, most sunglasses filter all UVB, but not necessarily all UVA.[12]

INDOOR AIR pollution causes illnesses and the "sick building syndrome" symptoms.[13] Ventilation can eliminate this.

• **Radon** is implicated in up to 20,000 deaths from lung cancer in the United States.[14] A person living in a house with an indoor radon level of 4 pica Curies/liter has the same risk of developing lung cancer as a person who smokes half a pack of cigarettes per day.[15] Coal miners who are exposed to radon and also smoke have a higher risk of lung cancer.[16]

• **Involuntary inhalation of tobacco smoke** doubles the lung cancer rate.[17] Seventeen percent of all lung cancers are found in people who never smoked but who inhaled smoke between ages of 3 and 15. There should be no smoking in public places.

• **Stoves** without chimneys and kerosene stoves produce many pollutants, several of which are carcinogenic.

• **Heat exchangers, cooling towers**, and **leaky showerheads** provide favorable culture media for many microorganisms. These bacteria and other organisms disperse in droplets and remain airborne via mechanical or thermal air movements. *Legionella premophilia* (Legionnaires' disease) and many other organisms have been detected airborne in closed indoor situations.

• **Other indoor pollutants** come from materials that are used in the construction of modern buildings, such as formaldehyde (associated with human cancer), isocyanates, solvents, and volatile synthetic organic compounds.

WATER POLLUTION

• **Synthetic organic chemicals** amount to over 700 in our drinking water.[18] Forty of these are carcinogens, and three (benzene, chloromethyl ether, and vinyl chloride) are associated with human cancer.[19] Drinking polluted water is said by the EPA to be one of the top four health hazards in America. The EPA allows municipalities to average their water toxicities over a year. For example, much more chlorine is added to water during summer months to hold down microorganisms. In some cities, the tap water level of chlorine carcinogens exceeds the standard by 20 percent during these months. The same spike of toxicity holds true for nitrates and pesticides, both used seasonally for lawn beautification and farming.

Chlorination produces trihalomethanes – chloroform and bromohalomethane – that double the risk for gastrointestinal and urinary bladder cancers.[19-24] The EPA's safety limit of chlorine and its harmful associated carcinogens is based on the consumption of two liters of water a day, and this does not take into account increased consumption in summer, or the fact that these compounds can be absorbed during bathing.

• **Inorganic chemicals** like arsenic, chromium (certain chemical form), nickel, and lead are toxic. Lead impairs children's IQ and attention span. One in six people in the United States drinks water with higher than acceptable levels of lead.

The amount of calcium and magnesium in water determines water "hardness." It appears that soft water, water containing lesser amounts of calcium and particularly magnesium, is correlated with a higher incidence of all cardiovascular diseases, osteoporosis, hypertension, and breast and colon cancer.

• **Radioactive materials** in water varies with geography, geology, industrial wastes, pharmaceutical use, and nuclear power generation.[25]

• **Living organisms** – bacteria, viruses, and protozoa –can resist water purification, and these are responsible for 33 percent of all gastrointestinal infections in the United States.

• **Solid particulates** include clays, asbestos particles, and organic particulates.

WHO IS TO BLAME FOR THE SHAMBLES OF THE WATER SUPPLY? Probably everyone. Most states do not comply with existing standards, or comply by way of loopholes. For example, a loophole permits water suppliers to flush lead-filled water out of plumbing before testing tap water. The EPA has been lax because it only recently has imposed restrictions for radon in the drinking water.

Eighty percent of the top 1,000 superfund sites, that is, those designated as containing toxic waste and chemical contaminants, are leaching these toxic substances into the ground water. In many geographic sites in the United States, well water has been contaminated. About 10 percent of all underground tanks, which store gasoline or other hazardous chemicals, leak. Too many pesticides and fertilizers are used by farmers and homeowners. Industries dump chemicals and other harmful pollutants into our water supply, and homeowners dump chemicals into household drains.

Addressing the Problem.   One of the major obstacles to clean up America's underground toxic wastes is the unrealistic requirement that has been set by government authorities throughout the nation. The problem is that the objectives are simply too difficult to be accomplished by existing technologies. If the requirement had been to reduce the contaminants from 2,000 parts per billion to, say, 10 parts, it would be possible to reduce the health hazard by 99.5 percent and leave limited funds available for twenty or thirty more of the same type of clean-up projects. It is better to clean up all the toxic sites by a significant factor like 99.5 percent than only a few sites by a factor of 99.99 percent and thereby propagate endless litigation.

A number of cities refuse to build costly processing plants and instead choose to pay less expensive fines. The EPA observes that small utilities tend to violate regulations the most, falsify documents, and even wash away evidence because of a thirty-day window given them by the state.

WATER DERIVED FROM DISTILLATION OR REVERSE OSMOSIS IS MORE PURE THAN TAP OR SPRING OR "BOTTLED"

CONCLUSION
There are documented airborne and waterborne carcinogens. It is essential for us to detect and clean our environment of as many carcinogens as possible.

Henry is doing all the right things and now includes the use of sunscreens and sunglasses.

15
Electromagnetic Radiation

Joe's History
Joe is 46 and received radiation to his face to treat acne. He remembers putting his feet in an X-ray machine to see his feet in his new shoes. He had multiple X-rays over the years and sleeps with an electric blanket and clock radio near his head.

The electromagnetic radiation spectrum includes gamma rays, X-rays, ultraviolet light, visible light, infrared, microwaves, FM radio waves, AM radio waves, and long radio waves. Electromagnetic radiation with wavelengths longer than the color red (ranging from infrared to radio waves) or shorter than the color violet (ranging from ultraviolet to X-rays and gamma rays) is not visible to the eye. Radiation exposure is another risk factor for developing breast cancer.

DIAGNOSTIC AND THERAPEUTIC RADIATION
Ionizing radiation causes cancer. Mammograms, CT scans, therapeutic radiation, and other radiation exposures increase the risk for developing cancer. Increased risk for breast cancer was first seen among women in Japan who were irradiated during the atomic bombings. More women who had exposure during ages 10 to 25 developed breast cancer from the radiation fall-out than women who were younger or women who were older.[1] Women with tuberculosis who had multiple serial chest X-rays to follow the course of the disease also had substantially increased rates of breast cancer.[2]

CT Scans.   Almost 85 percent of the radiation to which we are exposed in developed countries is from natural sources, but 15 percent is from human-made sources. Of these, about 97 percent is from diagnostic radiology – mainly CT scans. The dose for a single chest CT scan is the equivalent of 20 mammograms – about 2 to 3 cGy.

Children commonly receive an overdose of radiation when they have CT scans.[3,4] In fact, they receive doses that are at least five times greater than necessary. Radiologists can reduce the dose without compromising image quality but they do not. The number of indications CT scans are used for children has increased dramatically. Japanese children exposed to a single dose of 5 cGy during World War II have a four times greater risk for breast cancer. **So if a child today has two or three CT scans of the same area** – each giving 2 to 3 cGy per CT scan – over the long term, **the risk of cancer is increased significantly**.

The lifetime risk of developing cancer attributable to diagnostic X-rays is 1% to 2%, except in Japan where it is 3.2%.[5] Table 1 shows the actual number of cancers per year in various countries relative to the number of X-rays given per 1000 people.

Table 1. Number of Cancers per Year from Diagnostic X-rays				
	Annual X-rays per 1000 people	Number Cancers		Annual X-rays per 1000 people	Number Cancers
Australia	565	431	Netherlands	600	208
Canada	892	784	Norway	708	77
Croatia	903	169	Poland	641	291
Czech Rep	883	172	Sweden	568	162
Finland	704	50	Switzerland	750	173
Germany	1,254	2,049	United Kingdom	489	700
Japan	1,477	7,587	United States	962	5,695
Kuwait	896	40			

Therapeutic Radiation for Cancer Treatment.   Patients treated with radiation have a higher rate of cancers from it, often in sites remote from the treatment fields. There is also more sarcomas seen in heavily treated areas of the body. Patients who had radiation therapy for various diseases have a higher incidence of breast cancer if the radiation therapy was delivered to or near the breast, for example, chest radiation therapy to treat Hodgkin's disease.[6] The women or men who developed breast cancer secondary to radiation for Hodgkin's disease were all under the age of 40 and on average had the radiation about ten years prior to the diagnosis of breast cancer.

Prostate cancer. Men with early stage prostate cancers are being treated with Intensity-Modulated Radiation Therapy (IMRT) rather than the three-dimensional conformal radiation therapy. IMRT involves more fields and a larger volume of normal tissues is exposed to lower doses. Also, the number of monitor units of the radiation machine is increased by a factor of 2 to 3, thereby increasing the total body exposure due to leakage radiation. Both factors tend to increase the risk of a second cancer. **IMRT will likely double the incidence of second cancers to about 1.75% compared to conventional radiation treatments.**[7]

Breast cancer. Men with early stage breast cancers are being treated with breast-conserving surgery followed by radiation therapy. **On balance, it seems that there is a slight increase risk for developing breast cancer in the breast opposite the one that received radiation treatment for breast cancer** – Table 2. These patients should be watched closely.

Table 2. Risk of cancer in untreated breast from scatter radiation

Total Patients	Risk
97,346 [8,9]	Slight Increase
84,620 [10-23]	No Increase

However, breast cancer radiation therapy does increase the risk for developing leukemia (particularly in association with certain chemotherapies), lung cancer (especially in smokers), and sarcomas.[23]

THERAPEUTIC RADIATION FOR NONCANCEROUS LESIONS INCREASES CANCER RISK. In the past, radiation had been given for benign lesions. This is generally no longer done. Thymus gland, scalp, benign breast infections, and other sites were treated with radiation that later produced secondary cancers.

ELECTROMAGNETISM INCREASES RISK

Nonionizing electromagnetic radiation is generated largely through electrical and magnetic fields around us that include infrared rays, microwaves, radiowaves, and alternating electrical currents. All of these, except for infrared rays, penetrate the body readily. Such radiation is found in household wiring, appliances, high-tension wires, radio transmitters, television screens, video display terminals, electric blankets, and even the Earth, which has its own electromagnetic field. In fact, this electromagnetic field is responsible for making a compass needle point in the direction of north. However, the Earth's electromagnetic fields do a flip flop, the North and South Pole fields trading places at intervals of hundreds of thousands of years. Electromagnetism produces vague symptoms of fatigue, nausea, headache, loss of libido, and increases cancer risk.[24]

An electromagnetic field is created along wires when electricity flows and is measured in gauss. The electromagnetic field is made of two components: the electric field made from the strength of the charge that starts the flow, and the magnetic field that results from the motion of the alternating currents. The energy needed to make electricity flow is called voltage. More voltage is needed to make electricity go farther. Voltage is either stepped-up or stepped-down along transmission lines by transformers at substations or on utility poles near homes. The strength of the field is important for human health.

All electrically driven products have electromagnetic fields that, among other things, suppress melatonin, a hormone produced by the pineal gland in the brain. Melatonin regulates the immune system. Low levels of melatonin have been linked to breast and **prostate** cancer.[25] Postmenopausal women who use electric blankets have a higher risk of breast cancer.[26] The closer you are to a given appliance or other source, the higher is the strength of the electromagnetic field.

HIGH VOLTAGE WIRES INCREASE RISK

- Children living near the wires have a two times higher risk of developing cancer.[27-29]
- Men exposed to electrical and magnetic fields at work have an increased risk of leukemia (especially acute myeloid leukemia), brain tumors, and breast cancer.[30-34]

LOW VOLTAGE WIRES INCREASE RISK

- There are more childhood leukemia and childhood brain cancers, as well as adult cancers when homes have a large amount of house wiring or are close to telephone pole power lines.[35]
- Low-frequency electromagnetic fields produce weak electric fields in our bodies, affecting hormone levels, the binding levels of ions to cell membranes, certain genetic processes inside the cell such as RNA and protein synthesis, and calcium ions that play a major role in cell division.

COMPUTER MONITORS INCREASE RISK

The "extremely-low-frequency" magnetic fields produced by these monitors have been linked to cancers, breast disorders, spontaneous abortion (16 studies),[36] and other health problems. The US Environmental Protection Agency recommended that the radiation fields produced by these monitors be categorized as *probable* human carcinogens. Color monitors produce more radiation. The amount of radiation is always higher at the sides, back and top of the monitor. The more powerful the monitor, the more radiation is emitted. Workers should sit at least two feet away from the front of the monitor and stay at least four feet away from the back or sides of a co-worker's monitor. The same precautions for laser printers. Some computer makers already sell low-radiation monitors but do not advertise them as such, perhaps fearing that these would create concern and anxiety about other terminals that the company produces.

Table 3. Electromagnetic Fields of Various Sources

Source	Electromagnetic Field Strength (milligauss)*
Coffee makers	0.7-1.5
Crock pots	0.8-1.5
Refrigerators	0.1-3.0
Clothes dryers	0.7-3.0
Irons	1.0-4.0
Toasters	0.6-8.0
Garbage disposals	8-12
Dishwashers	7-14
Televisions	0.3-20.0
Washers	2-20
Desk Lamps	5-20
Blenders	5-25
Fans	0.2-40.0
Portable Heaters	1.5-40.0
Fluorescent Fixtures	20-40
Ovens	1-50
Ranges	3-50
Microwave ovens	40-90
Hair Dryers	1-100
Shavers	1-100
Mixers	6-150
Vacuum Cleaners	20-200
Can Openers	30-300
Electric wires on telephone pole	10-600
High tension electric wires	50-10,000

*At a distance of 30 centimeters

MAGNETIC RESONANCE IMAGING SCANS. Patients undergoing MRI scanning are exposed to three types of electromagnetic radiation: static magnetic fields, pulsed radiofrequency (RF) electromagnetic fields, and gradient (time-varying) fields. Atoms of all tissues resonate at specific frequencies within an electromagnetic field and produce signals that convert to images.

The fastest MRI scanners rely on the time-varying fields to obtain large amounts of information in milliseconds that produce a clearer image. However, time-varying fields produce electric currents in the body. These currents can cause cardiac arrhythmias or nerve stimulation. Further research is needed to determine the harm to the human body.

CELLULAR PHONES INCREASE THE RISK FOR CANCER SLIGHTLY because they produce radiofrequency radiation and therefore effect cells and tissues.[37-42]

OTHER HEALTH CONSEQUENCES.
Electromagnetic fields increase cortisol that suppresses the immune system. The fields can alter cancer cell membranes and make them resistant to the immune system.[43] Microwaves affect our circadian rhythms, which in turn affect our sleep patterns, growth, and repair mechanisms, and even IQ tests in animals.

ADDRESSING THE PROBLEM. New transmission lines should be routed to avoid developed areas and increase the distance from the lines to the houses. The problem is that little can be done to reduce the electromagnetic fields from the low-voltage lines within our cities.

Help yourself! Use computer monitors that have reduced electromagnetic radiation. Use electric blankets only to preheat the bed. Move electric alarm clocks as far away from your bed as is practical. Buy home appliances that have minimal fields. We obviously need to be wary about where we live, avoid high-tension wires, and take other common sense precautions.

Joe is making changes. He moved her clock radio, doesn't use the electric blanket, and began following the Ten Point Plan, including protective antioxidants. He will only get diagnostic X-rays if truly indicated.

16
Sedentary Lifestyle

Ric's History
Ric is 56 years old in middle management corporate America working a gazillion hours a week. He has two children in nearby colleges who he tries to visit on weekends. He "doesn't have time to exercise." Sound familiar?

We have all accepted that a sedentary lifestyle or lack of exercise is a risk factor for the development of cardiovascular illnesses. A sedentary lifestyle can also suppress the immune system and increase the risk for cancer and other diseases. Doctors preach about exercise and people generally are aware of it, sometimes even putting on their sneakers to do something about it. Sales of exercise equipment have risen over the past few years, but more often than not, these treadmills, stationary bicycles, and other very expensive devices remain unused in most people's basements. More than 90 percent of all Americans older than age 18 do not exercise. People who exercise are subsidizing the health-care costs for those who do not.

EXERCISE ENHANCES THE IMMUNE SYSTEM [1-12]

- Exercise increases the number and activity of T and B cells, natural killer cells, macrophages, and lymphokine activated killer cells and their regulating cytokines.
- Exercise slightly raises body temperature leading to an increase in the production of pyrogen, an interleukin that enhances lymphocyte functions. High temperatures kill viruses and cancer cells.[13-14]
- Exercise inhibits cancer growth.[15,16]

EXERCISE DECREASES PROSTATE CANCER RISK[17,18]

EXERCISE DECREASES PROSTATE CANCER PROGRESSION[19,20]

EXERCISE IMPROVES FUNCTION AND QUALITY OF LIFE FOR PATIENTS WITH PROSTATE CANCER[21-22]

EXERCISE LOWERS RISK FOR WOMEN'S CANCERS [23-30]
- Women who engaged in college sports had a lower incidence of cancers of the breast, ovary, cervix, vagina, and uterus.

EXERCISE DECREASES COLON CANCER RISK[31-33]
- Men who have sedentary jobs have a 1.6 higher risk of developing colon cancer, especially in the descending colon, than their colleagues who have more active jobs.
- People who work at a sedentary job for more than 40 percent of their work years developed colon cancer two times more frequently compared to those who never have.
- The risk of getting colon cancer was 1.3 times higher for those in sedentary jobs than for those in active jobs (1.1 million men in Sweden, 19 year study).
- Increased physical activity causes more motility of the gastrointestinal tract and more frequent evacuation of the colon. The longer the stool remains in the colon, the longer a carcinogen (fecapentaene) in the stool has to exert its effect on the colon. Consequently, the higher is the risk for cancer.

WALKING DECREASES CARDIOVASCULAR RISK [34,35]
- Brisk walking for 30 minutes a day most days of the week with dietary restraint or vigorous exercise each produce a similar and substantial decrease in cardiovascular disease among women. Even moderate walking speed decreases risk.

LIFESTYLE ACTIVITY vs STRUCTURED EXERCISE
- Lifestyle activity (household chores, stair climbing, and walking for 30 minutes a day) is as effective as structured ex-

ercise for weight loss, decreasing blood pressure and the risk of cardiovascular disease (500 women and men).[36,37]

EXERCISE DECREASES CARDIOVASCULAR RISK[38-43]

- Exercise performed at frequent intervals over a long period of time decreases cardiovascular risk and sudden heart attack by strenuous exertion. However, bouts of heavy exertion pose a significant threat for sedentary people who have coronary artery disease or risk factors for it (331,000 people).
- Small improvements in physical fitness produce a significantly lower risk of death (2014 men, 22 year follow-up).
- Exercise reduces borderline or mild hypertension.
- Exercise reduces triglycerides.

FUTURE PROJECTIONS. What will happen to future generations as our jobs become more service related? Children are less physically active and physically fit than their counterparts of twenty or even ten years ago. Forty percent of children aged 5-8 exhibit signs of obesity, elevated blood pressure, and high cholesterol levels, according to the American Alliance for Health, Physical Education, Recreation and Dance. Our schools must help get our children into shape. However, only four states require all students to take a specific amount of physical education in all grades, kindergarten through twelfth: Illinois, New Jersey, New York, and Rhode Island. Only Illinois requires that all students take physical education classes every day. With a decrease in exercise, an increase in obesity, an increase in junk food, and the other risk factors that we have already discussed and will discuss, the incidence of cancer and other diseases will continue to spiral with each succeeding generation unless we dramatically alter our lifestyles.

BEGINNING AN EXERCISE PROGRAM

The one most important factor likely to initiate and increase a person's physical activity is the physician's recommendation.[44] Physical activity promotes health, affords a longer life, and decreases the risk for cancer, cardiovascular disease, hypertension, diabetes, osteoporosis, obesity, mental health, musculoskeletal disorders, and immunological abnormalities.[45,46]

Everyone, young or old, should exercise and increase their lifestyle activities. People are more likely to engage in low-intensity activities since they are more comfortable, convenient, and affordable, as well as safer. However, you must begin your exercise program slowly working up to the desired level. You should not start a heavy physical exertion program particularly if you have been sedentary because you can have a heart attack.

Because of the risk of sudden death associated with beginning to exercise, anyone 35 or older, or less than 35 with cardiac risk factors, should be medically screened with a full history and physical exam, and an electrocardiogram (ECG). A stress test is indicated if you have symptoms of heart disease.

An exercise program should be individualized because abilities and motivations differ. Your heart rate should be monitored. Of course, you should be warned to stop exercising immediately if you experience chest pain, severe shortness of breath, palpitations, or other cardiac symptoms. You should contact your physician at once if any of these occur. And finally, it is well known that people who continuously engage in a heavy exercise program, like marathon runners, are more susceptible to getting upper respiratory infections. Heavy exercise can suppress the immune system and hence should be avoided.

New athletes often consult with their physicians about exercise and nutrition. Athletes realize that proper nutrition plays a major role in their performance. Over 7 million high-school athletes are in an age group that has the highest risk of nutritional deficiencies. An adequate diet, with the proper vitamin and mineral supplementation is a must for all athletes. Athletes who attain their ideal weight may require additional calories for the extra energy they need. They can monitor this by weighing themselves regularly. Athletes should not take steroids to increase muscle mass – these cause diseases including cancer. Exercising the muscles will increase muscle mass.

TAKE CONTROL

The benefits of exercise are huge. Exercise lowers the risk for cancer, cardiovascular disease, hypertension, stroke, diabetes, obesity, depression and other diseases.[47-49] The immune system is enhanced. Cancer patients can benefit from walking.[50]

My recommendations are simple: For 20-30 uninterrupted minutes 4 to 5 times a week, you should walk briskly, do everyday household chores, and/or climb stairs. These activities require no fancy warm-up suits, no fancy leotards, and no membership fees. In inclement weather, you simply go to a shopping mall to walk. Virtually everyone can walk. All age groups benefit from brisk walking. Climbing stairs for 15-20 minutes is also beneficial. During repetitive stair climbing, each individual step increases life by about four seconds.[51]

There is no excuse for not walking or stair climbing. Check with your physician first and gradually build an exercise program. Again, exercise is another risk factor over which you have absolute control.

Ric decided to walk briskly 20-30 minutes four times a week. After hearing the data, he knows he will live longer by making this small investment in time and effort.

17
Stress and Sexuality

Fred's History
Faced with being a 42 year-old single parent, working father, Fred came to me full of anxiety, stress, and loss of libido. He told me he was worried that he may develop prostate cancer. He was going through a contentious divorce.

STRESS

As early as the second century, Galen, the physician who systematized medical learning, said that psychological factors contributed greatly to the development of cancer. He believed that melancholic women were more likely to develop cancer than those who were not. Other physicians of the eighteenth and nineteenth centuries observed the same relationship between emotional trauma and the development of cancer.[1]

NERVOUS SYSTEM AND IMMUNE SYSTEM COMMUNICATE with each other by way of nerve chemicals and special proteins made by immune cells. Special neuroendocrine cells have been found in important immune structures, and specialized T cells have been found at the ends of large peripheral nerves.[2] The nervous system can influence the immune response and the immune response, in turn, can alter nerve cell activities. Cells from the immune system can send messages to the brain, relaying information about invading microorganisms or other problems that might not otherwise be detected by the classical nervous sensory system.

The nervous system sends fibers to the thymus gland, the immune organ in which T lymphocytes are matured. The nerve fibers form a very specific pattern in this organ.[3] The spleen, lymph nodes, and bone marrow also contain very specific patterns of nerve fibers. The nerves follow the blood vessels into the organ and branch out into areas that contain T cell lymphocytes and not in areas that contain B cells.

The immune system influences the nervous system with proteins and hormones. One of the hormones produced by the immune system, called thymosin alpha 1, acts on the hypothalamus and pituitary gland in the brain to increase production of cortisol. Cortisol depresses the immune system by decreasing the number of lymphocytes, decreasing the mass of the spleen, and decreasing the size of the peripheral lymph nodes, among other things.[4] Early in life, thymosins protect T lymphocytes from the immunosuppressive effects of cortisol and allow them to mature normally.

STRESS IMPAIRS HUMAN IMMUNE SYSTEM[5-25]

- **Stress + Inability to Cope = Impaired Immune System**
- Stress and depression inhibit the function of lymphocytes, helper T cells, natural killer cells, and antibody production. These studies were done on medical and dental students who are routinely under great stress.
- Hypnosis and meditation can suppress the immune response.
- We can condition ourselves to suppress our own immune system by a variety of triggers.

STRESS INCREASES CANCER RISK[26,27] FOR:

- Children who had a significant stressful change a year before, including personal injury and/or change in the health of a family member.[28]
- People who experience the loss of a loved one.[29]
- People who are widowed, divorced, or separated; individuals who express a sense of loss and hopelessness; and those who have an inability to cope with the stress of separation.[30-32]
- People who are unable to express negative emotions and who also have reduced aggressive behavior.[33-35]
- People with an inability to cope.[36-38] People with depression.

- People who have stress and a precancer.[39]
- Swedish people who had serious aggravation at work had a 5.5 times greater risk for colorectal cancer than those without such pressure. People who work in high pressure situations, over which they have little control, face the highest risks.[41]

Detection of a cancer occurs many years after the first cell changed into a cancer. When people are asked about a past stressful event after being told that they do have cancer, their perception of that stressful event may be very different from what actually happened.

STRESS IMPAIRS MEMORY[42] After several days of stress, some aspects of memory is impaired in healthy people.

STRESS IMPAIRS WOUND HEALING[43]

STRESS INCREASES NEURAL TUBE DEFECTS[44]
Severe emotional stress during pregnancy especially that related to death of a child, increases the risk for neural crest defects.

STRESS CONTRIBUTES TO DIABETES as a cause of it because it raises blood sugar and increases obesity.[45,46]

STRESS INCREASES ASTHMA ATTACKS [47]

A PERSONALITY PRONE TO CANCER
Is there a cancer-prone personality? The evidence suggests that a person who is unable to cope with stress may have a higher risk for the development of cancer. Those who can cope better have less of a risk. Therefore, learn to cope, learn relaxation techniques (see inset) and techniques like meditation and use other techniques that you think will help you to cope.

Relaxation Technique

Get into a very comfortable lounging position. Concentrate on "feeling" every part of your body with your mind. You can begin by thinking about your right foot, then your right ankle, right leg, right thigh, then left foot, etc. Then move to your hands up to your shoulders and neck, and so on. Now, start to tense specific muscle groups as hard as you can, hold them tense for twenty or thirty seconds, then relax them. Again, start with your feet muscles (tense, relax), the leg muscles (tense, relax), and so on. You may repeat the entire sequence once or twice. While you are doing this, tell yourself that you are tightening your muscles each time you do so, and, provided that your effort is exhausting, you will look forward to relaxing each muscle group. While this is happening, you can think of a pleasant place that invokes fond memories. This sequence should produce relief and relaxation, and decrease your anxiety levels. Stress is another risk factor over which you have a great deal of control. Seize control of stress!

CANCER CAUSES STRESS

Many people with cancer have pronounced anxiety, some are depressed, and some experience sexual dysfunction. Men with prostate cancer have to deal with many losses – health, erectile dysfunction, and confidence. They often focus on death anxiety; living with uncertainty; fear of recurrence; understanding complex treatments; body and self-image; sexuality; relationship with doctor, partner, family and friends; changes in lifestyle; and setting goals for the future.

STRESS REDUCTION PROLONGS SURVIVAL AND DECREASES RECURRENCES and also:

• Anger toward disease increases survival.
• Cancer patients who have at least one confidant live longer than those who do not. Patients who confided in a nurse or physician lived even longer.[48]
• Belief system is linked to survival. The deaths of 28,000 adult Chinese-Americans and 400,000 "white" Americans

were studied. Chinese-Americans, but not whites, die significantly earlier than normal (one to five years) if they have a disease, and their birth year is considered ill-fated by Chinese astrology and medicine.[49] The more strongly a person is attached to Chinese traditions, the more years of life are lost.

SEXUALITY

Being sexually active can enhance your immune system.[50] More than 100 undergraduates between the ages of 16 and 23 were asked how frequently they had sexual occurrences. An antibody (IgA) of the immune system was measured in their saliva and found to be the highest for those who had sexual occurrences one or two times per week. The antibody IgA was lower for those who had more sexual occurrences – three or more times a week. In another study, promiscuity actually impaired the immune system.[51]

Masturbation is a sexual occurrence that is practiced by 92% of men and 58% of women in the US, and 82% of men and 75% of women in Britain.[52,53] The percentages are probably even higher than reported. Self-masturbation is described as having sex with the person you love the most or having sex with the only person whose sexual history you can trust completely. It is safe. Masturbation has a very colorful history. It is written that the ancient Egyptians' Sun God, Atum, masturbated to create the first couple. Ancient Judaic teaching, however, was that it was a crime worth the death penalty. Onan, committed the Biblical sin by spilling his seed on the ground. St Thomas Aquinas said it was a sin worse than adultery or rape. The Kellogg Cereal Company developed a special breakfast cereal designed by Mr. Kellogg to prevent masturbation.

CONCLUSION

Constant depression, anxiety, and uncontrollable stress are risk factors for developing a cancer. Stress depresses the immune system If you develop a cancer and believe that you will do badly, studies show that you *will* do badly. If you develop a cancer and think that you will do well and you deny that you have the illness, studies show that you *will* do well.

You will learn in the chapter on Quality of Life and Ethics that physicians are obligated by law to tell the patient the life expectancy for his or her particular illness. A significant number of patients who, after hearing that they have a finite period of time to live – three or six or nine months – go home, circle a day on the calendar, and proceed to die on that day. Since psychological factors have a tremendous influence on overall survival, perhaps a physician should not pronounce an exact sentence for an individual based on statistics of thousands of similar patients who were simply treated "conventionally." Based on many studies, a modified lifestyle that includes psychological support, as in our Ten-Point Plan, will give a patient a better quality of life and increased survival.

Fred and I set goals for stress reduction and behavior guidelines for his children. The household settled down, Fred had less stress, and his immune system became enhanced.

18

Lack of Spirituality

Charles B. Simone, II

Bill's History

Bill is 37 years old, was raised in a religious household, but stopped attending religious services and praying years ago. He developed prostate cancer and turned to prayer.

SPIRITUAL TRENDS

When asked about religion, most Americans say they are religious, they do believe in heaven and hell, and they believe that prayer has healing power.[1-3]

April 1998 CBS News poll:

- 80% believe personal prayer can help medical treatment
- 22% say they have been cured by prayer
- 63% believe doctors should join their patients in prayer
- 34% believe prayer should be part of medical practice
- 60% say they pray at least once a day
- 64% say they pray for their own health and 82% say they pray for the health of others.

March 1997 CNN/USA TODAY/GALLUP POLL:

- 61% believe that religion can answer all or most of today's problems, but 20% believe that religion is old-fashioned
- 30% attend church or synagogue once a week, 13% almost every week, 17% about once a month, 30% seldom

February 1996 USA Weekend Faith and Health Poll:

- 79% believe faith can help people recover from illness
- 56% say their faith has helped them recover from illness
- 49% of 18 to 34 year olds say their faith helps them heal and that number rises to 62 percent in the 45-54 age group
- 63% want doctors to talk to patients about spiritual faith
- 10% say a doctor has talked to them about spirituality

June 1996 TIME/CNN poll:
- 82% believed in the healing power of prayer
- 73% said praying for someone else can help their illness
- 77% said God sometimes intervenes to cure people
- 64% said doctors should join their patients in prayer

SPIRITUALITY AND DISEASES

ARTHRITIS [4]
- Many arthritic patients believe that prayer reduces pain and improves their quality of life.

BLOOD PRESSURE [5]
- People who attend religious services regularly and prayed or studied the Bible at least daily had lower blood pressure than those who did so less frequently or not at all (4,000 people).
- Nine other studies demonstrate similar findings (thousands of people).

CANCER [6-11]
- 93% of 736 women with gynecological cancer said that their spirituality helped to sustain their hopes to fight the cancer.
- Over 75% of spiritual people are better able to cope with their deadly malignant melanoma.
- When told they have cancer, many people turn to God.
- Numerous studies find that for cancer patients, religious, spiritual, and quality of life are most important.
- Spirituality helps both the physical and mental well being of the terminally ill patient.

CARDIAC CONDITIONS [12-16]

- Spiritual patients heal more quickly after open heart surgery
- Patients who had heart attacks have less complications if others pray for them.

DEPRESSION AND MENTAL HEALTH [17-34]

- Among 1,900 women twins, those who were more religious had lower rates of depression, smoking, and alcohol abuse.
- The National Institute on Aging found that older adults who attended church weekly or more often, had half the depression rates compared to those who did not.
- Multiple other studies involving thousands of patients demonstrate similar results: those who used their religious faith to cope were significantly less depressed and had better mental health.
- Schizophrenics were less likely to be hospitalized if they continued religious worship.

IMMUNE SYSTEM [35]

- Elderly church goers (1,718 studied) have an enhanced immune system as measured by elevated levels of interleukin-6.

LIFE SPAN, GENERAL HEALTH, AND DECREASED HOSPITAL STAYS [36-55]

- Attending religious services and spirituality are associated with increased lifespan and better health (thousands of patients studied over decades).
- Hospitals stays are shorter for those who are spiritual.
- Coping skills are increased for those who are spiritual.
- Spirituality acts as a bridge between hopelessness and meaningfulness in life for terminally ill patients with AIDS.
- Attending religious services regularly increases life span by 7 to 14 years for African Americans – 24,000 adults.
- Those who never attend services have a 50 percent higher risk of mortality and are about four times as likely to die from respiratory disease, diabetes, or infectious diseases.

- Reviews and meta-analysis confirm that spirituality and religious involvement is a protective factor against disease.
- Death after heart surgery is 14 times less likely if the elderly patient is socially active and finds strength in her/his religious faith.

QUALITY OF LIFE [56-64]

- Multiple studies demonstrate that people who attend religious services weekly or read the Bible or pray daily have a better quality of life with or without an illness. These people include teenagers, divorcees, acutely ill persons, and others involved in stressful life events.

SMOKING [65]

- People who attend religious services weekly or read the Bible or pray daily are 990% less likely to smoke.

SUBSTANCE ABUSE [66]

- People who attend religious services weekly or read the Bible or pray daily are less likely to abuse alcohol or drugs.

Bill turned again to prayer and religious services in his time of need. During stressful times, some people make deals with their God, ..."if you let me live, I'll do this, this and this..." Bill found his religious strength and thereby enhanced his immune system and decreased his risks for disease.

19
Genetics

Tom's History
Tom is 39 years old and his father just died of prostate cancer at age 65 and his father's brother died of it at age 74. Does Tom have a genetic risk for prostate cancer?

Inherited genetic factors make a minor contribution to the causation of cancer.[1] About 7 percent of all prostate cancer patients have an inherited basis for this disease. There is no genetic basis for all other prostate cancer patients. Prostate cancer in other people is due to the risk factors that we have discussed. Chance alone may account for some clustering of prostate cancer cases seen in some families because prostate cancer is a very common malignancy, affecting one in six men. However, in other families, clustering of several cases of prostate cancer may be related to an inherited mutation in a specific gene.

ONCOGENES AND TUMOR SUPPRESSOR GENES
Every person has a set of oncogenes and tumor suppressor genes. Oncogenes promote tumor growth only when they are turned on. Tumor suppressor genes actually inhibit tumor formation when they are turned on. What activates these genes? Certain vitamins and minerals turn on tumor suppressor genes and, at the same time, suppress oncogene activity. Many other factors like dietary fat, tobacco, alcohol, etc. activate oncogenes. What we do to ourselves will determine whether oncogenes will be turned on or not.

However, certain people may have a predisposition to having the oncogene turned on more quickly than the tumor suppressor gene. For example, some people who smoke do not necessarily develop cancer. Hence, some exposed individuals may genetically resist the carcinogen effect. Other people, however, may show an increased susceptibility to a given carcinogen. The majority of people are in between those who are resistant and those who have an increased susceptibility. This situation, therefore, is not based on true genetics but simply on a predisposition for activating existing genes that can promote or suppress tumors.

HEREDITARY CANCER

Six features characterize most hereditary forms of cancer:
1. Early age when the cancer is found.
2. Multiple cancers occurring in the same person at the same time with specific patterns within families or patients.
3. Physical signs and markers in hereditary cancer syndromes.
4. Characteristic pathological features.
5. Longer survival when compared to people who develop the same cancers without a hereditary basis.
6. Mendelian inheritance patterns of cancer transmission.

These features do not all apply all the time to a specific patient because there are variable expressions and penetrance (degree of expression as time goes on) of the affected genes. However, these six features will help guide the clinician in identifying a hereditary variant of many hereditary cancer syndromes.

Besides strict Mendelian genetics, traits can be passed along by non-Mendelian genetics and by genomic imprinting.[2,3] Genomic imprinting is the phenomenon whereby the expression or nonexpression of a gene is determined by the parental origin of that gene. Many factors modulate genomic imprinting, non-Mendelian traits and genotypes: dietary factors including antioxidants, free radicals, fats; estrogens; androgens; environmental pollutants, and other factors.[4] Other than strict Mendelian genetics, all the other forms of genetic influences are rare and have little influence on the majority of our diseases.

PROSTATE CANCER GENETICS – HPC1

As has been stated, only about 7 percent of all prostate cancer patients have an inherited Mendelian basis for their cancer. These men are diagnosed before age 50 and may have as many as three or more affected family members. A major prostate cancer susceptibility locus was found on chromosome 1(1q24-q25), and studies have shown that men with prostate cancers linked to this gene have their initial diagnosis at a younger age and have higher grade and higher stage cancers. This gene is called **HPC1** and is thought to be involved in only 33% of inherited prostate cancers or 3% of all cases.

p53 GENE – THE PREVENTION GENE. On chromosome number 17, there is an area called the p53 region. The p53 protein is the leader in the body's antitumor army. When the p53 gene has been *mutated* or *changed* or *altered* by free radicals or other agents, cancers and other illnesses develop.[5] The p53 gene is the most commonly altered gene in human cancer. It is one of the most important members of the tumor suppressor oncogene family. Of the 7.5 million people worldwide who are annually diagnosed with cancer, about half of them have the p53 mutation in their tumors.[6,7] A mutated or altered p53 is found in about 25% of breast cancers, 12% of brain cancers, 12% of soft tissue sarcomas, 6% of leukemias, and 6% of osteosarcomas.

The P stands for Protein but really denotes Prevention because the action of p53 is to help prevent cancer by acting as a tumor suppressing gene. The p53 protein or suppressor gene puts the breaks on cell growth and division so when a cell starts to grow too rapidly or divides too many times, it will push that cell into a program of self-destruction and prevent multiplication of the cell. This is called apoptosis. Apoptosis is part of normal cellular development and is triggered by DNA damage from radiation, chemicals including chemotherapy, and free radicals. The p53 gene normally binds to other genes and thereby controls their expression.

BREAST CANCER GENETICS. Only about 5 percent of all breast cancer patients have an inherited basis for their cancer and those genes are **BRCA1 and BRCA2. BRAC 1 is associated with prostate cancer.**

Whether family members are genetically affected or unaffected, they experience tremendous psychological consequences. Unaffected family members often feel relief but, at the same time, tremendous guilt. After affected or nonaffected patients receive genetic information, they require intensive psychological support. In addition, once this information is known to the patient, insurance companies may use the information to deny that person life and health insurance.

SUMMARY

Inherited genetic factors make a minor contribution to the causation of cancer.[1] Only about 7 percent of all prostate cancer patients have an inherited basis for this disease. However, your existing normal genes, like p53, can be altered by free radicals or other means. Once these genes change, once the tumor suppressor genes no longer work, or once the oncogene gets turned on, a tumor cell can grow uninhibited.

It is important to modify your lifestyle early enough in life so that these changes in oncogenes and tumor suppressor genes never occur. Furthermore, if you do have prostate cancer, it is imperative to modify your lifestyle so that no further free radicals are formed and tumor promotion does not occur. Change your lifestyle factors now.

Tom learned that he did not have an inherited genetic basis for developing prostate cancer, but his poor lifestyle could alter his protective p53 gene. He decided to change his lifestyle to minimize any risk.

20
Cancer Angiogenesis

CANCER ANGIOGENESIS

Every day approximately 350 billion normal cells divide in your body to form new ones. Every time one of these cells goes through the reproductive cycle, there is always a possibility that it can transform into a cancer cell, especially if you have multiple lifestyle risk factors. But usually, if the immune system is working properly, these transformed cells are killed.

But if just one of these transformed, cancerous cells escapes the immune system, it starts to grow into a small colony of cancer cells. This is called an *in situ* cancer – it remains in one site. This is usually a cancer of a millimeter or so in diameter.

Avascular Cancer Mass

At this point, the cancer is usually harmless because it has no blood vessels to remove the cancer's wastes or to supply it with oxygen and nutrients. Hence, this *in situ* cancer cannot grow. Oxygen, nutrients, and wastes are diffused to and from blood vessels. So unless blood vessels are intimately in contact with the cancer cells, even the most aggressive cancer cells may remain dormant for months or years.

Vascularization of the Cancer

For the small colony of cancer cells to grow into a large detectable cancer, it must become vascularized – a process known as *angiogenesis* – the formation of (*-genesis*) new blood vessels (*angio-*). This happens when cancer cells release a chemical substance, called tumor angiogenesis factor (TAF), that induces new blood vessels to form.[1-3] Many substances induce or inhibit angiogenesis.

Inducers of Angiogenesis	Inhibitors of Angiogenesis
Estrogen	Tamoxifen, Medroxyprogesterone
Prostaglandins E1, E2	Aspirin
Interleukin 8	Interferon, Severe Infection
Vascular endothelial growth factor	Methotrexate, Bleomycin
Transforming Growth Factor-B	Mitoxantrone, Bisantrene
Angiotensis II	Retinoids, Vitamin D3 analogs
Plasminogen activator	Hyperthermia, Radiation Therapy
Substance P, Fibroblast growth factor	Minocycline, Suramin

Existing blood vessels that are near the small group of cancer cells are stimulated by TAF to produce and send to the cancer cells small new blood vessels, capillaries that penetrate the cancer.   These newly formed blood vessels feed the cancer with oxygen and nutrients, and, in addition, remove wastes. Now the cancer grows rapidly and becomes pink because it is being fed, oxygenated, and its wastes are removed.

Cancers can generally be detected by our technology only when they are the size of about a centimeter (half inch) diameter sphere or more (one cubic centimeter). This small spherical mass contains about one billion cancer cells.

Angiogenesis and Metastasis

As the vascularized cancer grows, it invades and destroys local tissues as well as more distant sites in the body. For a cancer to metastasize or spread to other parts of the body, it must first invade the local tissue and then the bloodstream, and finally land in a distant organ and begin the process of growth and angiogenesis all over again at that site. Cancer cells manufacture a complex series of enzymes and other proteins necessary to accomplish all this.[4,5]

Angiogenesis is an integral part of the ability of the cancer cells to gain access to the bloodstream initially and then flourish in distant organs. In fact, many studies have shown that if angiogenesis does not occur, the cancer cannot metastasize.[6]

This leads to a very important fact. **When a cancer is large enough to be detected in the primary site, it has already developed angiogenesis and hence its cells have already spread to other organs.** The colonies in these distant organs are usually not large enough to be detected but are capable of growth and angiogenesis.[7]

A high number of blood vessels in the cancer as seen under the microscope, correlates well with a high likelihood of spread to other organs at the time of biopsy, especially breast cancer, prostate cancer, lung cancer, and melanoma.[8-12]

Angiogenesis and Leukemias

Until recently, scientists thought that angiogenesis only played a role in the growth and spread of solid cancers like prostate, breast, colon and rectal, uterus, and many others. Leukemias also depend upon angiogenesis for growth. Patients with leukemia have high urine levels of an inducer of angiogenesis, and as the leukemia was successfully treated, these urine levels fell to normal.[13]

Age Alters Angiogenesis

Usually, young people have more aggressive cancers compared to older people because they have a greater and more rapid angiogenic response.[14] Also, older animals are unable to efficiently support the growth of the new blood vessels once the process started.

Severe Infection Inhibits Angiogenesis

Observation in humans and animals suggests that severe infection inhibits angiogenesis and thereby shrinks cancer.[15]

Steady State for Normal Blood Vessels

The vascular system in humans is designed to remain quite dormant for relatively long periods of time – weeks in women and decades in men.[16] The creation of new blood vessels occurs regularly every month as part of the menstrual cycle and also during the time of pregnancy. The placenta (tube connecting the fetus to the mother) manufactures a protein called placental proliferin that stimulates angiogenesis. This ensures that the fetus will be fed. And after a while, since *new* blood vessels are no longer needed because the existing blood vessels are adequate, the placenta manufactures another protein to inhibit angiogensis, called proliferin-related protein.[17] Men, however, do not have a need for new blood vessel formation regularly.

Jonathan decided to take one 325 mg aspirin every day to help prevent angiogenesis and look forward to the day when proteomic pattern profiling will be available commercially.

PART FOUR

Prostate Cancer: Detection to Conventional Treatment

21

Prostate Cancer Detection

Nicole L. Simone, M.D.

Digital rectal examination by physician after a thorough history, PSA (Prostate Specific Antigen), and a biopsy with a Gleason score are the main tests to detect a prostate cancer.

Does early detection of prostate cancer and therefore subsequent earlier treatment, increase the length of life?

DIGITAL RECTAL EXAMINATION (DRE) BY PHYSICIAN

Digital rectal examination (DRE) by a competent physician is a simple, non-invasive and inexpensive exam that aids in the detection of prostate cancer. Men older than 50 years should have a yearly DRE. It should be done with the patient in a standing position bent over at the waist. A gloved finger is inserted into the rectum to allow for direct physical exam of the prostate gland. The examiner will note the size of the prostate, the consistency of it, and whether there are any firm areas or nodules. A cancer is generally very hard and not raised from the surface of the gland. A firm area extending at the top of the prostate suggests that the seminal vesicles are involved with cancer. About 95% of prostate cancers arise in the periphery of the gland, and the rest are anteriorly located and cannot be easily palpated unless it is advanced. Benign prostatic hyperplasia arises in the central portions of the gland.

Not all firm nodules are cancer – they can be calcium deposits, infections, old prostatitis infection (granuloma), blood vessel infarcts, and firm nodules of benign prostatic hyperplasia. A biopsy of the prostate is the only way to absolutely determine if the abnormal nodule is cancer. **About 30% to 40% of nodules palpated on rectal exam are found to be cancers by biopsy**.[1]

At diagnosis, about 10% to 15% of prostate cancer cases found on digital rectal examination extend beyond the confines of the prostate capsule with no laboratory evidence of nodal or distant metastatic spread.[2]

THE DRE IS NOT RELIABLE. Disturbingly, as many as 25% of men with metastatic prostate cancer had a normal prostate examination.[3] A large study of 450 men who underwent DRE revealed that no statistically significant association could be found between the results of a DRE and presence of prostate cancer.[4] The digital rectal examination is still widely used in practice because it is inexpensive, and relatively noninvasive.

THE DRE DOES NOT EXTEND LIFE.

PSA – PROSTATE SPECIFIC ANTIGEN

In this section, we review PSA as a screening test of asymptomatic patients. However, if a man has signs or symptoms suggestive of a malignant process in the prostate, they certainly should have a PSA regardless of their age.

The objective of a screening test is to detect a cancer before it has a chance to spread to other organs of the body. While this is certainly a noble pursuit, does it work? And, importantly, what age groups should be screened by digital rectal examination and PSA.

The number of new cases of prostate cancer began to increase in 1987 largely as a result of the increase in routine screening of men with the PSA blood test.[5] The prostate makes a protein called PSA that is secreted into the blood in two forms: free PSA and PSA that is bound to proteins in the blood. A simple blood test can determine the total PSA. However, a normal blood value has been difficult to determine because both normal and abnormal prostates make it. Traditionally, 0 to 4 ng/ml has been assigned as the normal range. Values above 10 ng/ml are considered abnormal. For values falling between 4 to 10 ng/ml a decision must be made by both the patient and his physician to determine if a biopsy should be pursued. **It is alarming to learn that 20% of men with prostate cancer have a PSA less than 4 ng/ml. Only 25% of patients with PSA in the 4 to 10 ng/ml range, however, will have prostate cancer.**

Many attempts have been made to devise different normal ranges based on such characteristics as age and race. As a man ages, the prostate usually enlarges due to benign prostatic hyperplasia and consequently, the PSA rises as well. Table 1.

Table 1. Age-Adjusted Normal PSA Values[6]	
40 to 49 years old	0 to 2.5 ng/ml
50 to 59 years old	0 to 3.5 ng/ml
60 to 69 years old	0 to 4.5 ng/ml
70 to 79 years old	0 to 5.5 ng/ml

Many African-American men have prostate cancers when the PSA is lower. A study involving 400 African-American men at Walter Reed Army Medical Center showed that nearly 40% of prostate cancers were missed if the normal limit of 4 ng/ml was used.[7] Therefore, the normal range for PSA for African-American men over age 50 should be 0 to 3.5 ng/ml.

Research has shown that two methods of interpreting the PSA test can make the test more specific for prostate cancer.

- **PSA VELOCITY – HOW QUICKLY THE PSA CHANGES OVER TIME.** A change in PSA of 0.75 ng/ml per year might suggest cancer.[8,9]
- **FREE PSA.** PSA is found in the blood either by itself or bound to protein. When the normal PSA value is between 4 to 10 ng/ml, the measurement of free PSA makes the test more sensitive in detecting prostate cancer. For reasons that are not known, the amount of free PSA tends to be lower than the bound portion in patients who have prostate cancer.[10] **If the percentage of free PSA is less than 25%, cancer is unlikely and biopsy may be unnecessary.**[11]

CAUSES OF ABNORMAL PSA OTHER THAN CANCER

- Benign prostatic hyperplasia
- Prostatitis (inflammation of the prostate) – PSA should return to patient's normal after proper treatment
- Bike riding for extended periods of time; Marathon Running[12]
- Ejaculation
- Mechanical manipulation: Digital rectal exam, Biopsy, Cystoscopy, Foley catheter placement and TURP.
- Finasteride, 5-alpha-reductase blocker, to treat BPH, causes a 50% reduction in PSA[13]

PSA DOES NOT EXTEND LIFE. There is no conclusive evidence that routine use of PSA screening in all men decreases the death rate from the disease. This is because even if prostate cancer is detected early, aggressive management of prostate cancer provides little or no improvement in survival rates. Furthermore, prostate cancer develops over a long period of time. It is often said that men die with prostate cancer, not from it. Early detection will increase the number of prostate cancer cases resulting in anxiety, depression and fear for patients who are unlikely to suffer from any symptoms of the disease. In an effort to "do something" many patients will undoubtedly be treated resulting in unnecessary suffering from side effects and expenditure of health care dollars on unnecessary treatments.

PSA IS USED TO FOLLOW THE ACTIVITY OF PROSTATE CANCER in a person who was either observed or treated with radical prostatectomy or radiation, or hormones. The PSA is commonly elevated for men with benign prostatic hyperplasia, but usually less than in those with cancer.

Benign Prostate Hyperplasia	7 ng/ml
Cancer confined to prostate	12 ng/ml
75% have cancer	Greater than 10 ng/ml
Cancer spread beyond prostate	Greater than 100 ng/ ml

PROTEOMIC PATTERNS FOR EARLIER DETECTION OF CANCER [14,15] There has been no effective method

of early detection of cancers and consequently the great majority of patients with newly diagnosed cancer are detected too late. Since 1930, the lifespans for both men and women with cancer has not changed indicating little progress has been made. New technologies are critically needed to detect a cancer long before angiogenesis begins to feed the cancer.

Certain abnormal proteins (**proteomic**) may be secreted in unique patterns into the blood stream from pathological changes within an organ. We investigated several cancers.

First, serum from each patient with a prostate problem (cancer or non-cancer) is placed on a special surface that attracts specific proteins, in this case, hydrophobic proteins. Repeated washings with special chemicals remove unwanted proteins. Then a laser beam is used to hurl the remainder proteins from the surface into a chamber separating the lighter weight proteins from the heavier proteins. Hence, a unique Proteomic Pattern of lighter to heavier weighted proteins is created after Laser treatment for each serum specimen.

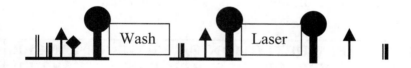

A large number of unique proteomic patterns may occur. Therefore, a bioinformatics tool, a special software program, was developed to recognize patterns and match subsequent test serum samples with known patterns from either cancer or non-cancer patient proteomic patterns. For example, let's say that the serum used in the diagram was from an ovarian cancer patient. Then proteomic patterns from other patients that are identical or very similar could suggest a cancer as well.

FINDINGS
- **For Prostate Cancer** proteomic patterns accurately identified 36 of 38 (95%) prostate cancer patients, while 177 of

228 (78%) patients were correctly classified as having benign conditions. For men with marginally elevated PSA (4-10 ng/ml, 137 men) the specificity was 71%. Serum proteomic pattern diagnostics could help decide whether to perform a biopsy on a man with an elevated PSA.

- **For Ovarian Cancer** this new technology accurately identified all 50 ovarian cancer cases that included 18 stage I cases. Of the 66 cases of non-cancer disease, 63 were recognized as non-cancer. This yielded a sensitivity of 100 percent, specificity of 95 percent, and a positive predictive value of 94 percent compared with a positive predictive value of only 34 percent for the blood test currently used to detect ovarian cancer, the CA-125 test

INTERPRETATION. Serum proteomic pattern profiling may constitute a sensitive and specific tool for earlier cancer identification.

ULTRASOUND can be used to help identify areas of the prostate that were abnormal by DRE. It can also be used to guide biopsy needles into the prostate for aspiration.

DOES EARLY DETECTION OF PROSTATE CANCER AND THEREFORE SUBSEQUENT EARLIER TREATMENT, INCREASE THE LENGTH OF LIFE? ANSWER: NO

This is the question posed at the start of the chapter. How could the answer be NO? If we detect a prostate cancer early why does it not increase the length of life? The answer is simple. By the time our technology can detect a cancer, it has already spread to other parts of the body by way of the bloodstream via angiogenesis.

SUMMARY
The emotionally charged widespread use of screening DREs and PSAs have cut into much needed health-care dollars for no gain. Clinical scientists should make recommendations and set policy based on scientific facts and not emotions or wishes. It

is a disservice to give false hope to men about the value of DRE and PSA. Only the truth should be given to people. Many men will advocate DRE and PSA no matter what – they erroneously believe that that these tests are "all they've got," or that these tests prevent prostate cancer. If these tests were a treatment, we would have to call them an unproven treatment.

WHAT TO DO? YOU CAN PREVENT PROSTATE CANCER BY FOLLOWING THE TEN POINT PLAN. CURRENT SCREENING TESTS ARE NOT THE ANSWER, PREVENTION IS. IF YOU DO HAVE A PROSTATE CANCER, YOU CAN EXTEND YOUR LIFE BY FOLLOWING THE SAME TEN POINT PLAN.

My recommendations for asymptomatic men:
- Physician Digital Rectal Examination – all men starting at age 50.
- Take the Self Test in Chapter 3 and follow the Ten Point Plan Modification. If overall prostate cancer risk assessment is high, then you should be followed based upon clinical judgment.

22
Establishing the Diagnosis and Stage

Charles B. Simone, II

Alan's History

Alan came to see me for a check-up. I obtained his blood, examined his prostate and felt a small nodule on the left side. His biopsy was positive. We proceeded to determine where else the disease might be.

If your physician feels a nodule in the prostate, you should have a biopsy. A pathologist establishes the diagnosis of prostate cancer after examining prostate tissue under the microscope. The PSA (Prostatic Specific Antigen) and the Gleason score that determine aggressiveness of the cancer are both important factors that must be assessed. The next step is to determine the "stage," i.e., find out with our limited technology if the cancer is confined to the prostate or has already **noticeably** spread. All this information can predict prognosis and determine treatment options.

BIOPSY PROCEDURE

■ NEEDLE BIOPSIES can be performed in the operating room with either a general or regional anesthetic. Six biopsies are obtained through needles that are inserted between the scrotum and the anus into the prostate. If there is a suspicious palpable nodule, then of course, this is specifically biopsied with an attempt to remove as much of the nodule as possible. If there is no palpable nodule, the surgeon attempts to sample the entire prostate with six biopsies in different locations.

■ **DELAY IN DIAGNOSIS BY FOUR TO SIX MONTHS DOES NOT AFFECT LIFESPAN** when findings are ambiguous or equivocal and a cancer is later proved. However, the news media, consumer groups, cancer charities, and ultimately the attorneys, force immediate biopsy. There has been no change in lifespan for prostate cancer since 1930, that means everything we have done to date – screening programs, early detection, hormonal treatment, radiation therapy, surgical techniques – has done nothing to increase the survival of any patient with prostate cancer. So waiting four to six months to repeat a PSA to ascertain whether there is progression, represents little or no time at all and, in fact, has no impact on survival. It takes about 4 to 6 months for a change.

Prostate biopsies are not emergencies. However, once a biopsy has been recommended and a man has made the decision to go ahead with the biopsy, somehow, emotionally, it has to be done yesterday. But waiting two or three weeks has absolutely no effect on the ultimate outcome. Once the diagnosis of cancer is established, the patient and family review the options with his physician.

DETERMINE IF CANCER HAS SPREAD
Three things need to be done: Digital rectal examination, PSA, and biopsy with a Gleason score determination. CT scans and ultrasounds have not been reliable to determine if the lymph nodes that drain the prostate are positive or negative. However, high-resolution MRI with magnetic nanoparticles allows the detection of small and otherwise undetectable lymph node metastases in patients with prostate cancer.[1]

PATHOLOGY – MICROSCOPIC CLASSIFICATION

PIN – PROSTATIC INTRAEPITHELIAL NEOPLASIA
This is not an invasive cancer but rather a collection of benign cells that are lined with cells that seem to be malignant. This

combination is a precursor to an invasive cancer of the prostate. PIN has two categories – Low-grade and High-grade.

■ **Low-grade PIN** – is not often associated with an invasive cancer.

■ **High-grade PIN** – is seen in 5% of biopsy specimens.

Prognosis. About 35% to 50% of men with high-grade PIN will develop an invasive cancer.[2,3]

Treatment. These men should be re-biopsied in 6 to 12 months.

ATYPICAL SMALL ACINAR PROLIFERATION

About 5% of prostate biopsies have atypical glands that are suspicious for but are not cancer. It is not high-grade PIN.

Prognosis. About 45% of men with this diagnosis will develop an invasive cancer.[4,5]

Treatment. These men should be re-biopsied in 6 to 12 months.

INVASIVE CANCER

■ **Invasive Adenocarcinoma** – 97% of all prostate cancers. It is difficult to diagnose prostate cancer and is often underdiagnosed. A second opinion is sometimes a good idea. In general, diagnosis of prostate cancer is made on the basis of architecture, cell appearances, and other findings on the slide[6] – a review of which is beyond the scope of this chapter. These cancers are quite hard and can metastasize to bone or other organs like lung, liver, and brain.

Some benign conditions can mimic prostate cancer:

Adenosis	Clear cell cribriform hyperplasia
Atrophy	Granulomatous prostatitis
Basal cell hyperplasia	Paraganglia
Cowper's glands	Prostate infarcts
Nephrogenic adenoma	Sclerosing adenosis
Radiation atypia	Signet ring cell lymphocytes
Seminal vesicles	Xanthoma

■ **Carcinosarcoma** – 0.1% of all prostate cancers, has a mixed pattern of adenocarcinoma and sarcoma.

■ **Sarcoma** – 0.1% of all prostate cancers that include leiomyosarcoma, rhabdomyosarcoma, or fibrosarcoma.

There are other rare invasive prostate cancers that include: Adenoid Cystic Carcinoma, Endometrioid cancers, Periurethral duct carcinoma, malignant Lymphoma, and several others.

PROGNOSTIC FACTORS (FACTORS THAT PREDICT OUTCOME) and the extent of disease (stage) determine the patient's treatment options and prognosis. We know, however, that by the time we can actually detect a prostate cancer, tumor cells have already spread to other parts of the body through the bloodstream.

■ **Gleason Score** is one of the most important prognostic factors because it indicates the biological aggressiveness of the cancer and correlates well with the stage and metastatic potential.

The Gleason scoring system is based solely on the appearance of the prostate biopsy under the microscope. Using a low-power microscope, one can see patterns ranging from small non-aggressive glands to larger aggressive glands. The pathologist will look for two distinct and dominant patterns of glands and then grade them based on how aggressive or non-aggressive they appear. The least aggressive looking pattern of glands is given the score of 1, the most aggressive is given a 5. Each of the two dominant patterns is then given a score of 1 to 5, and then the two numbers are added. For example, if the first most dominant pattern of glands looks very aggressive, the pathologist might score that group with a 5. If the second most dominant pattern of cells looks aggressive but less so than the first, the pathologist will score that group with a 4. The two numbers are added and the patient's Gleason score becomes a 9 – indicating an overall aggressive cancer. However subjective this seems, the Gleason score is the most powerful prognostic indicator.

A patient with a Gleason score of 7 or more will do poorly compared to a patient with a score of 2 through 6. A score of 2 to 4 is not very aggressive, 5 to 6 moderately aggressive, 7 is aggressive, and 8 to 10 very aggressive.

Often the Gleason score will influence the treatment offered to a patient. For example, a young man with a Gleason score of 5 or 6 would be offered all the treatment options for localized prostate cancer, but perhaps the option of observation would be encouraged. However, if he had a score of 7 or higher, more aggressive options would be encouraged even though the survival is the same for all options.

The type of treatment offered is also influence by the Gleason score. A man with a Gleason score of 6 would be offered brachytherapy, whereas a man with a Gleason score of 7 would be offered external beam therapy because there is a higher chance of cancer being outside the prostate gland. A man with a Gleason score of 8 to 10 might not be offered surgery because of the high probability that the cancer is already into the surrounding structures. On the other hand, lymph nodes may not even be removed if a man has a Gleason score of 6, normal rectal exam, and a PSA less than 10 ug/ml. There is a 15% chance of cancer spread into the lymph nodes with a Gleason score of 2 to 5; 100% chance if it is 8 to 10.

High-grade cancers produce less PSA per cancer cell, but generally have higher PSAs because these cancers tend to be larger in volume than low-grade cancers.

Best Prognosis: Gleason score 6 or less.

■ **PSA** (Prostatic Specific Antigen). The normal range is between 0 and 4 ng/ml. However, up to 20% of men with prostate cancer will have a PSA less than 4 ng/ml. And only 25% of men with a PSA between 4 and 10 ng/ml will have a positive biopsy.

Best Prognosis: PSA less than 4 ng/ml.

■ **Cancer Size.** The more cancer there is, the lower is the survival. There are multiple ways of trying to accurately assess the cancer volume based on the percentage of cancer is a needle biopsy, and imaging studies.

Best Prognosis: Small volume of cancer.

■ **Lymph Node Status.** Positive lymph nodes herald a poor prognosis. The chance of having positive lymph nodes increases with stage and Gleason score

Best Prognosis: Negative lymph nodes

	Chance of Lymph Node Metastases
Stage A	10%
Stage B	20%
Stage C	60%
Stage D	80%
Gleason Score 2-5	15%
Gleason Score 9-10	100%

■ **Perineural Invasion** (growth of cancer cells along the nerve sheath) increases the risk of cancer spreading through and beyond the prostate capsule. This finding generally does not influence a clinical or operative decision.

Best Prognosis: No perineural invasion.

■ **Prostate Lymphatic Vessel Cancer Invasion** heralds a high recurrence rate and eventual death from the disease.

Best Prognosis: No cancer cells in prostate lymphatics.

■ **Prostate Blood Vessel Cancer Invasion** heralds a high recurrence rate and eventual death from the disease.

Best Prognosis: No cancer cells in prostate blood vessels.

■ **Angiogenesis** is the growth of new blood vessels from existing blood vessels to feed a cancer and promote its spread.

Best Prognosis: No angiogenesis.

■ **Androgen Receptor** is not routinely assayed. However, often a patient with androgen receptor negative cancer has a higher rate of recurrence.

Best Prognosis: Positive androgen receptor

■ **Ploidy and S-Phase Fraction** are determinations of aggressiveness of cancer cells. Cancer cells with the normal amount of DNA are called diploid. An abnormally high DNA content is called aneuploidy, and the prognosis is usually poor. The S-phase fraction denotes how quickly the cells turn over. The higher the S-phase number, the more aggressive the cancer cells are. However, neither of these is generally helpful if the prostate Gleason score is accurate.

Best Prognosis: Diploid status; DNA index =1.0; S-phase < 7%.

■ **Neuroendocrine Differentiation** is the change of prostate cancer cells to a small cell carcinoma, or carcinoid-like cancer, or more commonly, to a focal area of neuroendocrine tissue. This change may have an adverse influence on men with hormone resistant prostate cancer and can be determined using the Chromogranin A test.

Best Prognosis: No neuroendocrine differentiation.

■ **Ki-67** is specific for all aggressive cells in a cancer.

Best Prognosis: No Ki-67 detected.

STAGING OF PROSTATE CANCER is done after a biopsy to determine whether the cancer has spread to other parts of the body. Treatment and prognosis are determined by the stage of the patient. There are two staging systems
– the ABCD or the T staging system.

■ STAGE A OR STAGE T 1 – Rectal exam is negative, but cancer is found in surgical specimen during operation for prostatic hyperplasia, or an elevated PSA prompts a biopsy that is positive.

STAGE A1 or STAGE T 1a – The cancer is limited to less than 5% of the prostate tissue removed at surgery, or an elevated PSA prompts a biopsy that is positive. Fewer than 2% have lymph node involvement. This stage produces no symptoms.

STAGE A2 or STAGE T 1b – The cancer involves more than 5% of the prostate tissue removed at surgery, or an elevated PSA prompts a biopsy that is positive. About 35% have lymph node involvement. This stage produces no symptoms.

STAGE T 1c –an elevated PSA prompts a biopsy that is positive.

■ STAGE B OR STAGE T 2 – disease can be felt during a rectal exam but still confined to the prostate. PSA is elevated.

STAGE B1 or STAGE T 2a – The cancer is a small discrete nodule limited to one lobe of the prostate. About 20% have lymph node involvement. This stage produces no symptoms.

STAGE B2 or STAGE T 2c – The cancer is a small discrete nodule limited to both lobes of the prostate and 35% have lymph node involvement. This stage produces no symptoms.

■ STAGE C or STAGE T 3 – palpable cancer extends beyond the prostate to nearby structures, but there are no distant metastases. A common symptom for this stage is difficult urination.

STAGE C1 or STAGE T 3b – Cancer has broken through the prostate capsule but there is no seminal vesicle involvement. About 50% have lymph node involvement.

STAGE C2 or STAGE T 3c – Seminal vesicles are involved and 80% have lymph node involvement.

The objective of treatment is to slow down the cancer's growth and relieve the urinary symptoms.

■ STAGE D –cancer has spread to other organs of the body that may include the bones, lungs, liver, or brain, etc, causing bone pain, weight loss, difficult urination and fatigue. The goal of treatment is to relieve pain and symptoms.

CONCLUSION

Now that you have all the information about your cancer including tissue type, nodal status, prognostic factors, extent or stage of disease, you can explore the best treatment options available for your case.

Alan had an early stage prostate cancer with an excellent prognosis. He modified his lifestyle according to the Ten Point Plan to improve and extend his life.

23

Localized Treatment Options for Prostate Cancer

Rudy's History

Rudy learned he has prostate cancer. He became depressed, angry, and for the first time contemplated his own mortality. He wanted the best treatment to maximize his lifespan.

Once the diagnosis of invasive prostate cancer has been made, treatments are considered. Staging should be confined to a serum PSA (Prostate Specific Antigen), a digital rectal examination, and a biopsy with a Gleason score that indicates aggressiveness. Localized treatment is intended to eradicate cancer that is presumably confined to the prostate itself. But by the time we find it and think it is confined to the prostate, it has already disseminated to other parts of the body by way of lymph node channels and also by way of the bloodstream.

The number of localized prostate cancers increased from about 50 percent of all cases in 1988 to more than 75 percent of cases by 1996 because of the prevalent use of the PSA.[1]

In 1983, the following were the treatment choices for men with localized prostate cancer: 50% had no treatment (observation only), 10% had radical prostatectomy, 27% had radiation therapy, and 13% had hormone treatment. By 1992, things changed dramatically. Radical prostatectomy was used for 37% of cases, radiation therapy in 32%, observation for 23%, and 8% received hormones. Since 1991 radical prostatectomy has been the most commonly used treatment. Radical prostatectomy rose 8-fold for men less than 60 years old, and 6 fold for men 60-69. More are done in the western states of the United States than in the eastern states.

Because of the PSA screening test more men are being diagnosed with early stage prostate cancer that will rarely cause a problem for them. **In 1995 the Prostate Cancer Panel of the American Urological Association reviewed a total of 12,501 published medical articles and concluded that all patients with newly diagnosed, clinically localized prostate cancer should choose one of the following options for treatment since no one treatment was better than the other for extending life**: (1) Observation – no treatment, (2) Radical prostatectomy, (3) External beam radiation therapy, and, (4) Radiation seed implant therapy (Brachytherapy).[2] In this chapter, we will also include (5) Cryosurgery [freezing] and (6) Hormones.

Before any therapies are offered, a man should consider his life expectancy without prostate cancer, his overall medical health, the Gleason score that indicates aggressiveness of the prostate cancer, and the stage of the cancer indicating where the cancer is located. He must explore of all his options and then determine his personal preference for a treatment after hearing about the various side effects. Also, he should be informed that since 1930 the lifespan of a prostate cancer patient has not changed.

1. OBSERVATION

Observation is frequently referred to as "watchful waiting" or surveillance. As a result of widespread PSA (prostate-specific antigen) screening, about 6 of 10 cases of early prostate cancer in the United States are now diagnosed when the tumor is still too small to be clinically detected or problematic. In fact, many prostate cancer patients die of causes other than prostate cancer. These findings suggest that observation alone is a perfectly acceptable choice. We will review the science that provides the foundation for this choice.

NATURAL HISTORY OF PROSTATE CANCER – that is, prostate cancer that is untreated.

In 1940, men with localized prostate cancer (Stage B) were observed without treatment. The 5-year survival was 19%, the 10-year survival was 4%, and the 15-year survival was 1%.[3] By 1976, for a similar group of patients, the survival rates were 71%, 51%, and 28% respectively.[4]

The Veterans Administration Cooperative Urology Research Group randomized men with Stage B prostate cancer to observation alone or radical prostatectomy.[5] The results were astounding: 5-year, 10-year, and 15-year survival rates for the observation group were 85%, 59%, and 39% respectively – essentially the same as for the radical prostatectomy group. These results continued to fuel the notion of observation only.

Six other studies were pooled together involving 828 men (mean age of 69) diagnosed with early prostate cancer. The aggressiveness of the cancer was examined using the grading of I, II, or III. Grade III is the most aggressive. The ten-year survival rates for patients under observation alone were 87%, 87%, and 34% respectively for grades I, II, and III.[6] These numbers exceed those treated with surgery.

In another study, fifty patients with cancer that penetrated the prostate capsule were observed – 58% had grade I, 38% had II, and 4% had III. The survival at 5 years was 88% and at 9 years, 70%.[7] Again, these numbers are better than those for patients who were treated in other studies with radiation or radical prostatectomy.

A prospective Swedish study of 642 men, 223 of whom (mean age 72 years) had localized prostate cancer (66% grade I, 30% II, 4% III) followed only by observation. The 15-year survival was 81% that was identical to those who received radical treatments.[8]

One of the best studies is from the Connecticut Tumor Registry of 767 men with untreated prostate cancers ages 55 to 74.[9] The important predictor of survival was found to be the aggressiveness of the cancer. Those with low-grade cancers (Gleason score 2 to 5) had a life expectancy comparable to the general population. Those with moderate-grade cancers (Gleason score 6 to 7) had a 3 to 5 year loss of life expectancy and those with high-grade cancers (Gleason 8 to 10) had a 6 to 8 year loss of life expectancy compared to the general population.

Using decision analysis based on the life expectancy of patients 60 to 75 years old, observation alone gave the same lifespan as did radical prostatectomy or radiation therapy.[10,11] A structured review of the medical literature showed the identical results: observation alone gave the same lifespan as did radical prostatectomy or radiation therapy.[12]

OBSERVATION VERSUS RADICAL PROSTATECTOMY

Two prospective randomized trials studied 95 men[13] and 142 men[14] with early stage prostate cancer who were treated either with radical prostatectomy or observation alone. In the first study, there was no difference in survival between the two groups at the end of 15 years. The second study showed the same results at the end of 23 years. Radical prostatectomy is no better than observation.

In another randomized trial, 695 men less than 75 years old with newly diagnosed prostate cancer (Gleason score of 5 to 7) were randomly assigned to watchful waiting or radical prostatectomy. After 7 years of follow-up there was no significant difference in overall survival between surgery and watchful waiting,[15] but the quality of life was better for the men in the watchful waiting group.[16] Another trial underway is called The Prostate Cancer Intervention versus Observation Trial (PIVOT).

A population-based study comparing prostate cancer treatments reviewed 59,576 patients in the National Cancer Institute's Surveillance, Epidemiology, and End Results Program. The patients were between ages 50 and 79. The results showed that for men with Gleason score 2 to 4, the 10-year survival was 98% for those treated with surgery, 89% for radiation therapy, and 92% for those observed with no treatment.[17]

Overall, the life expectancy of men being observed only (mainly older men with less aggressive prostate cancers) is the same or better compared to the life expectancy of men treated with surgery or radiation or, for that matter, of the general population.

In fact, as new studies evolve using PSA to detect recurrence of cancer for any age group, the results for surgery and radiation outcomes will decline.

2. RADICAL PROSTATECTOMY

Radical prostatectomy has been the standard surgical treatment for prostate cancer. The surgical treatment has been refined since 1980, thus somewhat reducing the side effects. The prostate and the seminal vesicles are removed and a bilateral lymph node dissection is done. Compared to what was expected before surgery by X-ray studies, more disease will usually be demonstrated after the pathologist examines the removed tissues.

Three studies involving close to 6,500 patients treated with radical prostatectomy show that the 5-year survival is about 74%, and the 10-year survival is about 59%.[18-20] Other studies show similar results. About 10% of patients who had surgery require an additional form of treatment because of local recurrence.[21]

It is important to realize that radical prostatectomy can disseminate prostate cancer cells to other parts of the body by way of the blood.[22]

Patients with high Gleason score (8 to 10), seminal vesicle involvement or lymph node metastases have the highest rates of failure and would be better served with another treatment modality.[23]

Salvage radical prostatectomy has been used sometimes for those patients who have failed radiation treatment. But this is not advisable because of the 10-fold higher risk of side effects afterwards.

The rates of postoperative and late complications are significantly reduced if the procedure is performed at a hospital that does a high volume (more than 100 per year) and by a surgeon who does a high volume of radical prostatectomies (more than 30 per year).[24]

Average cost for a radical prostatectomy: $20,000 (range from $18,000 to $22,000 depending on the location in the US).

3. RADIATION THERAPY – EXTERNAL BEAM

Localized prostate cancer can be effectively controlled using external beam radiation. The total radiation dose to the prostate is 65 to 70 Gray or higher given over 7 weeks or more. Even when cancer has spread beyond the prostate to nearby structures (Stage C), radiation can control the disease. Radiation (45 Gray) is delivered to the whole pelvis only when Stage C disease exists or when the lymph nodes are positive. If lymph nodes are removed surgically, the whole pelvis should not be radiated because there is a high chance (more than 25%) that the patient will develop penile, scrotal and leg edema. Overall, there are fewer side effects when the radiation is delivered using Three-Dimensional Conformal Radiation Therapy (3DCRT).

Average Medicare Global fees for 3D Conformal Radiation Therapy: $13,750.

More men with early stage prostate cancers are being treated with Intensity-Modulated Radiation Therapy (IMRT) rather than the three-dimensional conformal radiation therapy. IMRT involves more fields and a larger volume of normal tissues is exposed to lower doses. Also, the number of monitor units of the radiation machine is increased by a factor of 2 to 3, thereby increasing the total body exposure due to leakage radiation. Both factors tend to increase the risk of a second cancer. **IMRT will likely double the incidence of second cancers to about 1.75% compared to conventional radiation treatments** (see page 139).

Average Medicare Global fees for IMRT: $46,390.

4. BRACHYTHERAPY OR INTERSTITIAL RADIATION is the use of radioactive seeds placed into the body, in this case, into the prostate gland.

Many patients find this technique more desirable because it takes only about three hours or so in an outpatient surgical center compared to radical prostatectomy requiring weeks of recovery, or a daily radiation treatment for seven weeks or more, Monday through Friday.

Brachytherapy is most effective when there is a small cancer volume and the seeds are arranged homogenously. About 150 to 180 Gray are delivered to the prostate gland over the course of a year using Iodine-125 seeds. Usually, this technique is done only if the lymph nodes are free of cancer. When pelvic nodes are positive for cancer, some oncologists use brachytherapy if the lymph nodes have been removed or if the pelvis has been radiated. The side effects increase dramatically in this situation and there is no gain in survival. Brachytherapy may also be used if cancer recurs in the prostate after treatment with external beam radiation. In this case, brachytherapy can control about 98% of cases.[25]

Local control with brachytherapy is about 80% to 90% of cases, but some studies show less favorable local control at 40%. Impotence is seen in 25% to 30% of cases.

Average Medicare Global fees for brachytherapy: $12,240.

FATIGUE.   Many patients who undergo radiation treatment, either by external beam or brachytherapy experience fatigue. Fatigue is not due to radiation *per se*, but mainly to the fact that: (1) Patients have been told they may experience fatigue during radiation; (2) They travel to and from the radiation therapy unit daily, five days a week; (3) They have anxiety and depression associated with their newly diagnosed cancer and with seeing physically ill patients who have advanced cancers.

Surgery, external beam radiation, and brachytherapy have been shown to be equivalent options for early stage prostate cancer when one examines matched-pair analyses and retrospective analyses.[26-28]

5. CRYOSURGERY

The ancient Egyptians first used cold packs on wounds to relieve pain. Then in the mid 1800s, physicians in England used cryotherapy to treat cancer and nerve pain. During the early 1900's cryosurgery was used to treat dermatology diseases. Liquid nitrogen became available after World War II. Via insulated probes attached to a circulating pump, liquid nitrogen was used to treat skin disorders, brain cancers, Parkinson's disease, and some neuromuscular disorders.

Cryosurgical ablation of the prostate cancer was used in the 1960s with good survival results. But the procedure was abandoned because of technical difficulties until the late 1980s when ultrasound guided the freezing technique. In 1999 Medicare approved cryosurgery for reimbursement thus providing another modality to treat prostate cancer and further confounding the patient with yet another choice.

Cryosurgery kills cells by direct mechanical shock, osmotic shock (freezing and dehydration of the cell), and cellular hypoxia (no oxygen).

The patient is treated in the operating room with either a general or regional anesthetic. The ultrasound-guided needle insertion between the scrotum and the anus allows for proper placement of the needles into the prostate. This mechanical technique is the same as that for radioactive seed placement. There is no biological effect on structures adjacent to the frozen tissue, and the treatment is completed in a few minutes. The treatment can be repeated in the future.

The survival results from scores of published studies are similar to radical prostatectomy or radiation or observation.[29-34]

Cryosurgery is an option for: (1) those who have localized prostate cancer and decide not to have radical prostatectomy or radiation or observation, (2) those who have recurrent disease after having been treated with radical prostatectomy or radiation or prior cryosurgery, or (3) those who have a large prostate cancer that is obstructing the bladder or causing some other local complication.

Average Cost for Cryotherapy: $13,500.

Side Effects of Various Treatments and Costs				
	Radical Prostatectomy	External Radiation	Brachy-therapy	Cryotherapy
Death from Treatment	1%	< 0.5%		0
Erectile Dysfunction	50%-80%	30%-50%	20%-50%	30%-65%
Cardiopulmonary Complications	8% older than 65			
Cystitis	0	7%	4%-7%	
Rectal Injury	1.2%	1.7%		
Rectal Irritation	0	13%	6%-14%	8%
Urethral Strictures	6%-18%		6%-8%	3%
Urinary Incontinence	8%		13%-18%	1%
Requiring pads	8%-30%	7%		15%
COST	$20,000	$13,750 **3D** $46,390 **IMRT**	$12,240	$13,000

6. HORMONE TREATMENT TO SHRINK LOCALIZED PROSTATE CANCER BEFORE OTHER TREATMENTS BEGIN – IS IT WORTHWHILE? The prostate is a hormone sensitive organ. One can change its metabolism simply by reducing or blocking the effects of serum testosterone. Any of the following can change the effects of testosterone: estrogen, progesterone, go-nadotropin-releasing hormones analogues, adrenal enzyme synthesis inhibitors, and antiandrogens. Hormone treatment can cause hot-flushes, loss of libido or erectile function, weight gain, breast enlargement, liver inflammation, and osteoporosis.

In about 35% to 50% of cases, seemingly localized prostate cancers are actually not – they are spread beyond the prostate gland but our technology does not detect this. Therefore it seemed reasonable to shrink the cancer down so that localized treatments like surgery, radiation or cryosurgery would have a better chance to decrease the toxicity to adjacent normal tissues and help improve the effectiveness of the modality being used.

Preceding surgery, hormone treatment does not improve the surgery or the survival[35,36] and it does not improve survival when used before radiation therapy either.[37]

There is a downside to using hormone early in the course of a cancer illness. Let's use an analogy. Picture three people in a room that is being flooded with a lethal chemical. The weak people will die – let's say two die. One survives and will have children who learn how to thrive in spite of this chemical. They are resistant to the chemical. They, in turn, have their own children who are strong and very resistant to the chemical. This analogy is the same for cancer. Resistant cells emerge and that's why hormones or chemotherapy stop working. Therefore, if a hormone or chemotherapy is brought in too early in the illness, you essentially throw that drug away.

RISING PSA AFTER LOCAL THERAPY FAILURE

After treatment for localized prostate cancer an elevated PSA level is a sign of persistent cancer, but an undetected level does not necessarily mean there is no cancer. But what if the PSA was undetectable then becomes elevated and continues to rise. About 50,000 men each year have a cancer recurrence that is indicated only by a rising PSA. They are otherwise fine with no symptoms, pains, or other indications of cancer. Patients always want to know their PSA, and when it is rising, they panic with fear. This often triggers expensive and unnecessary testing and even treatments that can be more harmful than the disease itself.

First of all, a rising PSA does not signal an impending death.[38] Moreover, we sometimes lose sight of the fact that we need to treat the whole patient and not just a laboratory value. Treatment should be instituted only when metastases or symptoms of disease are documented,[38] and even then, one needs to judge whether the treatment will actually help the patient. Adherence to such a policy is difficult because patients pressure their physician to treat their "growing cancer." There is rarely a persistent or durable decline in PSA levels even if a patient with a rising PSA is treated with radiation after surgery or surgery after radiation ("salvage" treatment).[39,40]

Options for men with rising PSA after a treatment/observation:
- **Observation** only
- **Radiation** treatment for those who have had radical prostatectomy – **no increase in survival.**
- **Salvage surgery or cryosurgery** only for selected patients who had radiation treatment – **no increase in survival.**
- **Hormonal therapy** – **no increase in survival.**

WHO WILL DEVELOP METASTASES?
There have been multiple attempts, analysis, tables, and statistics at trying to precisely define who will develop metastases. The bottom line is this – the higher the Gleason score (indication of aggressiveness), the more organs that the cancer involved initially, and the sooner the PSA rises after a treatment, the higher the overall risk for metastases and death.

Risk of Metastatic Progression			
	3 years	5 years	7 years
Gleason Score 8 to 10	40%	60%	70%
Gleason Score 5 to 7 plus rising PSA sooner than 2 years	20%	65%	85%
Gleason Score 8 to 10 plus rising PSA sooner than 2 years	50%	70%	85%

CONCLUSION
Review this chapter with your own condition in mind remembering that since 1930 the lifespan of a prostate cancer patient has not changed. Previously held age cutoffs don't apply any longer to each modality. Take enough time before deciding upon a treatment so that years from now you will be comfortable with that decision. Turn to the next chapter to learn if you need systemic treatment.

Rudy had options. After careful consideration he made a choice and modified his lifestyle to optimize his lifespan.

24

Conventional Systemic Treatment for Prostate Cancer

Todd's History

Todd was treated with radical prostatectomy and now has metastatic spread to his bones and therefore needs systemic treatment. Can he improve his lifespan if he chooses hormonal therapy, chemotherapy, and/or modifies his currently poor lifestyle?

The medical profession had deluded itself for over a century in thinking that prostate cancer was a surgical disease and that more aggressive treatment would result in more men being cured. We now realize that there are certain prognostic factors that define low and high risk for recurrence and shortened life (Table 1). By the time a prostate cancer is detected and then either observed or locally treated with surgery, radiation, or cryotherapy, it has already disseminated to other parts of the body. Thus we turned our attention to systemic therapies that enter the bloodstream and travel throughout the body to theoretically kill cancer cells anywhere. Systemic therapy includes hormonal therapy, chemotherapy, treatment with biological response modifiers, and anti-angiogenic agents. These agents may be used once the cancer has spread to other organs.

Table 1. Prognostic Factors That Define Low- or High-Risk for Recurrence and Shortened Life in Patients	
Low-Risk	**High-Risk**
Digital Rectal Exam – Normal	Digital Rectal Exam - Abnormal
Gleason score 1 to 4	Gleason score 8 to 10
Low, stable PSA	Rising PSA
Age greater than 70	Age less than 60
Healthy Lifestyle	High-fat, Low-fiber, Obesity, No antioxidants or B vitamins, Smoker or inhales others' Alcohol: 3+/week, Sedentary lifestyle, Stress

WHO WILL DEVELOP PROSTATE METASTASES?

There have been multiple attempts, analysis, tables, and statistics at trying to precisely define who will develop metastases. The bottom line is this – the higher the Gleason score (indication of aggressiveness), the more organs that the cancer involved initially, and the sooner the PSA rises after a treatment, the higher the overall risk for metastases and death (Table 2).

Table 2. Risk of Metastatic Progression			
	3 years	5 years	7 years
Gleason Score 8 to 10	40%	60%	70%
Gleason Score 5 to 7 plus rising PSA sooner than 2 years	20%	65%	85%
Gleason Score 8 to 10 plus rising PSA sooner than 2 years	50%	70%	85%

HORMONAL THERAPY kills cancer cells that depend upon hormones to grow. Androgens, such as testosterone, are growth promoters for many cells including prostate cancer. Prostate cancer cells may have androgen receptors that act as doorways for testosterone to enter the prostate cancer cell and thereby feed it. Most prostate cancer cells have androgen receptors. The intent of hormonal therapy is to deprive prostate cancer cells of androgens (testosterone) that would otherwise make them grow.

- **If you change the hormonal milieu of the patient, you can expect to see a response.**
- **During the first few weeks of a hormonal treatment there may be a flare of pain in the areas of the body that have cancer – this indicates that the treatment is working.**
- **About 30% to 50% of patients who initially respond to a hormonal therapy and then become resistant may have continued disease regression if the therapy is abruptly stopped.**
- **Responses to hormonal therapy last 6-12 months or longer.**

Approximately 80 to 90 percent of men with advanced prostate cancer respond initially to androgen deprivation for a disease free survival of 12 to 33 months.[1] Androgen deprivation, or any other treatment, will lead to a resistant colony of cancer that gives an overall survival of 23 to 37 months from the time the treatment was first started.

Remember our analogy. Picture three people in a room that is being flooded with a lethal chemical. The weak people will die – let's say two die. One survives and will have children who learn how to thrive in spite of this chemical. They are resistant to the chemical. They, in turn, have their own children who are strong and very resistant to the chemical. This analogy is the same for cancer. Resistant cells emerge and that's why hormones or chemotherapy stop working.

Between the 1950s and the 1970s, men were treated with either estrogens, to overwhelm their testosterone and suppress the androgen receptor, or orchiectomy (removal of testicles), that stops the manufacturing of most testosterone. These men had a slightly longer life and a better quality of life when compared to those receiving no treatment at all. Multiple studies verify this.[2-5] Luteinizing hormone-releasing hormone (LHRH) agonists and antiandrogens were introduced in the 1980s.

■ **ORGAN REMOVAL of both Testicles** (castration) by surgery (orchiectomy) can be done as an outpatient and produces an

immediate depletion of almost 90 percent of testosterone.[6] Orchiectomy produces the same length of life when compared to DES, or orchiectomy plus DES treatment, or placebo.[7] There is almost immediate relief of bone pain from metastasis after surgical castration. **Almost 50 percent of men choose orchiectomy if they are told about it.**[8] **Also, men have fewer problems with sexual function if they choose orchiectomy over an LHRH agonist treatment.**[9]

■ **DES** – **DIETHYLSTILBESTROL** is an estrogen taken by mouth that overwhelms testosterone and suppresses the androgen receptor thus depriving prostate cancer cells of testosterone.   In large doses, DES can cause cardiovascular and leg blood clots.   DES at a dose of 3 mg to 5 mg per day caused a slightly higher death rate compared to orchiectomy because of more cardiovascular problems. However, at 1 mg per day DES produces the same lifespan as those treated with orchiectomy[10] and LHRH agonists[11-15] and was superior to flutamide.[16] At 3 mg per day, DES produces the same lifespan as those treated with estramustine (an estrogen compound with a nitrogen mustard alkylating agent) and cyproterone.[17,18]

DES is no longer readily available in the United States because of its limited use due to some side effects and because of higher reimbursement to physicians who prescribe LHRH agonists.   In its place, we use Premarin tablets that have the same benefits as DES.

■ **ESTROGEN** (fosfestrol) is less cardiotoxic than DES and is given intravenously. It is no more effective than other treatments.

■ **LUTEINIZING HORMONE-RELEASING HORMONE (LHRH) AGONISTS** promote the effects of luteinizing hormone-releasing hormone (LHRH). When LHRH is elevated in the body for a prolonged period of time, the production of testosterone drops to very low levels.   Initially, however, for a short period of time, testosterone production goes up resulting in a temporary growth of the prostate cancer and can worsen areas of the body that are involved with cancer. LHRH agonists have no cardiovascular side effects. They are injected or placed into the muscle in preparations that can last for one, three, four, or 12 months. **There is no difference in survival between LHRH agonists and orchiectomy.**[19]

▪ ANTIANDROGENS

STEROIDAL ANTIANDROGENS – (Cyproterone and Megestrol Acetate) reduce testosterone levels and block the androgen receptor. Cyproterone is not very effective, has cardiovascular side effects, and is not available in the US.

NONSTEROIDAL ANTIANDROGENS – NSAA – (Flutamide, Nilutamide, Bicalutamide) do not decrease testosterone levels but rather, inhibit the binding of testosterone and dihydrotestosterone to the androgen receptor. Orchiectomy is more effective than these agents.[20]

▪ ANTIAROMATASES block the conversion of cholesterol into

other hormones that can promote the growth of hormone dependant cancer cells. This is used effectively in breast cancer treatment and is now being tested for prostate cancer.

▪ PC-SPES, Prostate Cancer Hope (spes – Latin word for

hope), is an herbal preparation that has been popular. PSA levels drop in virtually all patients with hormone-sensitive disease and a majority of those with hormone refractory disease. It is composed of 8 compounds, and therefore the quality control for PC-SPES is difficult. It has estrogen properties, toxicities and biochemical actions – the same as for DES, an estrogen compound, and in fact, DES has been found in this preparation[21,22] as well as rat poison, warfarin.[23] It has other anti-tumor activity but overall, the clinical responses to PC-SPES are similar to second-line hormonal agents like estrogen and ketoconazole.[24-27] It is more expensive than DES and less reliable.

▪ MAXIMUM ANDROGEN BLOCKADE DOES NOT PROLONG
LIFE. Surgical or medical castration, results in a decline in tes-

tosterone by about 90 percent. The adrenal glands produce the other 10 percent and this amount could still fuel a prostate cancer. Therefore, it was reasoned that an antiandrogen should be added to inhibit the synthesis of testosterone in the adrenal glands, thus producing maximum androgen blockade in the hope of increasing lifespan.

To make a very long and costly story short, **maximum androgen blockade did not prolong life**. In 2000 the Prostate Cancer Trialists' Collaborative Group published a meta-analysis of 27 mature trials involving 8,275 men with advanced prostate cancer, the majority of whom had metastatic disease.[28] This study represented 98 percent of worldwide randomized evidence of men in trials of maximum androgen blockade versus single therapy. Those who received maximum androgen blockade had a five-year survival of 25.4 percent compared to 23.6 percent of those treated only with a single agent. This difference was not statistically significant and the authors of the study would not support the use of maximum androgen blockade over single therapy.

■ INTERMITTANT THERAPY is treatment given to patients when the PSA rises or when symptoms occur secondary to progressive prostate cancer. After symptoms decrease or the PSA falls, the treatment is discontinued and restarted only when symptoms appear or when the PSA rises again. Why does this work? The theory is this: Testosterone makes prostate cancer cells grow and regulates the number of cells in the prostate. When testosterone is withdrawn, many cells will program themselves to die naturally, a process called apoptosis. A certain percentage of the remaining cells still depend on testosterone for their growth and become resistant. When testosterone is withdrawn, the testicles begin to recover, produce more testosterone that in turn, re-harnesses these resistant cells and makes them again depend upon testosterone for growth. The cycle repeats itself when androgens are again withdrawn. Obviously, this does not go on forever. Survival using intermittent treatment is comparable to continuous treatment, but the advantage is that the side effects are intermittent.[29]

■ **STEROIDS** alone, like prednisone, hydrocortisone, or dexamethasone, can give a 30% to 50% response rate.[30,31]

■ **ABRUPT WITHDRAWAL OF HORMONES - ABOUT 30% to 50% of patients who initially respond to a hormonal therapy and then become resistant may have continued disease regression if the therapy is abruptly stopped.**

CHEMOTHERAPY might be considered when the hormone treatments have failed but **prostate cancer generally does not respond to chemotherapy and chemotherapy does not increase survival in any randomized study.**[32-36]
The following are the most commonly used chemotherapy drugs for prostate cancer treatment as single agents or in combination: cyclophosphamide, doxorubicin, mitoxantrone, vinblastine, etoposide, cisplatin, carboplatin, 5-FU, taxanes, suramin, ketoconazole, and estramustine, an estrogen/nitrogen mustard combination.

The standard chemotherapy for prostate cancer is prednisone plus mitoxanterone given at 10-14 mg/m^2 intravenously every 3-4 weeks. Estramustine is also commonly used as a single agent or in combination with others. The taxanes are being used more frequently. Suramin, an antiparasitic drug, has been used without success. Thalidomide, an anti-angiogenic agent, is being used with limited success. And finally, also with minimal success is the use of autologous dendritic cells that are loaded with recombinant fusion protein consisting of prostatic acid phosphatase and granulocyte-macrophage colony-stimulating factor.

The overall chemotherapeutic response rate, that is, the percentage of men who had some objective decrease in PSA or cancer size for at least 4 weeks, varied between 4% and 40%. Not very good. The quality of life on these agents is also poor because of the side effects of the drugs.

TOXICITY OF SOME CHEMOTHERAPIES

Table 3. Chemotherapy Toxicities

Organ	Commonly Used Prostate Cancer Therapies			
	Cyclophosphamide	5-FU	Adriamycin	Taxol
Eye	Yes	Yes	Yes	
Lung	Yes		Yes	Yes
Heart	Yes*	Possible	Yes	Yes
Liver	Yes	Yes		
Bone Marrow	Yes	Yes	Yes	Yes
Gastrointestine	Yes	Yes	Yes	Yes
Nausea/Vomiting	Yes	Yes	Yes	Yes
Nerve Damage				Yes
Brain Dysfunction	Yes	Yes		
Skin / Hair Loss	Yes	Yes	Yes	Yes
Leukemia Risk	Yes		Yes	
Bladder Cancer Risk	Yes#			

*Only with high doses   #Drink 8 to 10 large glasses of water a day to prevent bladder bleeding and decrease the risk of bladder cancer.

ANTI-ANGIOGENESIS – New Blood Vessel Inhibition

Normal cells do not have the capability to promote angiogenesis. They may secrete low amounts of molecules known to induce angiogenesis, but they secrete much greater amounts of anti-angiogenic molecules that inhibit the inducers. Production of high-levels of these anti-angiogenic substances is what is thought to maintain vascular quiescence in healthy tissue. In contrast to healthy cells, new cancer cells produce angiogenesis inducers but very little of the angiogenesis inhibitors.

Many substances have anti-angiogenic activity. Some neutralize the enzymes manufactured by the cancer cell that burrow a hole in the tissue to allow room for a new blood vessel. Others interfere with the building blocks of new blood vessels.

Mammals produce natural inhibitors of angiogenesis that include: interferons, steroids, proteins from platelets (thrombospondin and platelet factor 4), enzyme (protease) inhibitors, vitamin A, and metabolites of vitamin D_3. Several drugs that were developed for other purposes also have anti-angiogenic activity. Anti-angiogenic agents do not interfere with chemotherapy or radiation therapy.

Table 4. Anti-Angiogenic Agents

Anticancer Drugs	Cancer Treatment	Antibiotics
Antiestrogens – Tamoxifen	Radiation Therapy	Minocycline
Interferons, Retinoids	Hyperthermia	Suramin
Bleomycin, Methotrexate		Herbimycin A
Bisantrene, Mitoxantrone		D-Penicillamine

Other
Aspirin, other inhibitors of prostaglandin synthetase
Vitamin D_3 metabolites
p53 Suppressor gene
Captopril, Megace, Thalidomide

Table 5. Theoretical Comparison of Chemotherapy and Anti-Angiogenic Therapy

Variable	Chemotherapy	Anti-Angiogenic Therapy
Target	Cancer Cell	Blood Vessel Cells
Affects Primary & Mets	Yes	Yes
Specificity	Low	High
Resistance Develops	Yes	No
Duration of Therapy	Moderate	Long
? Chemoprevention	No	Yes

Anti-angiogenic agents have been used since 1970 without any significant successes so far.

MOST EFFECTIVE AND MOST COST EFFECTIVE SYSTEMIC TREATMENT

Orchiectomy is the most effective and most cost effective treatment for localized prostate cancer or for prostate cancer that has spread to other organs. Although the injectable and oral hormones may be more popular, they are more costly and less effective. The following analysis is based on a 65-year-old man with a prostate cancer that has recurred.[37] Six treatments were evaluated: diethylstilbestrol (DES); orchiectomy; a nonsteroidal antiandrogen (NSAA), nilutamide; a luteinizing hormone-releasing hormone (LHRH) agonist, Zoladex; and combinations of an NSAA with an LHRH agonist or orchiectomy. These results changed little when PSA was used to guide therapy. Orchiectomy is the most effective and most cost-effective treatment. All the others yield small health benefits at high costs. Table 6.

Table 6. Treatment, Life Expectancy, and Cost-Effectiveness			
Treatment	Life Years	Quality of Life Years	Cost
Orchiectomy	7.6	5.10	$7,000
Diethylstilbestrol (DES)	6.8	4.64	$3,600
NSAA, nilutamide	7.4	4.98	$16,000
LHRH agonist, Zoladex	7.5	5.08	$27,000
NSAA + orchiectomy	7.5	5.05	$20,700
NSAA + LHRH agonist	7.5	5.03	$40,300

TREATMENT OF METASTATIC DISEASE
Prostate cancer may metastasize to bone, liver, brain, lung, skin, and other sites. Treatment is directed to relieving the symptoms that are produced by these metastatic lesions.
* Radiation
    o Used to treat a single area of bone pain, cord compression, or the brain, etc. The usual dose for a single confined area is 30 Gray.
    o A patient may have numerous metastatic bone sites for which a radioactive material is injected into the veins and travels to the bones. Strontium-89 is somewhat effective for alleviating pain temporarily, but greatly compromises the patient's bone marrow.[38] Another radioactive material is Samarium-153 EDTMP that seems to be a little less toxic and produces the same temporary pain relief.[39]
* Hormonal treatment may be used for any site that has metastatic disease.
* Biphosphonates inhibit bone osteoclasts and prostate cancer cell adhesion to bone. They provide temporary bone pain relief with minimal bone marrow suppression[40] and should be used only when the usual treatments fail.
* Chemotherapy can be considered for patients who have liver metastases or disease that is unresponsive to hormonal treatments. Survival is unchanged in all cases.

SYSTEMIC THERAPY FOR METASTATIC PROSTATE CANCER PATIENTS. General conclusions can be made:

- **LIFESPAN** – same for any systemic choice of treatment.
- **DISEASE-FREE INTERVAL** – period of time in which there are no disease events –no difference between therapies.
- **HORMONAL THERAPY: ORCHIECTOMY, DES, LHRH AGONISTS AND ANY OTHER HORMONE MANIPULATION PRODUCE THE SAME LIFESPAN AND RECURRENCE RATES.**
- **THERE IS NO BENEFIT FROM ADDING AN ANTI-ANDROGEN TO ANDROGEN DEPRIVATION**
- **DELAYED TREATMENT – THERE IS NO BENEFIT FOR STARTING ANDROGEN DEPRIVATION IMMEDIATELY WHEN A DIAGNOSIS IS MADE COMPARED TO STARTING LATER, WHEN THERE ARE SYMPTOMS OF DISEASE.**
- **ANDROGEN SUPPRESSION ALONE IS AS EFFECTIVE AS ANDROGEN SUPPRESSION PLUS CHEMOTHERAPY** for lifespan and recurrence rate, has fewer side effects, better quality of life.
- **CHEMOTHERAPY DOES NOT PROLONG LIFE**
- **QUALITY OF LIFE** – better with hormonal treatment
- **BIOLOGICAL RESPONSE MODIFIERS** or other immune system enhancers have shown no benefit.

THERAPY FOR METASTATIC PROSTATE CANCER PATIENTS RESISTANT TO HORMONES. General conclusions can be made:

- **EXTERNAL BEAM RADIATION CAN REDUCE PAIN**
- **RADIOACTIVE MATERIAL INJECTED CAN DECREASE PAIN FOR SOME MEN, BUT PRODUCES SIDE EFFECTS**
- **CHEMOTHERAPY CAN MINIMALLY HELP WITH PAIN BUT DOES NOT PROLONG LIFE**
- **BISPHOSPHONATES – INSUFFICIENT EVIDENCE TO RECOMMEND**

FOLLOW-UP FOR PROSTATE CANCER PATIENTS

- **Laboratory and Imaging Studies** – these studies don't change the outcome. These include imaging studies like bone scans, chest X-rays, etc., blood work, PSA, and liver tests. Cost of these unnecessary tests is close to $1 billion per year.
- **History and physical examination** every 3 to 6 months for 3 years, then 6 to 12 months for 2 years, then annually.

Once patients develop metastases, they are incurable.[41] Complete remissions are rarely seen. And, curiously, the interval of time between initial management of the early prostate cancer and the diagnosis of metastases is just about the same whether the patient is undergoing follow-up or not. Therefore, follow-up after surgery and primary treatment does not lead to earlier detection of metastases nor does it affect the overall survival. Recurrences are detected 85% of the time by the patient or by the physician during examination.

Besides an erroneous belief system, patient desires, pressure from the media and various organizations that say early detection is best, the driving force behind intensive follow-ups may be the threat of malpractice suits. A malpractice case is composed of two issues: deviation from the standard of care and "proximate cause." Based on the hard scientific data, the standard of care must be minimal surveillance. Proximate cause simply asks the question: Does a potential delay in a diagnosis of metastases make any difference in the ultimate outcome or survival? Proximate cause also would not be applicable because a patient is incurable once a recurrence is detected.

PROSTATE CANCER TREATMENT BY STAGE

STAGE A OR STAGE T 1 – Rectal exam is normal, but cancer is found in surgical specimen during operation for prostatic hyperplasia, or an elevated PSA prompts a biopsy that is positive.

STAGE A1 or STAGE T 1a – The cancer is limited to less than 5% of the prostate tissue removed at surgery, or an elevated PSA prompts a biopsy that is positive. Fewer than 2%

have lymph node involvement. This stage produces no symptoms.

STAGE A2 or STAGE T 1b – The cancer involves more than 5% of the prostate tissue removed at surgery, or an elevated PSA prompts a biopsy that is positive. About 35% have lymph node involvement. This stage produces no symptoms.

STAGE T 1c –an elevated PSA prompts a biopsy that is positive.

- Observation
- Radiation
- Radical Prostatectomy
- Cryosurgery

STAGE B OR STAGE T 2 – disease can be felt during a rectal exam but still confined to the prostate. PSA is elevated.

STAGE B1 or STAGE T 2a – The cancer is a small discrete nodule limited to one lobe of the prostate. About 20% have lymph node involvement. This stage produces no symptoms.

STAGE B2 or STAGE T 2c – The cancer is a small discrete nodule limited to both lobes of the prostate and 35% have lymph node involvement. This stage produces no symptoms.

- Observation
- Radiation
- Radical Prostatectomy
- Cryosurgery

STAGE C – palpable cancer extends beyond the prostate to nearby structures, but there are no distant metastases. A common symptom for this stage is difficult urination.

STAGE C1 or STAGE T 3b – Cancer has broken through the prostate capsule but there is no seminal vesicle involvement. About 50% have lymph node involvement.

STAGE C2 or STAGE T 3c – Seminal vesicles are involved and 80% have lymph node involvement.

The objective of treatment is to slow down the cancer's growth and relieve the urinary symptoms.

- Radiation

- Radical Prostatectomy in rare circumstances
- Cryosurgery in rare circumstances
- Hormonal – Orchiectomy, or administered hormones

STAGE D –cancer has spread to other parts of the body causing bone pain, weight loss, difficult urination and fatigue. The goal of treatment is to relieve pain and symptoms.

- Hormonal – Orchiectomy, estrogens, or other administered hormones
- Palliative radiation
- Possibly chemotherapy

SURVIVAL BY STAGE   As the cancer involvement advances with each stage, survival decreases.

Table 7. Percent Survival Based on Stage

Stage	Local Control	Percent Survival 5 Year	10 Year
Stage A	95%	85%-95%	65%
Stage B	85%	60%-80%	45%
Stage C	78%	30%-55%	15%-40%
Stage D	N/A	30%-40%	0

FACTORS THAT IMPROVE SURVIVAL
- COMPETENT IMMUNE SYSTEM INCREASES LIFESPAN
- PROPER DIET AND LIFESTYLE (SIMONE TEN POINT PLAN) INCREASES LIFESPAN
- ANTIOXIDANTS AND OTHER NUTRIENTS ENHANCE IMMUNE SYSTEM.

"UNPROVEN" TREATMENT COMPARED TO CONVENTIONAL TREATMENT PRODUCE THE SAME LIFESPAN AND QUALITY OF LIFE[42]
- Patients from an unconventional cancer clinic in California were matched with patients treated conventionally at a traditional academic cancer center in Philadelphia, Pennsylvania.

The Philadelphia investigators hypothesized that survival time would be the same for both groups on the assumption that the unproved remedy is no more effective in patients with end-stage disease than conventional care, itself largely ineffective. Results: Lifespan and quality of life were the same for both.

People seek unproven treatment because it has little or no toxicity and conventional treatment produces toxicity without increasing lifespan. Many of the agencies and/or "benevolent" charities in the United States have developed a "hit list" of unproven therapies and their proponents without having the therapy investigated – the therapy is guilty of quackery until proven otherwise. I am convinced that ALL therapies, conventional or otherwise, should be put through the same rigors of science to the degree that they can, and then evaluate the findings.

TREATMENT: EFFECTIVE OR NOT EFFECTIVE, DOES IT WORK? Rather than classify treatment as conventional, or unproven, or alternative, treatments should have only two broad classifications: EFFECTIVE or NONEFFECTIVE therapy. Does the treatment prolong survival and improve the quality of life? **Is the treatment effective? Does it work?** And at the same time, does the treatment do little or no harm?

For example, options for the treatment of localized prostate cancer include observation alone, surgery, radiation, cryosurgery, or hormones – these all produce the same survival. Likewise, hormonal therapy, chemotherapy, and unproven therapy in the example above produce the same survival. Survival is the same for both examples, but which modality produces the fewest side effects – which one would you pick? The EFFECTIVE choices are obvious.

If there were a cure for cancer somewhere, in someone's hideaway clinic, it would not remain secret, and all the fuss about the correct cancer treatment would be over. A cure for cancer could never be kept a secret.

Patients considering any treatment must always ask, "What are the risks and what are the benefits?" If the risks are minimal and the benefit is great, there is no question that the treatment should be entertained. However, if the risks are great and the benefit is minimal, reject that treatment.

CONCLUSION

Hormonal therapy and chemotherapy afford the same survival benefit. Chemotherapy is no more curative than hormonal therapy, and it is much more toxic. So, why is chemotherapy still used?

Patients with cancer have grown up listening to organized cancer groups, physicians, and the media extolling the virtues of chemotherapy. The more often you hear it, the more you believe that if you have cancer, you must have chemotherapy. And patients want hope. For instance, over half of a group of patients receiving chemotherapy for metastatic (incurable) disease believed that they would be cured, and all of these patients believed that chances of "cure" were greater than 50% even when they were told the opposite.[43] And even when they were told what the cure rates were for their stage of disease, patients routinely discounted the facts.

American oncologists are more likely to advise more aggressive treatment over less aggressive treatment than their counterpart oncologists in Europe. Most oncologists believe aggressive treatment will improve survival when it actually does not.[44] And patients want their physicians to make the major decisions regarding what treatment is appropriate for them.[45]

Survival for prostate cancer patients has changed little since 1930 using conventional treatment. However, I am convinced, based on the data already reviewed, that men who follow an optimal lifestyle (Ten Point Plan) coupled to effective treatment using non-immunosuppressing agents when possible, will fare better and live longer (Figure 1). They will be more competent immunologically, and their cancers will not be fed by lifestyle factors that we know perpetuate cancer growth.

SURVIVAL (LIFESPAN) FOR PROSTATE CANCER PATIENTS

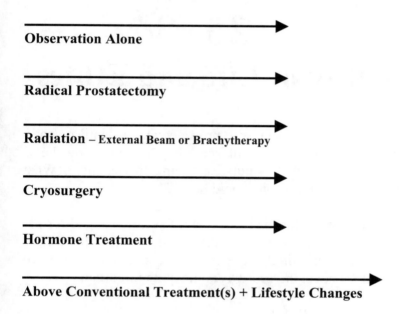

Observation Alone

Radical Prostatectomy

Radiation – External Beam or Brachytherapy

Cryosurgery

Hormone Treatment

Above Conventional Treatment(s) + Lifestyle Changes

Todd decided to have an orchiectomy and strictly adhere to the Simone Ten point Plan for lifestyle modification to extend his life.

25

Quality of Life and Ethics

Randy's History
Randy is 56 and has metastatic prostate cancer. Until recently his quality of life was alright according to him. Now he is faced with disease that is not responding to treatment. What should he be told and what should he do?

Since 1930, overall survival (life span) has not changed for patients with prostate cancer. In the ensuing years, treatments have become increasingly toxic. Issues concerning quality of life and ethics have, therefore, become quite important.

QUALITY OF LIFE is very important and should measure physical symptoms, psychological well-being, social functioning, daily activity levels, cognitive abilities, sexual dysfunction, and overall general life satisfaction. Quality of life assessments have been used for many illnesses including cardiovascular disease, strokes, and now cancer.

The National Cancer Institute has recommended that clinical trials include quality of life assessments and the U.S. Food and Drug Administration recognizes the benefit to quality of life as a basis for approval of new anticancer drugs.[1]

When two treatments yield similar disease-free survival and/or survival, the treatment that affords a better quality of life should be recommended. Conversely, if one treatment is effective but diminishes the quality of life so much that its use is unacceptable, that treatment is not worth undertaking.

Cancer treatments affect the quality of life. We demonstrated a better quality of life for 50 consecutive breast cancer patients who received radiation therapy and/or chemotherapy and who followed the Ten Point Plan that included certain vitamins and minerals. An international study showed substantial differences in quality of life scores between national groups. English-speaking patients in Europe were best able to cope with their cancer. German and Swedish patients, however, coped moderately well with their cancers. And the Italians were least able to cope.[2] This pattern fits with the conception that Northern Europeans are more reserved and complain less than Southern Europeans.

Studies of quality of life for patients receiving marrow transplants have not had clear-cut results. Some patients have an excellent quality of life following bone marrow transplant, but others do not fare as well.[3]

SEXUALITY AND BODY IMAGE

Any illness brings about changes in feelings of well being. Although rarely dealt with by the physician, sexual function is an integral part of an individual's well being.[4] Sexuality is important for all ages. In fact, 60% of cancer patients want more information on the impact of cancer on sexuality, and 55% want to discuss sexuality openly with their physicians – this rarely occurs.

Often a man recovering from a prostate disease or prostate cancer is worried about having to perform sexually. Knowing what to expect and finding out what you can do will help you. For most people, there are changes that mean they will need to adapt and develop new ways of giving and receiving sexual pleasure. Fatigue, the most common sexual difficulty experienced by cancer patients, can reduce interest in sexual activity. If fatigue is the problem, consider having sexual intercourse when you feel more energetic.

Sexuality also includes intimacy and emotional support. Being a cancer patient makes you feel vulnerable. Sometimes all you need is to be held by a loved one. It's easy to focus all your energies on treatment. But sexuality is important to a person's well being. And a patient's mental attitude can affect one's recovery. Feel free to talk with your doctor about any sexual problems you may have.

There are two physical phases of male sexuality, erection and ejaculation. Sexual arousal sends impulses down the nerves to engorge blood into the penis causing an erection. Erection is maintained by continued arousal and blood flow into the penis. Once there is no longer sexual arousal, with or without orgasm and ejaculation, the blood drains out of the penis and the erection ceases. Cancer treatment can affect both erections and ejaculation. But the mechanisms for each are different, so men can have an erection and achieve orgasm without ejaculation. A man who is unable to ejaculate (dry ejaculations) is infertile.

A NewsWeek article promoting testosterone enhancement as a risk for prostate cancer, claimed some surprising data:

Table 1. Orgasms According to Age as per NewsWeek				
Age	Orgasms Per Year	Age Bracket	Orgasms per 10 Yr.	Lifetime Total Orgasms
		0-20	500	500
20	104	20-30	1100	1600
30	121	30-40	1000	2600
40	84	40-50	650	3250
50	52	50-60	400	3650
60	35	60-70	280	3930
70	22	70-80	150	4080

Knowing the above information may influence what treatment options a man considers. If a man is 70 and lives until 80, he would have 150 orgasms left, and already had 4000! On the other hand, a man of 50 theoretically has another 800 orgasms, and might consider the treatment that would least likely affect potency.

MALE SEXUAL RESPONSE CYCLE as described in Masters and Johnson[5] is shown in Table 2. Systemic treatment, chemotherapy or hormonal treatment, decreases the sexual responses for both young and older men.

Table 2. Male Sexual Response Cycle		
	Young Men	**Older Men**
Excitement	Erection attained in 3-5 second Erection may be partially lost then rapidly regained intentionally. Erection diminishes easily with distractions like noise even though continuous stimulation	Erection attained in 15-20 seconds or longer Once erection lost, difficult to regain Erection maintained longer
Plateau	Increase in penis diameter and sometimes penis head Color change to red-purple	Just before ejaculation penis gets more elongated with increased girth
Orgasm	Ejaculation occurs by regular contractions (0.8 sec) of 3 sets of muscles forcing seminal fluid from the penis to a distance of 12-24 inches. After first 3 to 4 major expulsive efforts, there are minor ones occurring for several seconds.	Ejaculation the same as for young men except it is less forceful, sending the seminal fluid a distance of 6-12 inches. Fewer expulsive contractions.
Resolution	Two phases: 50% reduction in erection quite rapidly, then rest over many minutes.	Erection is completely lost within seconds of ejaculation.

TREATMENT OF ERECTILE DYSFUNCTION

- Phosphodiesterase type 5 inhibitors – these prescription drugs allow even small amounts of cGMP to effectively work to result in erections (Chapter 2).

- Vacuum pump is a hand- or battery-operated device that is placed over the penis. Air is pumped out, creating a vacuum that draws blood into the penis. A retaining band is then placed at the base of the penis to maintain the erection. After intercourse, the band is removed.

- Inflatable implants gives you the most natural erection of any implant. It's also the only implant that achieves the full girth of your natural erection and, in the flaccid state, is the most natural in appearance. The device does not affect sensation or the ability to achieve orgasm.

INFERTILITY - Removal of the prostate gland makes a man infertile. If both testes are removed, infertility results also.

Many men are very uncomfortable with the idea of this kind of surgery. Orchiectomy is an irreversible operation. Concerns about body image or self-image may lead men to choose a non-surgical option. Some men opt to have a *testicular prosthesis*, or artificial testicles, placed inside the scrotum to replace the testicles removed during an orchiectomy. The prosthesis makes the scrotum look much as it did before surgery.

QUESTIONS REGARDING SEXUALITY are rarely asked. However, one investigator is convinced that the following questions should be made part of any cancer questionnaire to determine the person's quality of life with regard to sexuality.
- How often does the man have sex with his partner?
- How often does he feel desire for sex?
- How often does he masturbate?
- What kinds of stimulation help him reach orgasm?
- What range of sexual practices is comfortable for him?
- Have his prostate cancer diagnosis and treatment changed his sexual frequency, function, or the types of touch used?

HOME CARE should be the principal setting for prostate cancer patients in the terminal stages because they will feel less anxious and more at ease at home than in a hospital or nursing-home setting. The older patient has more concerns regarding transportation, finances, and symptoms from other chronic illnesses in addition to the cancer. All the creature comforts that the patient is used to are there at hand. And truly the ideal setting for such a patient is in the home because a hospital setting can offer little that home care can't offer.

Family members must assume responsibility for physical and psychosocial demands of the patient with cancer. Everyone in the family has a new set of physical and psychosocial demands as care providers. The quality of life for both the patient and the family is a major issue and concern. A patient needs physical comforts and information. A care provider needs household management skills and information. When both groups are considered, the priority need is psychological. But the following must be addressed when caring for the terminal prostate cancer patient at home:[6] Hospice caregivers can help.

- Pain control and symptom management
- Communication with the physician
- Preparation for death
- Opportunity to achieve a sense of completion

QUALITY OF LIFE SUMMARY. Each of the qualities of life must be addressed and may determine the choice of treatment: physical symptoms, performance, general well-being, cognitive abilities, sexual dysfunction, and overall life satisfaction. Quality of life issues are now on equal footing with efficacy when the FDA considers a new drug.

ETHICS

Do patients with cancer really want to know the exact day they are going to die? And if a doctor does give them a range of time for life, how many patients then go home, mark the calendar, and proceed to die on that day? Most people who grow up in an industrialized society with multimedia communications are aware that patients who have cancer generally will die of it. This is not a revelation.

In my experience, all cancer patients who receive treatment, and, hence, interact with physicians and other patients in treatment areas, know their situation. Even very young people know. A six-year-old boy who I was treating for leukemia at the National Cancer Institute, asked me what it was like in heaven. A national survey found that 96% of Americans wanted to be told if they had cancer and 85% wanted to know how long they would live if their cancer usually led to death in less than a year.[7]

Moreover, a legal case involving ethical informed consent (*Arato v. Avedon*)[8] asked whether the law should force physicians to report statistical life expectancy information to patients. Mr. Arato had pancreas cancer that was treated surgically, then with experimental chemotherapy and radiation because there "is no effective treatment." The surgeon and oncologist never told Mr. Arato and his wife that only 5% survive for 5 years, nor did they give a prognosis or estimate of his life expectancy, nor were they asked. A recurrence occurred and the physicians knew he would die within a few months, but did not tell the patient about life expectancy.

The patient died and his wife sued the physicians claiming that the doctors were obligated under California's informed consent law to tell the patient about survival figures before asking him to consent to chemotherapy. The court decided Mr. Arato should have been informed. The physicians said if the patient knew of the high mortality rate, he would have no hope. And during the 70 visits, the patient did not ask questions about his life expectancy indicating to the physicians that he did not want to know. The patient's wife said had the patient known the facts, he would have declined all treatment and attended to his business affairs. His wife incurred tax losses due to poor business planning.

The lower court favored the physicians. The appeal court reversed the decision. The California Supreme Court upheld the decision in favor of the wife because of the doctrine of informed consent based on four tenets:

1. Patients are generally ignorant of medicine.
2. Patients have a right to control their own bodies and thus to decide about medical treatment.
3. To be effective, consent to medical treatment must be informed.
4. Patients are dependent upon their physicians for truthful information and must trust them (making the doctor-patient relationship a "fiduciary" or trust relationship rather that an arm's length business relationship).

The court concluded "the physician is under a legal duty to disclose all material information – information regarded as significant by a reasonable person in the person's position when deciding to accept or reject a recommended medical procedure – needed to make an informed decision regarding a proposed treatment."

The practice of medicine is an art as well as a science. It involves compassion and honesty. A good physician will always give a ray of hope as well as discuss the implications of a grave situation.

It is often easier to give another round of ineffective chemotherapy than to tell patients that there is nothing left in the anti-cancer arsenal. The clinician should sit with patients and families, hold their hands and tell them there is no way to control their cancer, but they will not be abandoned and will be made as comfortable as possible.[9]

Physicians are required to tell the patient about the probability that a proposed treatment will be successful and specifically define what the word "successful" means. A reasonable person should understand the probability of success from a particular treatment and then decide whether to accept that treatment or not. **We must tell patients of clinical trials but inform them that clinical trials do not improve the outcome.**[10] The poor results with conventional medicine are, of course, the whole basis for the ground swell concerning alternative medicine in the United States. Our culture emphasizes life and youth and vitality. We tend to shy away from talking about death and dying. Hope should always be given, but not false hope.

Sometimes there are financial conflicts that arise when one treatment is considered over another treatment. It has been said that the chief beneficiaries of cancer treatments that don't change survival and cause harm are often the oncology community and pharmaceutical companies and their stockholders.[11]

We really need to start thinking in terms of EFFECTIVE or NONEFFECTIVE treatment and tell patients about treatments in those terms. For instance, chemotherapy is noneffective for pancreas cancer. And perhaps, as I have said in the past, aggressive treatment to keep a person alive in the last several weeks of his or her life would stop if the patient and the family were truly informed about the futility of such efforts. The costs of health care provided to a patient in terminal stages in a hospital are enormous and consume anywhere from 20 to 30 percent of all the health-care dollars. The patient and the family may be responsible for this because they "want everything done." The physician is partly responsible because "our technology should help these patients." And the legal profession may, in part, be responsible as well; if everything is not done, will the family sue the physician?

Randy appreciated that he was told the truth about his terminal situation. This gave him "special time" with his family in his own home.

PART FIVE

Simone Ten-Point Plan for Prostate Disease Prevention and Cancer Life Extension

26

Simone Ten Point Plan for Prostate Disease Prevention and Cancer Life Extension

You can do many things to control the destiny of your life and the lives of your loved ones. A majority of men experience benign prostate disease causing symptoms that simply do not have to be. You can decrease the severity of these symptoms and the risk of developing prostate cancer. Prostate cancer affects one in six men, and those odds are getting worse. Eighty to ninety percent of all cancers are related to lifestyle factors: nutrition (high-fat, low-fiber diet, and lack of nutrients), tobacco smoke, alcohol, chemical carcinogens, ozone, air pollution, industrial exposure, some hormones and drugs, sedentary lifestyle, and lack of spirituality, etc. As we have learned, many of these cancer risk factors also put you at risk for developing and worsening cardiovascular diseases. Since we can now identify many of these factors, we should modify them to lessen our risks.

The likelihood of drastically increasing the number of cancer cures by conventional cancer therapies in the foreseeable future is not great, even though some of the very best minds and technologies are involved in cancer research. Cancer is the most complex group of diseases known, and there are many different causes. We must all do our part to *prevent* cancer in order to substantially reduce the number of new cancer cases. Americans need to know the risk factors for cancer and cardiovascular diseases. Adults who become aware of these risk factors and then modify their diets and lifestyles accordingly will reduce their risk of developing the diseases. Table 1 provides a list of the risk factors for cancer and heart disease that you can or cannot control. As you now know, you have direct control over virtually all of them except one – age.

Table 1. Risk Factors for Cancer and Heart Disease

Risk Factor	Controllable
• **Nutritional** – Fat Intake, Fiber Intake, Vitamin/Mineral Intake, Food Additives, Caffeine Intake	Yes
• **Obesity**	Yes
• **Tobacco Use**	Yes
• **Alcohol Use**	Yes
• **Drug Use**	Yes
• **Pesticides**	Yes
• **Environmental Factors** – Air Pollution (Outdoor, Ozone Depletion, Acid Rain), Indoor Pollution, Water Pollution and Treatment, Electromagnetic Fields	Yes
• **Radiation** – Sun exposure, Suntan Booths, Unneeded X-ray	Yes
• **Sexual-Social** – Female and Male Promiscuity, AIDS spread	Yes
• **Hormonal Factors** – Menarche*, First Pregnancy, Abortion or Miscarriage First Trimester of First Pregnancy, Benign Breast Disease, Failure to Repair Undescended Testicle, DES, Oral Contraceptive Use, Hormone Replacement Therapy, Androgen Use	Yes
• **Sedentary Lifestyle**	Yes
• **Stress**	Yes
• **Occupational Exposure Factors**	Yes
• **High Blood Pressure**	Yes
• **Lack of Comprehensive Physical Examination**	Yes
• **Age**	No

* A high-fat diet triggers early menarche.

Children will benefit the most from properly modified nutritional factors and daily habits. Information on nutrition should be part of a child's education throughout the school years, because nutritional practices and habits are easily modified in youth. If parents and teachers set the example of healthy lifestyle factors, children will continue these practices throughout their lives. There will be a consequent decrease in the incidence of cancer, cardiovascular and other diseases.

What can you do to help yourself?

Simply, I have presented the current body of scientific information concerning benign prostate disease, prostate cancer, and the factors that promote an existing prostate cancer. I now will discuss how those risk factors can be modified. Whether you have a benign prostate problem or prostate cancer, you will be better off when you closely adhere to my recommendations. As you have read, survival – lifespan – is positively affected mainly by proper lifestyle and not by existing conventional treatments. The preponderance of scientific information suggests that prostate health can be achieved by following our Ten-Point Plan. **Our Ten Point Plan can decrease the risk for cancer and increase the possibility of survival for those who have cancer.**

SIMONE TEN POINT PLAN FOR PROSTATE DISEASE PREVENTION AND CANCER LIFE EXTENSION

POINT 1. NUTRITION.

• **MAINTAIN AN IDEAL WEIGHT.** Decrease calories. Repeated fluctuations in your weight can increase the risk for heart attack and death.

• **LOW-FAT, LOW-CHOLESTEROL FOODS.** No four-legged animals, shellfish, or dairy products unless skim or non-fat products – not whole, 1%, or 2%. No farm-raised fish.

To reduce cholesterol, avoid:	To reduce triglycerides, avoid:
• Four-legged Animals	• Alcohol
• Dairy, except skim or non-fat	• Fruit, fruit juices
• Shellfish	• Cookie, candy, cake

Triglycerides are sugar-fats and are increased by anything that tastes sweet to your tongue. Triglycerides thicken the bloodstream and makes the LDL-cholesterol small, dense, and better able to block arteries.[1] Cholesterol takes about 6 months to come down, but triglycerides take only about 6 weeks. Remember, there are no fairies that sprinkle cholesterol or triglycerides into your blood while you are sleeping!

If your total dietary fats are less than 20 percent of your total calories, you will attain prostate health and decrease your risk of cancer and other health risks. It is also virtually impossible to gain weight on such a low-fat diet.

o *Poultry* cooked without the skin. White meat is best. Goose and duck are too fatty.

o *Fish* – all are fine except shellfish, sardines, mackerel, and fish canned in oil, all of which are high in fat or cholesterol.

o *Egg whites* are alright, not the yolk.

o *Eliminate saturated and polyunsaturated fats* – butter, margarine, meat fat, lard, and all oils.

o *Limit garnishes and sauces.* Ketchup and vinegar are fine. Unless they are fat-free, don't use salad dressings, prepared gravies and sauces, mayonnaise, sandwich spreads, or other products containing fats, oils, or egg yolks.

o *Food Labels* – you need to know how to read them to determine the percentage of fat calories from it. You need to know two numbers from the label: the total number of calories per ounce, and the number of fat grams per ounce, then add an imaginary zero to that number. Let's look at specific examples:

	Light Potato Chips	Pretzel
Total calories	120 per serving	100 per serving
Total fat grams	6	1
Imaginary zero to fat	60	10
Ratio	60 divided by 120	10 divided by 100
Percentage Fat	50%	10%

Eating these, you will:		
Gain weight	YES	NO
Decrease breast health	YES	NO
Increase risk for disease	YES	NO
Promote existing disease	YES	NO

What if there is no food label to read? Well, you already know which foods are good and which are not –Table 2.

Table 2. Percent Fat Calories in Foods			
Good		**Bad**	
Vegetables/Fruit	<10%	Beef and Lamb	50-80%
Breads	10-20%	Pork (the "white meat")	80%
Fish	10-20%	Dairy – non-skim	60-90%
Pasta, Grains, Cereals	10-20%	Eggs	70%
Poultry (no skin)	20-35%	Diet Margarine	100%

• **CONSUME** *SOLUBLE* **AND** *INSOLUBLE* **FIBER** (25-35 grams/day). Fruits, vegetables, cereals are mainly *insoluble* fibers. Pectins, gums, and mucilages have *soluble* fibers that can decrease cholesterol, trigylcerides, sugars, and carcinogens. Both increase fecal bulk and bowel movement frequency, slow an irritable bowel, or speed up a constipated bowel. Use a supplement of *soluble* fiber to insure a consistent amount each day.

Taken with water, soluble fiber supplements make you feel full due to longer time in stomach and, hence, can be used effectively to decrease your appetite so that you lose weight.

You can eat whole or lightly milled grains like rice, barley, and buckwheat. Whole-wheat bread and whole-wheat pasta, cereals, crackers, and other grain products can also be eaten as can unsweetened fruit juices and unsweetened cooked, canned, or frozen fruit.

• **AVOID BUTTER ROLLS, COMMERCIAL BISCUITS, MUFFINS, DOUGHNUTS, SWEET ROLLS, CAKES, EGG BREAD, CHEESE BREAD,** and commercial mixes containing dried eggs and whole milk.

• **SUPPLEMENT YOUR DIET WITH THE CORRECT NUTRIENTS, IN THE CORRECT DOSES, IN THE CORRECT CHEMICAL FORM, AND THE CORRECT RATIO OF ONE TO ANOTHER BASED ON YOUR LIFESTYLE.** Take high doses of all antioxidants (the carotenoids, vitamins C and E, selenium, cysteine, bioflavonoids, copper, zinc), and the B vitamins with food; calcium and its enhancing agents, at bedtime.

Simone Antioxidant – Nutrient Supplementation			
Carotene	30 mg	**Selenium**	200 mcg
Lutein	20 mcg	**Copper**	3 mg
Lycopene	20 mcg	**Zinc**	30 mg
Vitamin A	5500 IU	Iodine	150 mcg
Vitamin D	400 IU	Potassium	30 mg
Vitamin E	400 IU	Chromium	125 mcg
Vitamin C	350 mg	Manganese	2.5 mg
Folic Acid	400 mcg	Molybdenum	50 mg
Vitamin B1	10 mg	Inositol	10 mg
Vitamin B2	10 mg	PABA	10 mg
Niacinamide	40 mg	**Bioflavonoids**	10 mg
Vitamin B6	10 mg	Choline	10 mg
Vitamin B12	18 mcg	**L-Cysteine**	20 mg
Biotin	150 mcg	**L-Arginine**	5 mg
Pantothenic acid	20 mg		

*Antioxidants are bolded

Simone Calcium Formula		Simone Fiber Formula	
Calcium carbonate	1000 mg	Soluble Fiber	800 mg
Magnesium	280 mg	Pectin, Gums (Guar, oat)	
Potassium bicarbonate	200 mg	Mucilages (kelp, psyllium)	
Boron	4 mg	Insoluble Fiber	200 mg
L-Lysine	4 mg	**Simone Essential Fatty Acids**	
Silicon	4 mg	Linolenic Acid	2 to 8 grams
Threonine	4 mg	Linoleic Acid	3 to 9 grams

o Most nutrients should be taken with food. However, calcium and nutrients that enhance its metabolism should be taken at bedtime or on an empty stomach because most foods (fiber) will bind calcium and render it useless. Most supplements have calcium in the same tablet with the other nutrients, and, in effect, you get little or none of it when taken with food.

o Do not take supplements that contain iron because iron is associated with cancer promotion. There are many causes of anemia so unless you have a true iron deficiency anemia, there is no reason to take any supplemental iron, and this applies to menstruating women, too. If you do have a documented iron deficiency anemia you should be treated by a physician with therapeutic doses of iron in a thirty-day period. Patients who have a cancer and/or receive chemotherapy or radiation therapy usually have an anemia related to chronic disease and/or to therapy. No amount of iron will correct this anemia because it is not due to an iron deficiency.

- **ELIMINATE TABLE SALT.** Add only a minimal amount of salt while cooking. Most condiments, pickles, dressings, prepared sauces, canned vegetables, bouillon cubes, pot pies, popcorn, sauerkraut, and caviar have high amounts of salt in them.

- **AVOID FOOD ADDITIVES.** Avoid all foods containing nitrates, nitrites, or other harmful additives, or that were processed using a harmful technique (see Chapter 10). No pickled relish.

- **LIMIT SNACKS AND DESSERTS.** Healthy snacks or desserts include fresh fruit and canned fruit without added sugar, water ices, gelatin, and puddings made with skim milk. Do not eat commercially prepared cakes, pies, cookies, doughnuts, and mixes; coconut or coconut oil; frozen cream pies; potato chips and other deep-fried snacks; whole-milk puddings; ice cream; candy; chocolate; or gum with sugar.

- **BEVERAGES.** Distilled water, unsweetened fruit juices, and vegetable juices are great. Avoid caffeine-containing beverages – coffee, tea, cola, etc. Skim milk or non-fat products are OK – but remember dairy causes mucus production.

- **REMEMBER GOOD NUTRITION WHEN DINING OUT.** Call the restaurant to see if your needs as outlined here can be accommodated. Airlines and ocean liners will also help you. Request that your food be prepared without any salt products (Chinese food is high in sodium). Use lemon juice or vinegar on your salad.

- **TAKE 325 MG ASPIRIN EVERY OTHER DAY WITH FOOD IF YOU ARE ABLE.** Aspirin can decrease the risk of cardiovascular disease and also decrease the risk of cancer spread.

POINT 2. TOBACCO.

DO NOT SMOKE, CHEW, SNUFF, OR INHALE OTHER PEOPLE'S SMOKE. There is no easy, painless way to quit. The best way is simply to go "cold turkey" without tapering off or using any expensive smoke-ending courses. Remember, tobacco smoke also endangers the health of nonsmokers.   As a nonsmoker, demand that smokers not smoke in your presence, especially in public or work-related areas.

POINT 3. ALCOHOL and CAFFEINE.

AVOID ALL ALCOHOL, OR HAVE ONE DRINK OR LESS PER WEEK. AVOID CAFFEINE (COFFEE, TEA, CHOCOLATE).

POINT 4. RADIATION.

X-RAYS ONLY WHEN NEEDED. USE SUNSCREENS AND SUN-GLASSES. AVOID ELECTROMAGNETIC FIELDS from home appliances, office equipment, and outside electric fields.   All radiation is cumulative.

POINT 5. ENVIRONMENT.

KEEP AIR, WATER, AND WORKPLACE CLEAN, ESPECIALLY IN YOUR OWN HOUSEHOLD.   Avoid prolonged exposure to household cleaning fluids, solvents, and paint thinners. Some may be hazardous if inhaled in high concentrations. Pesticides, fungicides, and other home garden and lawn chemicals are also dangerous. Environmental protection standards should be rigorously observed. For instance, a person working with asbestos (insulation, brake lining, etc.) should wear a mask to protect the respiratory and gastrointestinal systems.

POINT 6. SEXUAL-SOCIAL FACTORS, HORMONES, DRUGS.

AVOID PROMISCUITY, HORMONES, AND ANY UNNECESSARY DRUGS.

POINT 7. LEARN THE SEVEN EARLY WARNING SIGNS

- Lump in breast
- Nonhealing sore
- Change in wart/mole
- Unusual bleeding
- Persistent cough/hoarseness
- Change in bowel/bladder habits
- Indigestion/trouble swallowing

POINT 8. EXERCISE

Brisk walking for 20 minutes four times a week or household chores, or weekend warrior activities are good forms of exercise. Exercise can enhance the immune system, decrease the risk of cancer, cardiovascular disease, and osteoporosis. Everyone should start a program of exercise, but see a physician before doing so if you are at risk for cardiovascular disease. Initially the exercising should start out slowly, then increase to a comfortable level. I stress fast walking because it is easier to do than other forms of exercise – no equipment to buy, no change of clothing, no one to rely on except yourself. You can walk in a shopping mall in inclement weather. Calisthenics should also be done to firm up abdominal-wall muscles and decrease that "spare tire." Five to ten sit-ups, with knees bent, can readily be done at home every day. Lower back pain is one of the most common pains in America. Simple stretching and flexing exercises will prevent and treat lower back pain.

Remember, the data show that some amount of exercise is better than none. Just a little exercise every day will benefit you enormously. Choose an exercise program that you are likely to follow, and stick with your exercise routine.

POINT 9. STRESS MODIFICATION, SPIRITUALITY, SEXUALITY

Stress is a risk factor for the development and promotion of prostate disease. To promote prostate health, you must modify your stress. Control stress by whatever means you can: meditation, self-hypnosis, spirituality, intimacy, or self-love, biofeedback, music, hot-water showers, or other methods you find relaxing. Stress is a killer! So find out what will help you relax.

Spirituality, or the Life Force, is what gives people hope and produces a calming and peaceful effect. Spirituality is often ignored by many people until they get into trouble with an illness or other aspects of life. Spirituality is comprised of many components. The scientific connection between the mind and body is inescapable. The mind has great control over the body and the immune system. So your attitude in dealing with any crisis is critical. Good spiritual attitude is important for good health and the proper functioning of the immune system. Having a good spiritual life is important for wellness and health. Lack of spirituality is a risk factor for illness. Remember the words of the Bible:

"Pleasant words are like a honeycomb, sweetness to the soul and health to the body" – Book of Proverbs (16:24)

"A man's spirit will endure sickness; but a broken spirit who can bear?" – Book of Proverbs (1.08:14)

Seek the psychological and emotional comfort of other people as well. Avoid loneliness.

Sexuality is also important. Re-read the section on Sexuality and Body Image. Do what makes you feel good; this will further relieve stress.

POINT 10. COMPREHENSIVE PHYSICAL EXAM.

CORRECT DIAGNOSIS IS IMPORTANT. PREVENTION IS THE KEY TO WELLNESS.

All men should have a comprehensive physical examination (combines a thorough history and a scalp-to-toe examination) with appropriate counseling and laboratory studies in order to prevent or detect early cancer or heart disease. If a physician is looking for early cancer and it is present, it then can probably be found.

A thorough history should include questions about all the risk factors for cancer listed in Chapter 3, as well as the questions at the end of this plan. The physical examination is important and should be complete, starting at the scalp and finishing at the toes. One capable, highly trained specialist should perform the entire examination, rather than your cardiologist checking the heart, your dentist looking in your mouth, and so on. The examining physician must be thorough in examining your prostate and breasts.

Laboratory tests are another part of an asymptomatic non-cancerous person's work-up. Little more than one ounce of blood and urine is taken and assayed. Table 3 lists the laboratory tests, the normal range of the tests, and the functions tested.

Table 3. Laboratory Tests for a Comprehensive Physical	
Laboratory Test	**Normal Range**
Stool for Occult Blood	Negative
Blood Counts: Hemoglobin	Female: 11.5-15 Male: 12.5-17
White Cell Count	3,700-10,500
Platelet Count	155,000-385,000
Cholesterol	130-200
Triglycerides	50-200
Glucose – blood sugar	65-115
Kidney Function: Creatinine	0.6-1.5
Blood Urea Nitrogen	5-25
Electrolytes: Calcium	8.5-10.8
Phosphate	2.4-4.5
Magnesium	1.3-2.1
Sodium	135-147
Chloride	96-109
Potassium	3.5-5.3
CO_2	23-33
Uric Acid	3.0-9.0
Liver Function : Total Protein	6.0-8.5
Albumin	3.5-5.5
Alkaline phosphatase	25-140
SGPT	0-45
SGOT	0-40
LDH	0-240
Total Bilirubin	0.1-1.2

Since prostate cancer patients have a higher incidence of colon cancer, testing the stool for trace amounts of blood is another important laboratory examination. Trace amounts of blood in the stool can result from some lesion(s) in the gastrointestinal tract, which can be a gastrointestinal cancer. Prior to and during the collection of the stool specimens, it is important to completely avoid red meat for three entire days, because red meat contains animal blood that will produce a positive result in the test. All other instructions must also be followed.

Certain fiberoptic procedures should be done when indicated. By using a fiberoptic laryngoscope, we have found many lesions of the nasopharynx and larynx when examining patients who have been exposed to passive smoke for several hours a day, patients who have been hoarse for two weeks or more, or other high-risk patients.

A colonoscopy is an examination of the colon with a fiberoptic flexible instrument, looking for abnormalities like lesions that may bleed. Indications for doing a fiberoptic colonoscopy:

1. To evaluate the colon when an abnormality was found with a barium enema.
2. To discover and excise polyps.
3. To evaluate unexplained bleeding: A positive occult blood stool test (detection of blood in the stool that could not be seen by the eye); Bleeding from the rectum.
4. To investigate an unexplained iron deficiency anemia.
5. To survey for colon cancer: A strong family history of colon cancer; To check the entire colon in a patient with a treatable cancer or polyp; A follow-up after resection of polyp or cancer at eighteen to thirty-six month intervals, depending on the clinical circumstances; In a patient with ulcerative colitis.
6. To investigate chronic inflammatory bowel disease.
7. To control bleeding.

An annual chest X-ray should be done in high-risk asymptomatic patients. If a cancer mass is found in the periphery of the lung, it can be surgically removed thereby affording the patient an excellent chance. A person's lung function can be readily assessed by pulmonary function testing – a series of tests that determine the quantity and speed of the air moving in and out of the lungs, the volumes of the lungs, etc.

You will feel better and stay well by following this
Simone Ten Point Plan

PROSTATE SURVEILLANCE: ASYMPTOMATIC MEN.
1. Digital Rectal Exam by Physician – all men at age 50.

SURVEILLANCE FOLLOW-UP: ASYMPTOMATIC PROSTATE CANCER PATIENTS (looking for recurrence or metastases)

Current Convention	Sufficient
Physical exam by physician	Physical exam by physician
First 2 years: every 3months	First 3 years: every 3-6 months
Years 2 to 4: every 4 months	Years 4 to 5: every 6-12 months
Years 5 to 6: every 6 months	6+ years: annually
6+ years: annually	
Laboratory tests	Laboratory tests – not needed
PSA, bone scan,	
liver function tests	

With these "routine" tests, an abnormality is found in less than 2 percent of all asymptomatic prostate cancer patients.

THE CANCER QUESTIONNAIRE below will help you work with your physician. If, after answering the questions, you find you have three or more of the possible "yes" answers in any one category, consult your physician.

CANCER QUESTIONNAIRE	NO	YES
General		
1. Have you been told by a doctor that you had cancer?	___	___
If yes, what kind?_____		
2. Have any of your blood relatives had cancer?	___	___
If yes, what kind?_____		
3. Have you lost 10-15 pounds over the past 6 months without knowing why?	___	___
Lungs		
4. Have you coughed up blood in the past several weeks?	___	___
5. Have you had a chronic cough daily?	___	___
6. Have you been told that you have emphysema?	___	___
7. Have you had pneumonia twice or more in the past year?	___	___
8. Have you ever smoked?	___	___
9. Did you quit smoking less than 15 years ago?	___	___
10. Do you smoke now?	___	___
Cigarettes: Number packs/day ___ Number of years___		

	NO	YES
Cigars Number cigars/day ___		
Pipe Number bowls/day ___		
11. Do you inhale others' smoke for one or more hours/day? ___	___	___

Larynx (voice box)

12. Have you had persistent hoarseness? ___ ___

Mouth and Throat

13. Have you had the following lasting more than 1 month?
      Pain or difficulty swallowing ___ ___
      Pain or tenderness in the mouth ___ ___
      A sore or white spot in your mouth ___ ___
14. Do you drink more than 4 oz of wine, 12 oz beer,
      or 1.5 oz whiskey every day? ___ ___

Stomach

15. Have you vomited blood in the past month? ___ ___
16. Have you had black stools in the past 6 months? ___ ___
      Does this happen when you are not taking iron? ___ ___
17. Have you had stomach pains several times a week? ___ ___
18. Has a doctor said that you had an ulcer or stomach polyps? ___ ___

Large Intestine and Rectum

19. Have you had a change in your usual bowel habits? ___ ___
20. Has your stool become narrow in diameter? ___ ___
21. Does this happen with every bowel movement? ___ ___
22. Have you had bleeding from the rectum? ___ ___
23. Have you had mucus in your stool every time? ___ ___
24. Have you been told that you have a polyp in the colon? ___ ___
25. Have you had ulcerative colitis? ___ ___

Breasts

26. Do you self-examine your breasts? ___ ___
27. Do you have a lump in either breast? ___ ___
28. Have you had breast pain recently? ___ ___
29. Has there been discharge or bleeding from your nipples,
      or have they begun to pull in (retract)? ___ ___
30. Are there any changes in the skin of your breasts? ___ ___
31. Have you ever had a breast biopsy? ___ ___

34. Have you ever had sexual intercourse? ___ ___
35. Did your mother take DES when pregnant with you? ___ ___

Skin

36. Has there been bleeding or change in a mole on you? ___ ___
37. Do you have a mole on your body where it may be
      irritated by underwear, a belt, etc? ___ ___
38. Do you have a sore that does not heal? ___ ___

	NO	YES
39. Do you have a severe scar from a burn?	___	___
40. Do you have fair skin and sunburn easily?	___	___
41. Do you sunbathe for hours or use a suntanning booth?	___	___
Thyroid		
42. Can you see or feel a lump in the lower front of your neck?	___	___
43. Have you had X-ray treatment to your face for acne, tonsil enlargement, or other reasons?	___	___
Kidney and Urinary Bladder		
44. Have you had blood in your urine?	___	___

CONCLUSION

The Cancer Questionnaire is only good if you take the time to answer the questions. Similarly, the points in my plan are only good if *you* follow them. The decision is yours.

Now after reading **The Truth About Prostate Health – Prostate Cancer** you already understand some of the ways in which you can attain prostate health, and reduce your risk for prostate cancer and risk of prostate cancer recurrence. Start by following the Ten-Point Plan presented here. And turn the page to find out what comes next.

27
Now What?

This may be the ending of my book, but it should be just a beginning for you. I hope the book has given you the information you need to understand what health is all about. Armed with this information, there are things you can and *should* do.

The responsibility for health does not lie with other people. It falls directly in your hands. It's up to you to do something. Start by taking care of yourself. Modify your lifestyle with your optimum health in mind. And if you should feel a lump, don't let fear immobilize you. See your health-care practitioner.

Next, take care of those close to you. Tell them to do something. If you want to take it one step further, join an organization or group. Work with others in support groups that aid and educate cancer patients and their families. Join with others to lobby against such cancer risks as second-hand smoke, air pollution, and toxic wastes. Anything can be accomplished if we work together.

Afterword

You have read quite a bit of information. But you should come away with a single important thought: **You have almost total control over the destiny of your health.** More and more people realize that by controlling risk factors – especially the major ones like nutrition, tobacco use, and alcohol consumption – you can control your well-being.

You now have the knowledge and the tools to modify your lifestyle to optimize your health and the health of your loved ones. You have the chance for a rendezvous with your well-being. Determine your own health's destiny. Seize this opportunity! Do it now!

For more information, please write to:

Charles B. Simone, M.D.
Simone Protective Cancer Institute
123 Franklin Corner Road • Lawrenceville, NJ 08648
609-896-2646
DrSimone.com

Books by Charles B. Simone, M.D.

- **Cancer and Nutrition** (1981, 1994, 2005)
- **The Truth About Breast Health – Breast Cancer,** *Prescription for Healing* (2002)
- **The Truth About Prostate Health – Prostate Cancer,** *Prevention and Cancer Life Extension* (2005)
- **How To Save Yourself From a Terrorist Attack** (2002)
- **KidStart**
- **Shark Cartilage and Cancer** (1994)

Medical and Scientific References

Introduction

1. Cancer statistics, 2004. *CA - Cancer J Clin.* 2004; 54:8-29.
2. Bailar J, E Smith. Progress against cancer? *NEJM.* 1986; 314:1226-32.
3. Boyd J, ed. NCAB approves year 2000 report. *The Cancer Letter.* 2000; 11(28):1-6.
4. Kolata G. Is the war on cancer being won? *Science* 1985; 29:543-44.
5. Boffey P. Cancer progress: Are the statistics telling the truth? *New York Times* Sept 18 1984; C1.
6. Bush H. Cancer cure. *Science.* 1984; 84:34-35.
7. Blonston G. Cancer prevention. *Science.* 1984; 84:36-39.
8. Marshall E. Experts clash over cancer data. *Science.* 1990;250:900-902.
9. Simone, CB. Cancer and Nutrition. McGraw-Hill.1983; revised 1995. Pages 1-237.
10. National Academy of Sciences, National Research Council, Food and Nutrition Board. 1989. *Diet and health: Implications for reducing chronic disease risk.* Washington, D.C.: National Academy Press.
11. The Surgeon General's Report on Nutrition and Health. 1988.
12. Butrum, et al. NCI dietary guidelines: Rationale. *Am J Clin Nutrition.* 1988; 48:888-95.
13. U.S. Bureau of Vital Statistics from 1900 to present.
14. *CA- A Cancer J for Clinicians.* 1962 – present.
15. Perception of cancer risks. *JNCI.* Sept 1,1993.

Chapter 1
The Scope of Cancer

Cancer statistics, 2004. *CA Cancer J Clin..* 2004; 54:8-29.

Chapter 2
Benign Prostate Syndrome, and Erectile Dysfunction

1. Barry, MJ, et al. 1992. The American Urological Association Symptom Index for benign prostatic hyperplasia. *J Urol* 148:1549-57.
2. Lepor H, Williford W, Barry M, et al. Efficacy of terazosin, finasteride, or both in benign prostatic hyperplasia. *NEJM.* 1996; 335:533-9.
3. Brown CT, Nuttall MC. Dutasteride: 5-alpha reductase inhibitor for lower urinary tract symptoms secondary to benign prostatic hyperplasia. *Int J Clin Pract.* 2003; 57: 705-9.
4. Wilt TJ, et al. Saw palmetto extracts for treatment of benign prostatic hyperplasia: A systematic review. *JAMA.* 1998; 280: 1604-1609.
5. Berges RR, et al. Randomized, placebo-controlled, double blind clinical trial of beta-sitosterol in patients with does not work by inhibiting 5 alpha reductase. *Lancet.* 1995; 345: 1529-1532.
6. Schuultz V, et al. *Rational Phytotherapy.* 3rd Ed, NY. Springer-Verlag; 1998; 232-233.
7. Andro MC, Riffaud JP. *Pygeum africanum* extract for the treatment of patients with benign prostatic hyperplasia: A review of 25 years of published experience. *Curr Ther Res.* 1995; 56: 796-817.
8. Preuss H. Use of natural products to treat BPH: emphasis on cernitin. *Original Internist.* 2000, June: 8-12.
9. Christensen, MM, et al. Transurethral resection versus transurethral incision of the prostate: a prospective randomized study. *Urol Clin North Am.* 1990; 17:621-30.
10. Dorflinger, T, et al. 1987. Transurethral prostatectomy or incision of the prostate in the treatment of prostatism caused by small benign prostates. *Scand J Urol Nephrol Suppl.* 1987; 104:77-81.
11. Oesterling, JE. Benign prostatic hyperplasia. *NEJM.* 1995; 332:99-109.
12. Kearse, WS, et al. 1993. The long-term risk of development of prostate cancer in patients with benign prostatic hyperplasia: correlation with stage A1 disease. *J Urol* 150: 1746-48.
13. Kapdi CC, Parekh. The male breast. *Radiol Clin North Am.* 1983; 21:137.
14. Nuttal FQ. Gynecomastia as a physical finding in normal men. *J Clin Endocrinol Metab.* 1979; 48:338.
15. Carlson HE. Current concepts: Gynecomastia. *NEJM.* 1980; 303:671.
16. Carlsen, B, et al. Evidence for decreasing quality of semen during the past 50 years. *BMJ.*1992; 305: 609-13.
17. Auger, J, et al. Decline in semen quality among fertile men in Paris during the past 20 years. *NEJM* 1995; 332: 281-85.
18. Irvine, DS. Falling sperm quality. *BMJ* 1994; 309: 476.
19. Colborn, T., et al. Chemically-induced alterations in sexual and functional development: the wildlife/human connection. 1992. Princeton: Princeton Scientific Publishing.
20. Ministry of Environment and Energy, Denmark. Male reproductive health and en-

vironmental chemicals with estrogenic effect. *Miljoprojekt nr* 290 1995. Copenhagen: Danish Environmental Protection Agency.

21. Leitzmann MF, Platz EA, et al. Ejaculation frequency and subsequent risk of prostate cancer. *JAMA*. 2004; 291:1578-1586.

22. Thompson IM, Goodman PJ, Tangen CM, et al. The influence of finasteride on the development of prostate cancer. *NEJM*. 2003; 349:215-224.

Chapter 3
An Overview of Risk Factors

1. The National Academy of Sciences. 1982. Nutrition, diet, and cancer.

2. Wynder EL, GB Gori. Contribution of the environment to cancer incidence: An epidemiologic exercise. *JNCI*. 1977; 58:825.

3. Workshop on Fat and Cancer. September Supplement to *Cancer Res*. 1981; 41(9):3677.

4. Mulvihill J. Genetic repertory of human neoplasia. In Genetics of human cancer. 1977 Ed. JJ Mulvihill, RW, Miller, and JF Fraumeni. New York: Raven Press, 137.

5. Armstrong B, R Doll. Environmental factors and cancer incidence and mortality in different countries, with special reference to dietary practices. *Intl J Cancer*. 1975; 15:617.

6. Bjarnason O, N Day, G Snaedal, Tilinuis. The effect of year of birth on the breast cancer age incidence curve in Iceland. *Intl J Cancer*. 1974; 13:689.

7. Miller AB. Nutrition and cancer. *Prev Med* 1980; 9:189.

8. Eskin BA. Iodine and mammary cancer. In: Inorganic and nutrition aspects of cancer, ed. G.H. Schrauzer. 1978; New York: Plenum Press, 293-304.

9. Upton AC. Future directions in cancer prevention. *Prev Med* 1980; 9:309.

10. Shank RC, GN Wogan, JB Gibson, et al. Dietary aflatoxins and human liver cancer.II. Aflatoxins in market foods and foodstuffs of Thailand and Hong Kong. *Food Cosmet Toxicol*. 1972; 10:61.

11. Tomatis L, C Agthe, H Bartsch, et al. Evaluation of the carcinogenicity of chemicals: A review of the monograph program of the International Agency for Research on Cancer. *Cancer Res*. 1982; 38:877.

12. Dargie H. Calcium channel blockers and the clinician. *Lancet*. 1996; 348:488.

13. Horton R. Do calcium antagonists cause cancer? *Lancet*. 1996; 348:49.

14. Correa A, Jackson L, Mohan A, et al. Use of hair dyes, hematopoietic neoplasms, and

lymphomas: A literature review. *Cancer Investigation*. 2000; 18(5): 467-479.

15. Wattenberg LW. Inhibitors of chemical carcinogenesis. *Adv Cancer Res* 1978; 26:197.

16. Pierce RC, M Katz. Dependency of polynuclear aromatic hydrocarbons on size distribution of atmospheric aerosols. *Environ Sci Technol* 1975; 9:347.

17. U.S. Environmental Protection Agency. Preliminary assessment of suspected carcinogens in drinking water. Report to Congress. Environmental Protection Agency, Washington, D.C.1975.

18. Harris RH, Page, Reiches. Carcinogenic hazards of organic chemicals in drinking water. In: Incidence of cancer in humans, ed. H.H. Hiatt, et al. Cold Spring Harbor Lab, 1977.

19. Dixon AK, Dendy P. Spiral CT: how much does radiation dose matter? *Lancet*. 1998; 352:1082-83.

20. deGonzalez A, Darby. Risk of cancer from diagnostic X-rays: estimates for the UK and 14 other countries. *Lancet*. 2004; 363:345-51.

21. Gardner MJ, et al. Results of case-control study of leukemia and lymphoma among young people near Sellafield nuclear plant in West Cumbria. *BMJ*. 1990; 300:423-29.

22. Wing S, et al. 1991. Mortality among workers at Oak Ridge National Laboratory: Evidence of radiation effects in follow-up through 1984. *JAMA*. 1991; 265:1397-1408.

23. Jablon S, et al. Cancer in people living near nuclear facilities. *JAMA*. 1991; 265:1403-8.

24. Mawson AR. Breast cancer in female flight attendants. *Lancet*. 1998; 352:626.

25. Gundestrup M, Storm HH. Radiation-induced acute myeloid leukaemia and other cancers in commercial jet cockpit crew: a population-based cohort study. *Lancet*. 1999; 354:2029-31.

26. Pukkala E, Aspholm R, Auvinen, et al. Cancer incidence among 10,211 airline pilots: a Nordic study. *Aviat Space Environ Med*. 2003;74:699-706

27. International Agency for Research on Cancer. 1980. Annual Report. World Health Organization. Lyon, France.

28. Miller, D.G. On the nature of susceptibility to cancer. *Cancer* 1980; 46:1307.

29. Walford, R.L. The immunological theory of aging. Munksgaard, Copenhagen, 1969.

30. Kahn, HA. The Dorn study of smoking and mortality among US veterans: Report on eight years of observation. In: Epidemiological study of cancer and other chronic diseases.

NCI Mono. 19. Washington, D.C. US Gov Printing Office. 1966.

31. Lichtenstein P, Holm N, et al. Environmental and heritable factors in the causation of cancer. *NEJM*. 2000; 343:78-85.

32. Weber GL, Garber JE. Family history and breast cancer: probabilities and possibilities. *JAMA;* 1993; 270:1602-1603.

33. Benditt EP, JM Benditt. Evidence for a monoclonal origin of human atherosclerotic plaques. *Proc Natl Acad Sci.* 1973; 70:1753.

34. Pero RW, C Bryngelsson, F Mitelman, et al. High blood pressure related to carcinogen induced unscheduled DNA synthesis, DNA carcinogen binding, and chromosomal aberrations in human lymphocytes. *Proc Natl Acad Sci* 1976; 73:2496.32.

35. de Waard F, EA Banders-van Halewijn, J Huizinga. 1964. The bimodal age distribution of patients with mammary cancer. *Cancer.* 1964; 17:141

36. Dyer AR, J Stamler, AM Berkson, et al. High blood pressure: A risk factor for cancer mortality. *Lancet.* 1975; i:1051.

37. Cotton T, et al. Breast cancer in mothers prescribed DES in pregnancy. *JAMA.* 1993; 269(16):2096-2100.

38. Wobbes T, Koops, Oldhoff. The relation between testicular tumors, undescended testes, and inguinal hernias. *J Surg Onc.* 1980; 14:45

39. IARC monographs on the evaluation of carcinogenic risks to humans 1994-1999. Geneva: WHO Publications.

40. Sharp DW. Gastric cancer: A new role for *Helicobacter pylori Science Watch.* 1993; 4:5.

41. Hjalgrim H, Askling J, Rostgaard K, et al. Characteristics of Hodgkin's lymphoma after infectious mononucleosis. *NEJM* 2003; 349:1324-1332.

42. Vilchez R, Madden C, Kozinetz C, et al. Association between simian virus 40 and non-Hodgkin lymphoma. *Lancet* 2002; 359:817-823.

43. Brooks J, Rud E, Pilon R, et al. Cross-species retroviral transmission from macaques to human beings. *Lancet* 2002: 360:387-388.

44. Diringer H. Proposed link between transmissible spongiform encephalopathies of man and animals. *Lancet.* 1995; 346:1208-10.

Chapter 4
Nutrition, Immunity, and Cancer

1. Cannon PR. Antibodies and protein reserves. *J Immunol.* 1942; 44:107.

2. Chandra R. Nutrition and immunology. New York: Alan R. Liss, Inc. Press. 1989; 3.

3. Rous P. The influence of diet on transplanted and spontaneous mouse tumors. *J Exp Med.* 1914; 20:433.4.

4. Tannenbaum A. The initiation and growth of tumors. Introduction I. Effects of underfeeding. *Am J Cancer.* 1940; 38:335.

5. Simone CB, Henkart. Permeability changes induced in erythrocyte ghost targets by antibody-dependent cytotoxic effector cells: Evidence for membrane pores. *J Immunol.* 1980; 124:954.

6. Burnet FM. Immunological surveillance. Oxford: Pergamon Press.1970.

7. Kersey JH, Spector, and R.A. Good. Primary immunodeficiency diseases and cancer: The immunodeficiency-cancer registry. *Intl J Cancer.* 1973; 12:333.

8. Spector G, Perry III, Good RA, Kersey. Immunodeficiency diseases and malignancy. The immunopathology of lymphoreticular neoplasms. 1978. ed. JJ Twomey, and RA Good. New York: Plenum Publishing, 203.

9. Penn. Malignant tumors in organ transplant recipients. New York: Springer-Verlag.

10. Birkeland SA, Kemp E, Hauge M. Renal transplantation and cancer. The Scandia transplant material. *Tissue Antigens.* 1975; 6:28.

11. Chandra R. Nutrition and immunology.

12. Delafuente, Panush. Potential of drug-related immunoenhancement of the geriatric patient. *Geriatric Med* 1990; 9:32-40.

13. Jeevan A, Kripke. Ozone depletion and the immune system. *Lancet.* 1993; 342:1159-1160.

14. Cooper KD, et al. UV exposure reduces immunization rate and promotes tolerance to epicutaneous antigens in humans. *Proc Natl Acad Sci.* 1992; 89:8497-8501.

15. Peters E, et al. Vitamin C supplementation reduces post-race symptoms of upper respiratory tract infection in ultramarathon runners. *Am J Clin Nutr.* 1993; 57:170-171.

16. Heath GW. Exercise and incidence of upper respiratory tract infections. *Med Sci Sports Exerc.* 1991; 23:152-157.

17. Aschekenasy A. Dietary protein and amino acids in leucopoiesis. *World Rev Nutri Diet.* 1975; 21:152.

18. Jose DG, Good RA. Absence of enhancing antibody in cell-mediated immunity to tumor homografts in protein deficient rats. *Nature.* 1971; 231:807.

19. Passwell JH, Steward, Soothill. The effects of protein malnutrition on macrophage function and the amount and affinity of antibody response. *Clin Exp Immunol.* 1974; 17:491.

20. Van Oss CJ. Influence of glucose levels on the *in vitro* phagocytosis of bacteria by human neutrophils. *Infect Immunol.* 1971; 4:54.

21. Perille PE, Nolan, Finch. Studies of the resistance to infection in diabetes mellitus: Lo-

cal exudative cellular response. *J Lab Clin Med.* 1972; 59:1008.

22. Bagdade JD, Root, Bulger. Impaired leukocyte function in patients with poorly controlled diabetes. *Diabetes.* 1974; 23:9.

23. Stuart AE, Davidson. Effect of simple lipids on antibody formation after ingestion of foreign red cells. *J Pathol Bacteriol.* 1976; 87:305.

24. Santiago-Delpin E, Szepsenwol. Prolonged survival of skin and tumor allografts in mice on high fat diets. *JNCI.* 1977; 59:459.

25. DiLuzio N, Wooles. Depression of phagocytic activity and immune response by methyl palmitate. *Am J Physiol.* 1964; 206:939.

Chapter 5
Antioxidants and Other Cancer-Fighting Nutrients

1. Pietrzik, K. Concept of borderline vitamin deficiencies. *Int J Vit Nutr Res* 1985; 27:61-73.

2. Brin M. Dilemma of marginal vitamin deficiency. *Proc 9th Int Cong Nutrition,* Mexico 1972; 4:102-115.

3. Werback MR. Marginal nutrient deficiencies. In: Textbook of Nutritional Medicine. Third Line Press. Tarzana, CA. 1999; Pp:32-41.

4. US Depart of HEW. HANES: Health and Nutrition Examination Survey 1994. Rockville, MD.

5. Baker H, Frank O. Sub-clinical vitamin deficits in various age groups. *Int J Vit Nutr Res.* 1985; 27:47-59.

6. US Dept. of Agriculture, Human Nutrition Information Service, 1985. Continuing Survey of Food Intakes by Individuals. CSFII Report No. 85-4.

7. Popkin B, Siega-Riz A, Haines P. A comparison of dietary trends among racial and socioeconomic groups in the US. *NEJM.* 1996; 335:716-20.

8. Ideas for better eating. Menus and recipes to make use of the dietary guidelines. Sci and Ed Admin/Human Nutrition. U.S. Dept. of Agriculture January 1981.

9. Dietary intake source data: US 1976-80. National Health Survey: 11, No. 231, DHHS Pub (PHS) 83-1681.March '83.

10. US Dept. of Agriculture. Nationwide Food Survey. 1980

11. Kant, et al. National Health and Nutrient Examination Survey II. *JADA.* 1991; 91:1526-32.

12. Pao E, Mickle. 1981. Problem nutrients in the United States. *Food Technology* September.

13. Krehl WA. The role of nutrition in preventing disease. Davidson Conference USC School of Dentistry. Feb. 29, 1981

14. Roe D. Drug-induced nutritional deficiencies. 1976.Connecticut: The AVI Publishing, Co.

15. Lieber C. Alcohol and malnutrition in the pathogenesis of liver disease and nutrition. VA Hospital. Mt. Sinai School of Medicine. New York, Bronx, NY. Sept.1975.

16. Baker H, Frank, Zetterman, et al. Inability of chronic alcoholics with liver disease to use food as a source of folates, thiamine and vitamin B6. *Amer J Clin Nutr* 1975; 28:1377-80.

17. Payne I, Lu G, Meyer K. Relationships of dietary tryptophan and niacin to tryptophan metabolism in alcoholics and non-alcoholics. *Am J Clin Nutr* 1974; 27:572-579.

18. Lumeng L, Li TK. Vitamin B6 metabolism in chronic alcohol abuse. *J Clin Invest.* 1974; 53:57-61.

19. Lieber C, Baraona, Leo, and Garro A. Metabolism and metabolic effects of ethanol, including interaction with drugs, carcinogens and nutrition. *Mutat Res* 1987;186:201-233.

20. Halsted C, Heise C. Ethanol and vitamin metabolism. *Pharmac Ther.* 1987; 34:453-64.

21. Aoki K, Ito Y, Sasaki, et al. Smoking, alcohol drinking and serum carotenoids levels. *Jpn J Cancer Res Gann.* 1987; 78:1049-56.

22. Fazio V, Flint D, Wahlqvist M. Acute effects of alcohol on plasma ascorbic acid in healthy subjects. *Am J Clin Nutr.* 1981; 34:2394-96.

23. Pelletier O. Vitamin C and cigarette smokers. *Ann NY Acad Sci.* 1975; 258:156-166.

24. US Department of Health, Education and Welfare. The health consequences of smoking. January 1973.

25. Hornig D, Glatthaar B. Vitamin C and smoking: Increased requirement of smokers. *Int J Vit Nutr Res.*1985; 27:139-155.

26. Menkes M, Constock G, Vuilleumier J, et al. Vitamin C is lower in smokers. *NEJM.* 1986; 315:1250-4.

27. Chow C, Thacker R, Changchit C, et al. Lower levels of vitamin C and carotenes in plasma of cigarette smokers. *J Am Coll Nutr.* 1986; 5:305-312.

28. Witter F, Blake D, Baumgardner R, et al. Folate, carotene, and smoking. *Am J Obstet Gynecol.* 1982; 144:857.

29. Gerster H. Beta-carotene and smoking. *J Nutr Growth Cancer.* 1987; 4:45-49.

30. Pacht E, Kaseki H, Mohammed J, et al. Deficiency of vitamin E in the alveolar fluid of cigarette smokers. *J Clin Invest* 1986; 77:789-96.

31. Serfontein W, Ubbink J, DeVilliers J, and Becker. Depressed plasma pyridoxal-5'-

phosphate levels in tobacco-smoking men. *Atherosclerosis.* 1986; 59:341-346.

32.   Who's dieting and why. 1978. A.C. Nielsen Co.

33.   Welsh S, Marston R. Review of trends in food used in the United States, 1909 to 1980. *J A Dietetic Assn.* 1982; August.

34.   Kasper H. Vitamins in prevention and therapy: Recent findings in vitamin research. *Fortschritte der Medizin* 1964; 82:22.

35.   Horo E, Brin M, Faloon W. Fasting in obesity: Thiamine depletion as measured by erythrocyte activity changes. *Arch Int Med.* 1983; 117:175-81.

36.   Fisher M, Lachance P. Nutrition evaluation of published weight-reducing diets. *J Am Diet Assoc.*1985; 85:450-454.

37.   Leevy C, Cardi L, Frank O, et al. Incidence and significance of hypovitaminemia in a randomly selected municipal hospital population. *Am J Clin Nutr* 1965;17: 259.

38.   Bristrian, Bruce, et al. Prevalence of malnutrition in general medical patients. *JAMA.* 1976; 235:15-18.

39.   Lemoine, et al. Vitamin B1, B2, B6 and status in hospital inpatients. *Am J Clin Nutr.* 1980; Dec 33-37.

40.   Driezen S. Nutrition and the immune response – a review. *Internat J Vit Nur Res.* 1979; 49.

41.   Beisel, et al. Single-nutrient effects on immunologic functions. JAMA. 1981; 245.

42.   Pollack SV. Nutritional factors affecting wound healing. *J Dermatol Surg Oncol.* 1979; 5:8.

43.   Kaminsky M, Windborn A.1978. Nutritional assessment guide. Midwest Nutrition, Ed and Res Foundation, Inc.

44.   Nationwide Food Consumption Survey, Spring 1980. U.S. Dept of Agriculture, Science and Education Administration, Beltsville, MD.

45.   Dietary intake source data. United States 1976-80.

46.   Kirsch A, Bidlack W. Nutrition and the elderly: Vitamin status and efficacy of supplementation. *Nutr* 1987; 3:305-314.

47.   Baker H, Jaslow S, Frank O. Severe impairment of dietary folate utilization in the elderly. *J Am Geriatrics Soc.* 1978; 26:218-221.

48.   First Health and Nutrition Examination Survey. 1971. U.S. Public Health Service. Vol. 72.

49.   Connelly TJ, Becker A, McDonald J. Bachelor scurvy. *Intl J Dermatol.* 1982; 21:209-211.

50.   Schorah CJ. Inapproprate vitamin C reserves: Their frequency and significance in an urban population. In: The importance of vitamins to health. Ed. T.G. Taylor. 1978. Lancaster, England: MTP Press, 61-72.

51.   Garry PJ, Goodwin J, Hunt, et al. Nutritional status in a healthy elderly population: Dietary and supplemental intakes. *Am J Clin Nutr.* 1982; 36:319-331.

52.   Roe DA. Drug-Induced Nutritional Deficiencies, 2nd ed. 1985. Westport, CT: AVI Publishing Co. 1-87.

53.   Brin, M. Drugs and environmental chemicals in relation to vitamin needs. In: Nutrition and Drug Interrelations. 1978. Ed. JN Hathcock and J. Coon. NY: Academic Press, 131-50.

54.   Driskell JA, Geders J, Urban M. Vitamin B6 status of young men, women, and women using oral contraceptives. *J Lab Clin Med* 1976; 87:813-821.

55.   Prasad A, Lei K, Oberleas, et al.Effect of oral contraceptive agents on nutrients. *Am J Clin Nutr* 1975; 28:385-91.

56.   Rivers JM, Devine M. Plasma ascorbic acid concentrations and oral contraceptives. *Am J Clin Nutr.*1972; 25:684-89.

57.   Truswell AS. Drugs affecting nutritional state. *Br Med J.* 1985; 291:1333-37.

58.   Clark A, Mossholder, Gates R. Folacin status in adolescent females. *Am J Clin Nutr.* 1987; 46:302-306.

59.   Sumner SK, Liebman M, Wakefield. Vitamin A status of adolescent girls. *Nutr Rep Intl.* 1987; 35:423-431.

60.   Saito N, Kimura M, Kuchiba, Itokawa. Blood thiamine levels in outpatients with diabetes mellitus. J Nutr Sci Vitaminol. 1987; 33:421-430.

61.   Mooradian AD, Morley J. Micronutrient status in diabetes mellitus. *Am J Clin Nutr.* 1987; 45:877-895.

62.   Vobecky JS, Vobecky J. Vitamin status of women during pregnancy. In: Vitamins and minerals in pregnancy and lactation. Ed. H. Berger. Nestle Nutrition Workshop Series, Vol. 16. NY: Vevey/Raven Press, Ltd., 1988; 109-111.

63.   Peterkin BB, Kerr R, Hama M. Nutritional adequacy of diets of low-income households. *J Nut Ed.* 1987;14(3):102.

64.   Shenai JP, Chytil F, Jhaveri, Stahlman. Plasma vitamin A and retinol-binding protein in premature and term neonates. *J Pediatr.* 1981; 99:302-305.

65.   Heinonen K, Mononen I, Mononen T, et al. Plasma vitamin C levels are low in premature infants fed human milk. *Am J Clin Nutr.* 1986; 43:923-924.

66. Vitamin E status of premature infants. *Nutr Rev.* 1986; 44:166-167.

67. Dietary intake source data. United States 1976-80.

68. First Health and Nutrition Examination Survey. U.S. Public Health Service.

69. Schoenthaler SJ, Bier ID. Vitamin-mineral intake and intelligence: A macrolevel analysis of randomized controlled trials. *J Alternative Complementary Med: Research on Paradigm, Practice, Policy.* 1999; 5:125-134.

70. Schoenthaler SJ, Bier ID. The effect of vitamin-mineral supplementation on the intelligence of American school children in grades one to six: A randomized double-blind placebo-controlled trial. *J Alternative Complementary Med: Research on Paradigm, Practice, Policy.* 1999; 6:19-30.

71. Eysenck HJ Schoenthaler SJ. Raising IQ level by vitamin mineral supplementation. In: Sternberg R, Grigorenko E, eds. *Intelligence, Heredity and Environment.* Cambridge, UK. Cambridge Univ Press. 1997; 363-392.

72. Schoenthaler SJ, Bier ID. The impact of enhancing nutrition using vitamin-mineral tablets on academic performance among school children: A randomized double-blind placebo-controlled trial. Paper submitted

73. Schoenthaler SJ, Doraz WE, Wakefield. The impact of a low food additive and sucrose diet on academic performance in 803 New York City public schools. *Intl J Biosocial Res.* 1986; 8:185-195.

74. Schoenthaler SJ, Amos SP, Doraz WE, et al. Controlled trial of vitamin mineral supplementation on intelligence and brain function. *Personality Individual Differences.* 1991; 112:343-350.

75. Benton and Roberts. Effect of vitamin and mineral supplementation on intelligence of a sample of school children. *Lancet.* 1988; Jan.:140-144.

76. Campbell, et al. Vitamins, minerals, and I.Q. *Lancet.* 1988; Sept:744-745.

77. Letter to the Editor. Vitamin/mineral supplementation and non-verbal intelligence. *Lancet.* 1988; Feb:407-409.

78. Grantham-McGregor SM, et al. Nutritional supplementation, psychosocial stimulation, and mental development of stunted children: The Jamaican study. *Lancet.* 1991; 338:1-5.

79. Brown, et al. J Pediatrics. 1972; 81:714.

80. Webb and Oski. Iron deficiency and IQ. *J Pediatr.* 1973; 82:827-30.

81. Benton, et al. Glucose improves attention and reaction. Biol Psychol. 1972; 24:95-100.

82. Benton. Influence of vitamin C on psychological testing. *Psychopharmacology.* 1982; 75:98-99.

83. Pfeiffer C, Braverman E. Zinc, the brain and behavior. *Biol Psychiat.* 1982; 17:513-31.

84. Godfrey P, et al. Enhancement of recovery from psychiatric illness by methylfolate. *Lancet.* 1990; 336:392-394.

85. Schoenthaler SJ, Bier ID. The effect of vitamin-mineral supplementation on juvenile delinquency among American school children: A randomized double-blind placebo-controlled trial. *J Alternative Complementary Med: Research on Paradigm, Practice, Policy.* 2000; 6:7-18.

86. Schoenthaler SJ, Amos SP, Hudes. A randomized trial of the effect of vitamin mineral supplementation on serious institutional rule violations. Submitted 2001.

87. Schoenthaler SJ, Bier ID. The effect of randomized vitamin-mineral supplementation on violent and non-violent antisocial behavior among incarcerated juveniles. *J Nutr Environmental Med.* 1997; 7:343-352.

88. Schoenthaler SJ. Diet and crime: An empirical examinatin of the value of nutrition in the control and treatment of incarcerated juvenile offenders. *Intl J Biosocial Res.* 1983; 1:25-39.

89. Schoenthaler SJ. Diet and delinquency: A multi state replication. *Intl J Biosocial Res.* 1983; 5:70-78.

90. Schoenthaler SJ. Diet and delinquency: Empirical testing of seven theories. *Intl J Biosocial Res.* 1986; 7:108-131.

91. Nazrul Islam SK, Jahangir Hossain K, Ahsan M. Serum vitamin E, C, and A status of the drug addict undergoing detoxification: influence of drug habits, sexual practice and lifestyle factors. *Eur J Clin Nutr.* 2001; 55:1022-7.

92. *Vitamin C in Health and Disease.* Packer L, Fuchs J, Eds. 1997. Marcel Dekker, Inc. New York.

93. *Natural Antioxidants in Human Health and Disease.* Frei B, Ed. 1994. Academic Press, San Diego, CA..

94. *Vitamin E in Health and Disease.* Packer L, Fuchs J, Eds. 1993. Marcel Dekker, Inc. New York.

95. *Beyond Deficiency: New Views on the Function and Health Effects of Vitamins.* Sauberlich HE, Machlin LJ, Eds. 1992. New York Academy of Sciences, New York, NY.

96. Newberne PM, Locniskar M. Roles of micronutrients in cancer prevention: recent evidence from the laboratory. *Prog Clin Biol Res.* 1990; 346: 119-134.

97.   Beckman KB, Ames BN.   Oxidative decay of DNA. *J Biol Chem.* 1997; 272:19633-36.

98.   Ames BN, Shigenaga MK, Park EM. DNA damage by endogenous oxidants as a cause of aging and cancer. In: *Oxidative Damage and Re-pair: Chemical, Biological, and Medical Aspects.* Davies KJA, Ed.   1991. pp 181-187. Perga-mon Press, NY.

99.   *Oncology Overview: Free Radicals and Peroxides in the Etiology of Cancer.* Pryor WA and National Cancer Institute, Eds.   1987. Government Printing Office, Washington, DC.

100.   *Free Radicals in Biology and Medicine.   Third Edition.* Halliwell B, Gutteridge JM, Eds. 1999; Oxford University Press. Oxford.

101.   Kaul A, Khanduja KL. Polyphenols inhibit promotional phase of tumorigenesis: Rele-vance of superoxide radicals. *Nutr Cancer.* 1998; 32:81-85.

102.   Cerutti P. Oxy-radicals and cancer. *Lancet.* 1994; 344:862-3.

103.   Cerutti PA, Ghosh R, et al. The role of the cellular antioxidant defense in oxidant car-cinogenesis.   *Environ Health Perspect.* 1994; 102:123-30.

104.   Marnett LJ. Peroxyl free radicals: potential mediators of tumor initiation and promotion. *Carcinogenesis.* 1987; 8:1365-73.

105.   Shigenaga MK, Park JW, et al. *In vivo* oxi-dative DNA damage: measurement of 8-hydroxy-2-deoxyguanosine in DNA and urine by high-performance liquid chromatography with electrochemical detection. *Methods Enzy-mol.* 1990; 186:521-30.

106.   Ames BN. Dietary carcinogens and anti-carcinogens. *Science.* 1983; 221:1256-64.

107.   Cooney RV, Kappock TJ et al. Solubiliza-tion, cellular uptake, and activity of beta-carotene and other carotenoids as inhibitors of neoplastic transformation in cultured cells. *Methods Enzymol.* 1996; 214: 55-68.

108.   *Antimutagenesis and Anticarcinogenesis Mecha-nisms II.* Kuroda Y, et al. Eds. 1990. Plenum Press. New York.

109.   Block G, Schwarz R.   Ascorbic acid and cancer: animal and cell culture data. In: *Natu-ral Antioxidants in Human Health and Disease.* Frei B, Ed.   1994; pp129-155.   Academic Press, San Diego, CA.

110.   Block G. The data support a role for anti-oxidants in reducing cancer risk. *Nutr Rev.* 1992; 50:207-213.

111.   Krinsky NI. Carotenoids and cancer: basic research studies. In: *Natural Antioxidants in Human Health and Disease.*   Frei B, Ed.   1994; pp239-261. Academic Press, San Diego, CA.

112.   Onogi N, Okuno M, et al. Antiproliferative effect of carotenoids on human colon cancer cells without conversion to retinoic acid. *Nu-trition and Cancer.* 1998; 32: 20-24.

113.   Rock CL, Flatt SW, Wright, et al. Respon-siveness of serum carotenoids to a high-vegetable diet intervention designed to pre-vent breast cancer recurrence.   *Cancer Epid Biomarkers Prev.* 1997; 6: 617-23.

114.   Menkes MS, Comstock GW, et al.   Serum beta-carotene, vitamins A and E, selenium and the risk of lung cancer.   *NEJM.* 1986; 315:1250-54.

115.   Wattenberg LW. Inhibition of carcinogene-sis by minor nutrient constituents of the diet. *Proc Nutr Soc.* 1990; 49:173-83.

116.   Knekt P. Vitamin E and cancer prevention. In: *Natural Antioxidants in Human Health and Disease.*   Frei B, Ed.   1994; pp199-238.   Aca-demic Press, San Diego, CA.

117.   Fontham ETH. Vitamin C, vitamin C rich foods, and cancer: epidemiologic studies. In: *Natural Antioxidants in Human Health and Dis-ease.* Frei B, Ed.   1994; pp 157-197. Academic Press, San Diego, CA.

118.   Patterson RE, White E, Kristal AR, et al. Vitamin supplementation and cancer risk: the epidemiological evidence. *Cancer Causes Control.* 1997; 8: 786-802.

119.   Bostick RM, Potter JD, et al. Reduced risk of colon cancer with high intakes of vitamin E: the Iowa women's health study. *Cancer Res.* 1993; 53:4230-37.

120.   Hunter DJ, et al. 1993. A prospective study of the intake of vitamins C, E, A and the risk of breast cancer. *NEJM.* 1993; 329:234-240.

121.   Ennever FK, Pasket. 1993. Vitamins and breast cancer. *NEJM.* 1993; 329:1579-1580.

122.   Jumann A, Holmberg L, et al. Carotene intake and the risk of postmenopausal breast cancer. *Epidemiology.* 1999; 10:49-53.

123.   Bohlke K, Spiegelman D, et al. Vitamins A, C, and E and the risk of breast cancer. *Br J Cancer.* 1999; 79:23-29.

124.   Verhoeven DTH, Asses N, et al. Vitamin C and E, retinal, carotene, and dietary fibre in relation to breast cancer risk. *Br J Cancer.* 1997; 75: 149-55.

125.   Negri E, LaVecchio C, et al. Intake of selected micronutrients and the risk of breast cancer. *Int J Cancer.* 1996; 65: 140-44.

126.   Punnonen R, et al. Activities of antioxidant enzymes and lipid peroxidation in endometrial cancer. *Eur J Cancer.* 1993; 29:266-269.

127.   Palan PR, et al. Beta-carotene levels in exfoliated cervical vaginal epithelial cells in cervical intra-epithelial neoplasia and cervical

cancer. *Am J Obstet-Gynecol.* 1992; 167:1899-1903.

128. Gridley G, et al. Vitamin supplement use and reduced risk of oral and pharyngeal cancer. *Am J Epidemiol.* 1992; 135:1083-092.

129. Zheng W, et al. Serum micronutrients and subsequent risk of oral and pharyngeal cancer. *Cancer Res.* 1993; 53:795-98.

130. Barone J, et al. Vitamin supplement use and risk for oral and esophageal cancer. *Nutr Cancer.* 1992; 18(1):31-41.

131. Shibata A, et al. Intake of vegetables, fruits, beta-carotene, vitamin C, and vitamin supplements and cancer incidence among the elderly: A prospective study. *Br J Cancer.* 1992; 66:673-679.

132. LeMarchand L, et al. Intake of specific carotenoids and lung cancer risk. *Cancer Epidemiol Biomarkers Prevent.* 1993; 2:183-187.

133. Knekt P, et al. Dietary antioxidants and the risk of lung cancer. *Am J Epidemiol.* 1991; 134(5): 471-479.

134. Stahelin HB, et al. Plasma antioxidant vitamins and subsequent cancer mortality in the 12-year follow up of the prospective Basel Study. *Am J Epidemiol.* 1994; 133(8):766-775.

135. Comstock GW, Alberg AJ, et al. The risk of developing lung cancer associated with antioxidants in the blood: Ascorbic acid, carotenoids, tocopherol, selenium, and total peroxyl radical absorbing capacity. *Cancer Epidemiol Biomarkers Prev.* 1997; 6: 907-16.

136. Prestin-Martin S, Pogoda JM, et al. Prenatal vitamin supplementation and risk of childhood brain tumors. *Int J Cancer.*1998; 11:17-22.

137. Eichholzer M, Stahelin HB, et al. Prediction of male cancer mortality by plasma levels of interacting vitamins: 17 year follow-up of the prospective Basel study. *Int J Cancer.* 1996; 66:145-50.

138. Gann PH, Ma J, et al. Lower prostate cancer risk in men with elevated plasma lycopene levels: results of a prospective analysis. *Cancer Res.* 1999; 59:1225-30.

139. Maramag C, Menon M, et al. Effect of vitamin C on prostate cancer cells *in vitro.* The *Prostate.* 1997; 32:188-95.

140. Chen J, et al. Antioxidant status and cancer mortality in China. *Int J Epidemiol.* 1992; 21(4):625-635.

141. Blot WJ, et al. Nutrition intervention trials in Linxian, China: Supplementation with specific vitamin-mineral combinations, cancer incidence, and disease specific mortality in the general population. *JNCI.* 1993; 85(18):1483-1492.

142. Smigel K. Dietary supplements reduce cancer deaths in China. *JNCI.* 1993; 85(18):1448-1450.

143. Jaakkola, et al. Treatment with antioxidant and other nutrients in combination with chemotherapy and irradiation therapy in patients with small cell lung cancer. *Anticancer Research.* 1992; 12(3):599-606.

144. Li JY, et al. Nutrition intervention trials in Linxian, China: Multiple vitamin and mineral supplementation, cancer incidence, and disease-specific mortality among adults with esophageal dysplasia. *JNCI.* 1993; 85:1492-1498.

145. Lippman S, et al. Comparison of low dose isotretinoin with beta-carotene to prevent oral carcinogenesis. *NEJM.* 1993; 328:15-20.

146. Toma S, et al. GI Treatment of oral leukoplakia with beta-carotene. *Oncology.* 1992; 49:77-81.

147. Benner S, et al. Regression of oral leukoplakia with alpha-tocopherol. *JNCI.* 1993; 85:44-47.

148. Benner and Hong. Clinical chemoprevention: developing a cancer prevention strategy. *JNCI.* 1993; 85:1446-47.

149. Paganelli, et al. Effect of vitamin A, C, and E supplementation on rectal cell proliferation in patients with colorectal adenomas. *JNCI.* 1992; 84:47-51.

150. Riemersma, et al. Risk of angina pectoris and concentrations of vitamins A, C, E, and carotene. *Lancet.* 1991; 337:1-5.

151. Fairburn K, et al. Alpha-Tocopherol, lipids, and lipoproteins in knee joint fluid and serum from patients with inflammatory joint disease. *Clinical Science.* 1992; 83:657-664.

152. Scheen AJ. Antioxidant vitamins in the prevention of cardiovascular diseases. First part: epidemiologic studies. *Rev Med Liege* 2000;55:11-8.

153. Scheen AJ. Antioxidant vitamins in the prevention of cardiovascular diseases. 2nd part: results of clinical trials. *Rev Med Liege* 2000;55:105-9.

154. Boaz M, Smetana S, et al. Secondary prevention with antioxidants of cardiovascular disease in endstage renal disease (SPACE): randomized trial. *Lancet.* 2000; 356:1213-18.

155. Giugliano D. Dietary antioxidants for cardiovascular prevention. *Nutr Metab Cardiovasc Dis* 2000;10:38-44

156. Marchioli R, Negri M, et al. Antioxidant vitamins and prevention of cardiovascular disease: laboratory, epidemiological and clinical trial data. *Pharmacol Res* 1999; 40:227-38.

157. Nappo F, et al. Impairment of endothelial function by hyperhomocystein and reversal by antioxidants. *JAMA*. 1999; 281:2113-18.

158. Monnier L , Avignon A , Colette C , Piperno M. Primary nutritional and drug prevention of atherosclerosis. *Rev Med Interne* 1999; 3:360-370.

159. Faggiotto A, Paoletti R. State-of-the-Art lecture. Statins and blockers of the renin-angiotensin system: vascular protection beyond their primary mode of action. *Hypertension* 1999; 34:987-96.

160. Yla-Herttuala S. Oxidized LDL and atherogenesis. *Ann N Y Acad Sci* 1999; 874:134-7.

161. Carrasquedo F, Glanc M, Fraga C. Tissue damage in acute myocardial infarction: selective protection by vitamin E. *Free Radic Biol Med* 1999; 26:1587-90.

162. Navarro-Alarcon M, Serrana H, et al. Serum and urine selenium concentrations in patients with cardiovascular diseases and relationship to other nutritional indexes. *Ann Nutr Metab* 1999;43:30-6.

163. Stamper M, et al. Vitamin E consumption and the risk of coronary disease in women. *NEJM* 1993; 328:1444-49.

164. Rimm E, et al. Vitamin E consumption and the risk of coronary heart disease in men. *NEJM*. 1993; 328:1450-56.

165. Steinberg D. Antioxidant vitamins and coronary heart disease. *NEJM*. 1993; 328:1487-1489.

166. Dieber-Rotheneder, et al. Effect of oral supplementation with D-alpha-tocopherol on the vitamin E content of human low-density lipoproteins and its oxidation resistance. *J Lipid Res*. 1991; 32:1325-32.

167. Graziano, et al. Beta-carotene therapy for chronic stable angina. *Circulation*. 1990; 82:201.

168. Gey, et al. Plasma levels of antioxidant vitamins in relation to ischemic heart disease and cancer. *Am J Clin Nutr*. 1987; 45:1368-77.

169. Gey, et al. Poor plasma status of carotene and vitamin C is associated with higher mortality from ischemic heart disease and stroke: Basel Study. *Clin Investig*. 1993; 71:3-6.

170. Mialal and Grundy. Effect of dietary supplementation with alpha-tocopherol on the oxidative modification of low density lipoprotein. *J Lipid Res*. 1992; 33:899-906.

171. Kok, et al. Serum selenium, vitamin antioxidants, and cardiovascular mortality: A 9 year follow-up study in the Netherlands. *Am J Clin Nutr*. 1987; 45:462-468.

172. Kardinal, et al. Antioxidants in adipose tissue and risk of myocardial infarction: the EURAMIC study. *Lancet*. 1993; 342:1379-82.

173. Hertog, et al. Dietary antioxidant flavonoids and risk of coronary heart disease: the Zutphen Elderly Study. *Lancet*. 1993; 342:1007-11.

174. Enstrom, et al. Vitamin C intake and mortality among a sample of the U.S. population. *Epidemiology*. 1992; 3:194-202.

175. Block, G. Vitamin C and reduced mortality. *Epidemiology*. 1992; 3:189-191.

176. Princen, et al. Supplementation with vitamin E but not beta-carotene *in vivo* protects low-density lipoprotein from lipid peroxidation *in vitro*. *Arteriosclerosis & Thrombosis*. 1992; 12:554-562.

177. Reaven, et al. Effect of dietary antioxidant combinations in humans. Protection of LDL by vitamin E but not by beta-carotene. *Arteriosclerosis & Thrombosis*. 1993; 13: 590-600.

178. Riemersma, et al. Risk of angina pectoris and plasma concentrations of vitamins A, C, and E and carotene. *Lancet*. 1991; 337:1-5.

179. Trout. Vitamin C and cardiovascular risk factors. *Am J Clin Nutr*. 1991; 53:322S-325S.

180. Salonen, et al. Relationship of serum selenium and antioxidants to plasma lipoproteins, platelet aggregability, and prevalent ischaemic heart disease in eastern Finnish men. *Atherosclerosis*. 1988; 70:155-160.

181. Murphy, et al. Antioxidant depletion in aortic cross clamping ischemia. *Free Rad Biol Med*. 1992; 13:95-100.

182. Christen W, Gaziano J, Hennekens CH, et al. Design of Physicians' Health Study II--a randomized trial of beta-carotene, vitamins E and C, and multivitamins, in prevention of cancer, cardiovascular disease, and eye disease, and review of results of completed trials. *Ann Epidemiol* 2000;10:125-34.

183. Cumming R, Mitchell P, Smith W. Diet and cataract: the Blue Mountains Eye Study. *Ophthalmology* 2000;107:450-6.

184. The age-related eye disease study: a clinical trial of zinc and antioxidants-age-related eye disease study report no. 2. *J Nutr*. 2000;130(5S Suppl):1516S-9S

185. Christen WG. Antioxidant vitamins and age-related eye disease. *Proc Assoc Am Physicians*.1999;111:16-21.

186. Brown L, Rimm EB, Seddon JM, et al. A prospective study of carotenoid intake and risk of cataract extraction in US men. *Am J Clin Nutr* 1999;70:517-24.

187. Chasan-Taber L, Willett WC, Seddon JM, et al. A prospective study of carotenoid and vitamin A intakes and risk of cataract extraction in US women. *Am J Clin Nutr* 1999; 70:509-16.

188. Garrett S, McNeil J, Silagy C, et al. Methodology of the VECAT study: vitamin E intervention in cataract and age-related maculopathy. *Ophthalmic Epidemiol* 1999; 6:195-208.

189. Stahelin HB. The impact of antioxidants on chronic disease in ageing and in old age. *Int J Vitam Nutr Res* 1999; 69:146-9.

190. Lyle BJ, Mares-Perlman JA, Klein BE, et al. Antioxidant intake and risk of incident age-related nuclear cataracts in the Beaver Dam Eye Study. *Am J Epidemiol* 1999;149:801-9.

191. Delcourt C, Cristol J, Leger C, et al. Associations of antioxidant enzymes with cataract and age-related macular degeneration. The POLA Study. Pathologies Oculaires Liees a l'Age. *Ophthalmology*. 1999;106:215-22.

192. The Age-Related Eye Disease Study (AREDS): design implications AREDS report no. 1. The Age-Related Eye Disease Study Research Group. *Control Clin Trials* 1999; 20:573-600.

193. Sperduto R, et al. Linxian cataract studies. Two nutritional intervention trials. *Arch Ophthalmol*. 1993; 111:1246-1253.

194. Hankinson S, et al. Nutrient intake and cataract extraction in women: A prospective study. *BMJ*. 1992 305:335<196>339.

195. Taylor, A. Cataract: Relationships between nutrition and oxidation. *J Am Coll Nutr*. 1993; 12:138-146.

196. Jacques and Chylack. Vitamin C plasma level inversely related to cataract incidence. Am J Clin Nutr. 1991; 53:352-55.

197. Seddon J.M., et al. The use of vitamin supplements and the risk of cataract among U.S. male physicians. *Am J Public Health*. 1994; 84:788-792.

198. Vitale S, et al. Plasma antioxidants and risk of cortical and nuclear cataract. *Epidemiology*. 1993; 4:195-203.

199. Robertson, et al. Ann NY Acad Sci. 1989; 570:372-382.

200. Knekt, et al. Serum antioxidant vitamins and risk of cataract. *BMJ*. 1992; 305:1392-1394.

201. Berkson BM. A conservative triple antioxidant approach to treatment of hepatitis C. *Med Klin*. 1999; 94:Supp III:84-89.

202. Hemila. Vitamin C and lowering of blood pressure. *J Hypertension*.1991; 9:1076-78.

203. Guilliano T. Ed. Free Radicals, Antioxidants, and Eye Disease. 1999; The Standard Publishing Co. Plover, WI.

204. Snow KK, Seddon JM. Do age-related macular degeneration and cardiovascular disease share common antecedents? *Ophthalmic Epidemiol* 1999; 6:125-43.

205. West S, et al. Are antioxidants or supplements protective for age-related macular degeneration? *Arch Opthalmol*. 1994; 112:222-227.

206. Seddon JM, et al. Vitamins, minerals, and macular degeneration. *Arch Opthalmol*. 1994; 112:176-179.

207. Seddon JM, et al. Dietary carotenoids, vitamins A, C, and E, and advanced age-related macular degeneration. *JAMA* 1994; 272:1413-1420.

208. Zandi PP, Anthony JC, Khachaturian et al. Reduced risk of Alzheimer disease in users of antioxidant vitamin supplements. *Arch Neurol*. 2004; 61:18-19.

209. Sano M, Ernesto C, et al. Controlled trial of selegiline, vitamin C, or both for Alzheimer's. *NEJM*. 1997; 336:1216-22.

210. Lethem R, Orrell M. Antioxidants and dementia. *Lancet*. 1997; 349:1189-91.

211. Levy, S., et al. The anticonvulsant effects of vitamin E. *Can J Neurol Sci*. 1992; 19:201-203.

212. Mutations in the copper-zinc containing superoxide dismutase gene are associated with Lou Gehrig's Disease. *Nutr Rev*. 1993; 51:243-245.

213. Yapa S. Detection of subclinical ascorbic deficiency in early Parkinson's disease. *Public Health*. 1993;106:393-395.

214. Fahn S. A pilot trial of high dose alpha-Tocopherol and ascorbate in early Parkinson's disease. *Ann Neurol*. 1992; 32:S128-S132.

215. The Parkinson's Study Group. Effects of Tocopherol and Deprenyl on the progression of disability in early Parkinson's Disease. *NEJM*. 1993; 328:176-183.

216. Shriqui C, et al. Vitamin E in the treatment of Tardive Dyskinesia: A double blind placebo controlled study. *Am J Psychiatry*. 1992; 149:391-393.

217. Bower B. Vitamin E may ease movement disorder. *Science News*. 1992; 141:351.

218. Adler L, et al. Vitamin E treatment of tardive dyskinesia. *Am J Psychiatry*. 1994.

219. Perrig W, Perrig P, Stahelin. Antioxidants enhance memory in the old and very old. *J Am Geriatr Soc*. 1997; 45:718-24.

220. Cooper DA, Eldridge AL, Peters JC. Dietary carotenoids and certain cancers, heart disease, and age-related macular degeneration: a review of recent research. *Nutr Rev*. 1999; 57:201-14.

221. Faure H, Fayol V, Galabert C, et al. Carotenoids: 2. Diseases and supplementation studies. *Ann Biol Clin*. 1999; 57:273-82.

222. Ascherio A, Rimm EB, Hernan MA, et al. Relation of consumption of vitamin E, vitamin C, and carotenoids to risk for stroke

among men in the United States. *Ann Intern Med.* 1999;130:963-70.

223. Bendich, A. Antioxidant vitamins and their function in immune responses. 1989. New York: Plenum Publishing Corp.

224. Brown L, Rimm ER, et al. A prospective study of carotene intake and cataracts. *Am J Clin Nutr.* 1999; 70:509-24.

225. Bendich A. Safety of beta-carotene. Review. *Nutr Cancer.* 1988; 11:207-214.

226. Pryor WA. Letter to Editor. Beta-carotene, vitamin E and lung cancer. *NEJM.* 1994; 612.

227. Pryor WA, Stahl W, Rock CL. Beta-carotene: From biochemistry to clinical trials. *Nutr Rev.* 2000;

228. Riboli E, Gonzalez CA, Lopez-Abente G, Errezola M Diet and bladder cancer in Spain: A multi-centre case-control study. *Intl J Cancer* 1991;49:214-219.

229. Bohlke K, Spiegelman D, Trichopoulou A, et al. Vitamins A, C and E and the risk of breast cancer: results from a case-control study in Greece. *Br J Cancer.* 1999;79:23-9.

230. Zhang S, Hunter DJ, Forman MR, et al. Dietary carotenoids and vitamins A, C, and E and risk of breast cancer. *JNCI.* 1999;91:547-556.

231. Torun M, Akgul S, Sargin H. Serum vitamin E level in patients with breast cancer. *J Clin PharmTherapeutics* 1995;20:173-178.

232. Favero A, Parpinel M, Franceschi S. Diet and risk of breast cancer: Major findings from an Italian case-control study. *Biomed Pharm* 1998;52:109-115.

233. Mezzetti M, La Vecchia C, Decarli A, et al. Population attributable risk for breast cancer: Diet, nutrition, and exercise. *JNCI* 1998;90:389-394.

234. Mannisto S, Pietinen P, Virtanen M. Diet and risk of breast cancer in a case-control study: Does the threat of disease have an influence on recall bias? *J Clin Epidem* 1999;52:429-439.

235. Cuzick J, Destavola BL, Russell MJ. Vitamin A, vitamin E, and the risk of cervical intraepithelial neoplasia. *BritJCanc* 1990;62:651-652.

236. Ho GYF, Palan PR, Basu J, et al. Viral characteristics of human papillomavirus infection and antioxidant levels as risk factors for cervical dysplasia. *Intl J Cancer* 1998; 78:594-599.

237. Verrault R, Chu J, Mandelson M. A case-control study of diet and invasive cervical cancer. *Intl J Cancer* 1989; 43:1050-1054.

238. Roncucci L, Di Donato P, Carati L, et al. Antioxidant vitamins or lactulose for the pre-

vention of the recurrence of colorectal adenomas. *Diseases Colon Rectum* 1993; 36:227-234.

239. Whelan RL, Horvath KD, Gleason NR, et al. Vitamin and calcium supplement use is associated with decreased adenoma recurrence in patients with a previous history of neoplasia. *Diseases Colon Rectum* 1999; 42:212-217.

240. Bostick RM, Poter JD, McKenzie DR, et al. Reduced risk of colon cancer with high intake of vitamin E: The Iowa Women's Health Study. *Cancer Res* 1993;53:4230-4237.

241. La Vecchia C, Braga C, Negri E, et al. Intake of selected micronutrients and risk of colorectal cancer. *Intl JCancer* 1997; 73:525-530.

242. White E, et al. Vitamin E lowers colon cancer risk. *Cancer Epidemiology Biomarker Prev.* 1997; 6:769-74.

243. Knekt P, Jarvinen R, Seppanen R, et al. Dietary antioxidants and the risk of lung cancer. *Am J Epidem* 1991; 134:471-479.

244. Yong L-C, Brown CC, Schatzkin A, et al. Intake of vitamins E, C, and A and risk of lung cancer. The NHANES I epidemiologic followup study. *Am J Epidem* 1997; 146:231-243.

245. Knekt P. Vitamin E and smoking and the risk of lung cancer. *Ann NY Acad Sci* 1993; 686:280-288.

246. Woodson K, Tangrea J, Barrett M ,et al. Serum alpha-tocopherol and subsequent risk of lung cancer among male smokers. *JNCI.* 1999; 91:1738-1743.

247. Le Gardeur B, Lopez S, Johnson WD. A case-control study of serum vitamins A, E, and C in lung cancer patients. *Nutr and Cancer* 1990; 14:133-140.

248. Harris R, Key T, Silcocks P, et al. A case-control study of dietary carotene in men with lung cancer and in men with other epithelial cancers. *Nutr and Cancer* 1991;15:63-68.

249. Barone J, Taioli E, Herbert JR, Wynder EL. Vitamin supplement use and risk for oral and esophageal cancer. *Nutr and Cancer* 1992;18:31-41.

250. Gridley G, McLaughlin JK, Block G,et al. Vitamin supplement use and reduced risk of oral and pharyngeal cancer. *Am JEpidem* 1992;135:1083-1092.

251. Negri E, Franceschi S, Bosetti C, et al. Selected micronutrients and oral and pharyngeal cancer. *Intl J Cancer* 2000; 86:122-127.

252. Heinonen OP, et al. Vitamin E supplements lower prostate cancer risk by one third. *JNCI.* 1998; 90:440-46.

253. Stryker WS, Stampfer MJ, Stein EA, et al. Diet, plasma levels of beta-carotene and alpha-tocopherol, and risk of malignant melanoma. *Am J Epidem* 1990; 131:597-611.

254. Blot WJ, Li J-Y, Taylor PR, et al. Nutrition intervention trials in Linxian, China: Supplementation with specific vitamin/mineral combinations, cancer incidence and disease-specific mortality in the general population. *JNCI.* 1993; 85:1483-1492.

255. Buiatti E, Palli D, Decarli A,et al. A case-control study of gastric cancer and diet in Italy. *Intl J Cancer* 1989; 44:611-616.

256. Charpiot P, Calaf R, DiCostanzo J, et al. Vitamin A, vitamin E, retinal binding protein (RBP) and prealbumin in digestive cancers. *Intl J Vitamin Nutri Res.* 1989; 59:323-328.

257. Shklar G, Oh S. Basis for cancer prevention by vitamin E. *Cancer Invest.* 2000; 18:214-22.

258. Gonzalez M, Mora E, et al. Vitamins C and E and cancer: An update on nutritional oncology. *Cancer Prev Intl.* 1998; 3:215-24.

259. Rimm E, Stampfer M, et al. Vitamin E consumption and the risk of coronary heart disease in men and women. *NEJM.* 1993; 328:1444-56.

260. Takamatsu S, et al. Effects on health of dietary supplementatin with 100 mg of d-alpha-tocopheryl daily for 6 years. *J Intl Med Res.* 1995; 23:342-57.

261. Stephans N, et al. Randomized controlled trial of vitamin E in patient with coronary disease: CHAOS Study. *Lancet.* 1996; 347:781-86.

262. Rapola J, et al. Effect of vitamin E and carotene on incidence of angina pectoris. *JAMA.* 1996; 275:693-98.

263. Hodis H, Mack W, et al. Serial coronary angiographic evidence that antioxidant vitamin intake reduces progression of coronary artery disease. *JAMA.* 1995; 273:1849-54.

264. Pryor W. Can vitamin E protect humans against the pathological effects of ozone in smog? *Am J Clin Nutr.* 1991; 53:702-722.

265. London R, Sundaram G, et al. Alpha-tocopherol, mammary dysplasia and steroid hormones. *Cancer Res.* 1981; 4:249-253.

266. Ceriello, et al. Vitamin E reduction of protein glycosylation in diabetics. *Diabetes Care.* 1992; 14:68-72.

267. Fogarty A, et al. Vitamin E, IgE, and atopy. *Lancet.* 2000; 356:573-74.

268. Kappus H, Diplock A. Tolerance and safety of vitamin E. *Free Rad Biol Med.* 1992; 13:55-74.

269. Bendich and Machlin. Safety of oral intake of vitamin E: A Review. *Am J Clin Nutr.* 1988; 48:612-19.

270. Vitamin E. 1989. Tenth Edition of Recommended Dietary Allowances. National Research Council. National Academy Press. Washington D.C.

271. Henning S, et al. Glutathione blood levels and other oxidant defense indices in men fed diets low in vitamin C. *J Nutr.* 1991; 121:1969-75.

272. Kamat AM, Lamm DL. Chemoprevention of urological cancer. *J Urol* 1999;161:1748-60.

273. Young KJ, Lee PN. Intervention studies on cancer. *Eur J Cancer Prev* 1999;8:91-103.

274. Shibata A, Paganini-Hill A. Intake of vegetables, fruit, beta-carotene, vitamin C and vitamin supplements and cancer incidence among the elderly: A prospective study. *Brit Journal Canc* 1992; 66:673-679.

275. Zhang S, Hunter DJ, Forman MR, et al. Dietary carotenoids and vitamins A, C, and E and risk of breast cancer. *JNCI.* 1999;91:547-556.

276. Zaridze D, Evstifeeva T, Boyle P. Chemoprevention of oral leukoplakia and chronic esophagitis in an area of high incidence of oral and esophageal cancer. *Annals of Epidemiology* 1993;3:225-234.

277. Landa M-C, Frago N, Tres A. Diet and the risk of breast cancer in Spain. *Europ J Cancer Prevent* 1994;3:313-320.

278. Yuan J-M, Wang Q-S, Ross RK. Diet and breast cancer in Shangai and Tianjin, China. *Brit J Cancer* 1995; 71:1353-1358.

279. Ronco A, De Stefani E, Boffetta P,et al. Vegetables, fruits, and related nutrients and risk of breast cancer: A case-control study in Uruguay. *Nutri and Cancer* 1999; 35:111-119.

280. Verrault R, Chu J, Mandelson M, Shy K. A case-control study of diet and invasive cervical cancer. *Intl J Cancer* 1989; 43:1050-1054.

281. Herrero R, Potischman N, Brinton LA,et al. A case-control study of nutrient status and invasive cervical cancer. I. Dietary indicators. *Am J Epidem* 1991; 134:1335-1346.

282. Van Eenwyk J, Davis FG, Bowen PE. Dietary and serum carotenoids and cervical intraepithelial neoplasia. *Intl J Cancer* 1991; 48:34-38.

283. Shibata A, Paganini-Hill A. Intake of vegetables, fruit, beta-carotene, vitamin C and vitamin supplements and cancer incidence among the elderly: A prospective study. *Brit J Cancer* 1992;66:673-679.

284. La Vecchia C, Negri E, Decarli A,et al. A case-control study of diet and colorectal can-

cer in northern Italy. *Intl J Cancer* 1988;
41:492-498.

285. Freudenheim JL, Graham S, Marshall JR. A case-control study of diet and rectal cancer in Western New York. *Am J Epidem* 1990; 131:612-624.

286. Ferraroni M, et al. Selected micronutrient intake and the risk of colorectal cancer. *Br J Cancer*.1994; 70:1150-1155.

287. La Vecchia C, et al. Intake of selected micronutrients and risk of colorectal cancer. *Intl J Cancer* 1997; 73:525-530.

288. Knekt P, Jarvinen R, et al. Dietary antioxidants and the risk of lung cancer. *Am J Epidem* 1991; 134:471-479.

289. Bandera EV, Freudenheim JL, et al. Diet and alcohol consumption and lung cancer risk in the New York State Cohort (United States). *Cancer Causes and Control* 1997; 8:828-840.

290. Ocke MC, Bueno-de-Mesquita HB, et al. Repeated measurements of vegetables, fruits, beta-carotene, and vitamins C and E in relation to lung cancer. The Zutphen Study. *Am J Epidem* 1997;145:358-365.

291. Yong L-C, Brown CC, et al. Intake of vitamins E, C, and A and risk of lung cancer. The NHANES I epidemiologic followup study. *Am J Epidem* 1997;146:231-243.

292. Voorrips LE, Goldbohm RA, et al. A prospective cohort study on antioxidant and folate intake and male lung cancer risk. *Cancer Epidem, Biomarkers Prevent* 2000;9:357-365.

293. Fontham ETH, Pickle LW, et al. Dietary vitamins A and C and lung cancer risk in Louisiana. *Cancer* 1988; 62:2267-2273.

294. Le Marchand L, et al. Vegetable consumption and lung cancer risk: A population-based case-control study in Hawaii. *JNCI.* 1989; 81:1158-1164.

295. McLaughlin JK, Gridley G, et al. Dietary factors in oral and pharyngeal cancer. *JNCI* 1988;80:1237-1243.

296. De Stefani E, et al. Diet and risk of cancer of the aerodigestive tract - II. Nutrients. *Oral Oncology* 1999;35:22-26.

297. Negri E, Franceschi S, et al. Selected micronutrients and oral and pharyngeal cancer. *Intl J Cancer* 2000; 86:122-127.

298. Eichholzer M, Stahelin HB, et al. Prediction of male cancer mortality by plasma levels of interacting vitamins: 17-year follow-up of the prospective Basel study. *Intl J Cancer* 1996; 66:145-150.

299. Deneo-Pellegrini H, et al. Foods, nutrients and prostate cancer: A case-control study in Uruguay. *Br J Cancer* 1999; 80:591-597.

300. Correa P, et al. Chemoprevention of gastric dysplasia: Randomized trial of antioxidant supplements and anti-*Helicobacter pylori* therapy. *JNCI* 2000; 92:1881-1888.

301. Botterweck AM, van den Brant PA, Goldbohm. Vitamins, carotenoids, dietary fiber, and the risk of gastric carcinoma. *Cancer* 2000; 88:737-748.

302. You W-C, Blot WJ, et al.. Diet and high risk of stomach cancer in Shandong, China. *Cancer Res* 1988; 48:3518-3523.

303. Buiatti E, Palli D, et al.. A case-control study of gastric cancer and diet in Italy. *Intl J Cancer* 1989; 44:611-616.

304. Boeing H, Frentzel-Beyme R, Berger M, et al. Case-control study on stomach cancer in Germany. *Intl J Cancer* 1991; 47:858-864.

305. La Vecchia C, Ferraroni M, et al. Selected micronutrient intake and the risk of gastric cancer. *Cancer Epidem, Biomark Prevent* 1994; 3:393-398.

306. Kaaks R, Tuyns AJ, et al. Nutrient intake patterns and gastric cancer risk: A case-control study in Belgium. *Intl J Cancer* 1998; 78:415-420.

307. Ekstrom AM, et al. Dietary antioxidant intake and the risk of cardia cancer and non-cardia cancer of the intestinal and diffuse types: A population-based case-control study in Sweden. *Intl J Cancer* 2000; 87:133-140.

308. You W-C, Zhang L, et al. Gastric dysplasia and gastric cancer: Helicobacter pylori, serum vitamin C, and other risk factors. *JNCI* 2000; 92:1607-1612.

309. Cameron E. In: Hyaluronidase and cancer. 1966; New York: Pergamon Press.

310. Pauling L. Preventive nutrition. *Medicine on the Midway.* 1972; 27:15.

311. Duffy S, Gokce, et al. Treatment of hypertension with ascorbic acid. *Lancet.* 1999; 354:2048-49.

312. Hall and Greendale. The relation of dietary vitamin C to bone mineral density. *Calcif Tissue Intl.* 1998;63:183-89.

313. US NHANES III. *Arch Int Med.* 2000; 160:931-36.

314. Bendich. Antioxidant vitamins and their function in immune response.

315. Hoffer A. Ascorbic acid and toxicity. *NEJM.* 1971; 285:635.

316. Klenner FR. Vitamin C and toxicity. *J Appl Nutr.* 1971; 23:61.

317. Hollman PC, Feskens EJ, Katan MB. Tea flavonols in cardiovascular disease and cancer epidemiology. *Proc Soc Exp Biol Med* 1999;220:198-202.

318. Hertog M, Feskens et al. Dietary antioxidant flavonoids and risk of heart disease. *Lancet.* 1993; 342:1007-11.

319. Rayman MP. The importance of selenium to human health. *Lancet.* 2000; 356:233-41.

320. Young VR, Richardson. Nutrients, vitamins, and minerals in cancer prevention. Facts and fallacies. *Cancer.* 1979; 43:2125.

321. Sakurai H, Tsuchiya K. A tentative recommendation for the maximum daily intake of selenium. *Environ Physiol Biochem.* 1975; 5:107.

322. Magalova T, Bella V, Brtkova A, et al. Copper, zinc and superoxide dismutase in precancerous, benign diseases and gastric, colorectal and breast cancer. *Neoplasma* 1999;46:100-4.

323. Frost,P, Chen JC, Rabbini I, et al. The effects of zinc deficiency on immune response. *Proc Clin Biol Res.* 1977; 14:143.

324. Ziegler D, Reljanovic M, et al. Alpha-lipoic acid in the treatment of diabetic polyneuropathy in Germany: current evidence from clinical trials. *Exp Clin Endocrin Diabetes.* 1999; 107:421-30.

325. Ziegler D, Hanefeld M, et al. Treatment of symptomatic diabetic peripheral neuropathy with antioxidant lipoic acid. A three week multicenter randomized controlled trial (ALADIN Study). *Diabetologia.* 1995; 38: 1425-33.

326. Reljanovic M, Reichel C, et al. Treatment of diabetic peripheral neuropathy with alpha-lipoic acid. A two tier randomized multicenter double-blind placebo-controlled trial. (ALADIN II). *Free Radical Res.* 1999; 31:171-79.

327. Ziegler D, Hanefeld M, et al. Treatment of symptomatic diabetic peripheral neuropathy with antioxidant lipoic acid. A 7 month multicenter randomized controlled trial (ALADIN III Study). *Diabetes Care.* 1999; 22:1296-1301.

328. Ruhnau KJ, Meissner HP, et al. Effects of three weeks oral treatment with the antioxidant alpha lipoic acid in symptomatic diabetic polyneuropathy. *Diabetes Med.* 1999; 16:1040-43.

329. Ou P, Nourooz ZJ, et al. Activation of aldose reductase in rat lens and metal-ion chelation by alpha lipoic acid. *Free Radical Res.* 1996; 25:337-46.

330. Filina AA, Davydova N, et al. Lipoic acid as a means of metabolic therapy of open angle glaucoma. *Vestn Oftalmol.* 1995; 111:6-8. Prehn JH, Karkoutly C, et al. Lipoic acid reduces neuronal injury after cerebral ischemia. *J Cereb Blood Flow Metabol.* 1992; 12:78-87.

331. Prehn JH, Karkoutly C, et al. Lipoic acid reduces neuronal injury after cerebral ischemia. *J Cereb Blood Flow Metabol.* 1992; 12:78-87.

332. Speizer FE, Colditz GA, Hunter DJ, et al. Prospective study of smoking, antioxidant intake, and lung cancer in middle-aged women (USA). *Cancer Causes Control.* 1999;10:475-82.

333. Virtamo J. Vitamins and lung cancer. *Proc Nutr Soc* 1999; 58:329-33.

334. Young KJ, Lee PN. Intervention studies on cancer. *Eur J Cancer Prev.* 1999;8:91-103.

335. Watkins ML, Erickson JD, Thun MJ, et al. Multivitamin use and mortality in a large prospective study. *Am J Epidem.* 2000;152:149-62.

336. Ohno Y, Wakai K, Dillon DS, et al. Dietary macro/micro-nutrients as a breast cancer risk: findings from nutritional case-control study in Jakarta, Indonesia. *Gan To Kagaku Ryoho.* 2000; 2:412-9.

337. Bogden JD, Louria DB. Aging and the immune system: the role of micronutrient nutrition. *Nutrition* 1999;15:593-5.

338. Chasan-Taber L, Willett WC, Seddon JM, et al. A prospective study of carotenoid and vitamin A intakes and risk of cataract extraction in US women. *Am J Clin Nutr* 1999; 70:509-16.

339. Lefebvre P, et al. Retinoic acid stimulates regeneration of mammalian auditory hair cells. *Science.* 1993; 260:692-95.

340. Rosenberg H, Felzman AN. In: The Book of Vitamin Therapy. 1974. New York: Berkley Publishing Corp.

341. Goodman LS, Gilman A, eds. A Pharmacological Basis of Therapeutics. 1977. 5th ed. New York: Macmillan.

342. Bendich and Langseth. Safety of vitamin A. *Am J Clin Nutr.* 1989; 49:358-371.

343. Lipkin M, Newmark HL. Vitamin D, calcium and prevention of breast cancer: a review. *J Am Coll Nutr* 1999;18:392S-397S.

344. Janowsky EC, Lester GE, Weinberg CR. Association between low levels of 1,25-dihydroxyvitamin D and breast cancer risk. *Public Health Nutr.* 1999;2:283-91.

345. Garland, et al. Serum vitamin D and colon cancer- 8 year prospective study. *Lancet.* 1989;18:1176-78.

346. Reitsma, et al. Regulation of myc gene expression. *Nature.* 1983; 306:492-495.

347. Mariani E, Ravaglia G, Forti P, et al. Vitamin D, thyroid hormones and muscle mass influence natural killer (NK) innate immunity in healthy nonagenarians and centenarians. *Clin Exp Immunol.* 1999;116:19-27.

348. Ross JA, Davies SM. Vitamin K prophylaxis and childhood cancer. *Med Pediatr Oncol.* 2000;34:434-7.

349. Boros LG. Population thiamine status and varying cancer rates between western, Asian

and African countries. *Anticancer Res* 2000;20:2245-8.

350. Rosenblatt KA, Thomas DB, Jimenez LM. The relationship between diet and breast cancer in US men. *Cancer Causes Control* 1999;10:107-13.

351. Elam M, Henninghake, et al. Effect of niacin on lipids and glycemic control. *JAMA.* 2000; 284:1263-70.

352. Wu K, Helzlsouer KJ, Comstock GW, et al. A prospective study on folate, B12, and pyridoxal 5'-phosphate (B6) and breast cancer. *Cancer Epidemiol Biomarkers Prev* 1999;8:209-17.

353. Zhang S, Hunter DJ, Hankinson SE, et al. A prospective study of folate intake and the risk of breast cancer. *JAMA* 1999; 281:1632-7.

354. Giovannucci, et al. Multiple vitamins reduce cancer risk. *JNCI.* 1993; 85:875-84.

355. Lipkin M, Newmark HL. Vitamin D, calcium and prevention of breast cancer: a review. *J Am Coll Nutr* 1999;18:392S-397S.

356. Cascienu S, et al. Effects of calcium and vitamin supplementation on colon cancer. *Cancer Invest.* 2000; 18:411-16.

357. Garland, et al. Dietary vitamin D and calcium and risk of colorectal cancer: A 19 year prospective study in men. *Lancet.* 1985; i:307.

358. Newmark H. Teens' low-calcium diets may increase breast cancer risk. *Oncology News Intl.* 1993; 2(11):2.

359. Baron JA, Beach, et al. Calcium supplementation for the prevention of colorectal adenomas. *NEJM.* 1999; 340:101-7.

360. V Matkovic, JZ Ilich, et al.Urinary calcium, sodium, and bone mass of young females. *Am J Clin Nutr* 1995; 62: 417-425.

361. Weaver CM, Peacock M, et al. Adolescent nutrition in the prevention of postmenopausal osteoporosis. *J Clin Endocrinol Metab.* 1999; 84: 1839-43.

362. Rodan GA. Therapeutic approaches to Bone Diseases. *Science.* 2000; 289:1508-14.

363. Bonjour et al. Gain in bone mass in prepubertal girls 3-5 years after discontinuation of calcium supplementation. *Lancet.* 2001; 358:1208-12.

364. Bendich A, Leader S, Muhuri P. Supplemental calcium for the prevention of hip fracture: potential health-economic benefits. *Clin Ther.* 1999;21:1058-72.

365. Ullom-Minnich P. Prevention of osteoporosis and fractures. *Am Fam Physician* 1999;60:194-202.

366. Marci CD, Viechnicki MB, et al. Bone mineral densitometry substantially influences

367. Cohen AJ, Roe FJ. Review of risk factors for osteoporosis with particular reference to a possible aetiological role of dietary salt. *Food Chem Toxicol* 2000;38:237-53.

368. Swaminathan R Nutritional factors in osteoporosis. *Int J Clin Pract* 1999;53:540-8.

369. O'Connell MB. Prevention and treatment of osteoporosis in the elderly. *Pharmacotherapy* 1999;19:7S-20S.

370. Hernandez-Avila M, et al. Caffeine, moderate alcohol intake and risk of fractures of the hip. *Am J Clin Nut.* 1991; 54:157-63.

371. Wong CA, Walsh L, et al. Inhaled corticosteroid use and bone-mineral density in patients with asthma. *Lancet.* 2000; 355:1399-403.

372. Liu B, et al. Use of selective serotonin-reuptake inhibitors or tricyclic antidepressants and risk of hip fractures in elderly people. *Lancet.* 1998; 351:1303-07.

373. Staessen JA, et al. Environmental exposure to cadmium, forearm bone density and risk of fractures: prospective population study. *Lancet.* 1999; 353:1140-44.

374. Bucher HC, Cook R, et al. Effects of dietary calcium supplementation on blood pressure. *JAMA.* 1996; 275:1016-1022.

375. Deary, et al. Calcium and Alzheimer's disease. *Lancet.*1986; (May 24):1219.

376. Pak, CY. Kidney stones. *Lancet.* 1998; 351:1797-801.

377. Curhan, G., et al. A prospective study of dietary calcium and the risk of symptomatic kidney stones. *NEJM.* 1993; 328:833-838.

378. NIH Consensus Development Panel on Optimal Calcium Intake. Optimal calcium intake. *JAMA.* 1994; 272:1942-1948.

379. Dawson-Hughes B, et al. Effect of calcium and vitamin D supplementation on bone density in men and women 65 years or older. *NEJM.* 1997; 337:670-6.

380. Khosla S, Riggs L. Treatment options for osteoporosis. *Mayo Clinic Proc.* 1995; 70:978-82.

381. Recommended Dietary Allowances. 1989. 10th Edition. National Research Council. National Academy Press. Washington, D.C.

382. Bigg, et al. Magnesium deficiency: Role in arrhythmias complicating acute myocardial infarction. *Med J Aust.* 1981; i:346-48.

383. Heptinstall, et al. Letters to the Editor. Lancet. 1986; 8:551-552.

384. Witteman J, et al. Reduction of hypertension with oral magnesium supplementation in women. *Am J Clin Nutr.* 1994; 60:124-31.

385. Britton J, et al. Dietary magnesium, lung function, wheezing in a randomized population. *Lancet*. 1994; 344:357-62.

386. Myers, Gianni, Simone. Oxidative destruction of membranes by doxorubicin-iron complex. *Biochemistry*. 1982; 21:1707-13.

387. Stevens R, et al. Body iron stores and risk of cancer. *NEJM*. 1988; 319:1047-1052.

388. Nelson R, et al. Body iron stores and risk of colonic neoplasia. *JNCI*. 1994; 86:455-60.

389. Simone CB, Simone NL, Simone CB II. Fibre supplementation. *Lancet*. 2001; 357:393.

390. Simone CB II, Simone NL, Simone CB. Consumption of fiber reduce the risk of colorectal cancer: A review. *J Ortho Mol Med*. 2000; 15:96-102.

391. Simone CB, Simone NL, Simone CB II. Fiber supplementation reduces the risk of colorectal cancer: A review. *Int J Integr Med*. 2000; 7:38-43.

392. Burkitt DP. Large-bowel cancer: An epidemiological jigsaw puzzle. *JNCI*. 1975; 54:3.

393. Stoll BA. Essential fatty acids, insulin resistance, and breast cancer risk. *Nutr Cancer*. 1998; 31:72-7.

394. Eynard AR. Does chronic essential fattyy acid deficiency constitute a pro-tumorigenic condition? *Med Hypotheses*. 1997; 48:55-62.

395. Stahl W, Sies H. Food sources of lycopene. *Arch Biochem Biophys*. 1996; 336:1-9.

396. Proceedings of the First International Conference on Chemoprevention of Prostate Cancer. *J Urol*.2004; 171(2):Part 2 of 2.

397. Ripple MO, Henry WF, Rago RP, et al. Prooxidant-antioxidant shift induced by androgen treatment of human prostate cancer cells. *JNCI*. 1997; 89:40.

398. Miller Ec, Giovannucci E, Erdman J, et al. Tomato products, lycopene, and prostate cancer risk. *Urol Clin North Am*. 2002; 29:83.

399. Vogt TM, Mayne St, Graubard BI, et al. Serum lycopene, other serum carotenoids, and risk of prostate cancer in US Blacks and Whites. *Am J Epidemiol*. 2002; 155:1023-32.

400. The effect of vitamin E and beta-carotene on the incidence of lung cancer and other cancers in male smokers. The Alpha Tocopherol Beta-Carotene Cancer Prevention Study Group. *NEJM*. 1994; 330:1029.

401. Chan JM, Stampfer MJ, et al. Supplemental vitamin E and prostate cancer risk in a large cohort of men in the US. *Canc Epidemiol Bio Prev*. 1999; 8:893.

402. Clark LC, et al. Decreased incidence of prostate cancer with selenium supplementation: results of a double blind cancer prevention trial. *Br J Urol*. 1998; 81:730.

403. Combs GF, Clark LC, et al. Reduction of prostate cancer risk with an oral supplement of selenium. *Biomed Environ Sci*. 1997; 10:227.

404. Most don't take daily vitamins. *USA Today*. March 15, 2001.

405. Woods R. Nutrient intake patterns. VNIS Health Communications Conference. "Vitamins in Women's Health: New Roles, New Directions." March 1994. Page 16.

406. Greenwald P, Kelloff G, et al. Chemoprevention. *CA – A Cancer J Clin*. 1995; 45:31-49.

Chapter 6
Nutritional and Lifestyle Modification in Oncology Care
AMIFOSTINE (WR-2721)

1. Brizel DM, Wasserman TH, Henke M, et al. Phase III randomized trial of amifostine as a radioprotector in head and neck cancer. *J Clin Oncol*. 2000;15:2850-2857.

2. Capizzi RL. Clinical status and optimal use of Amifostine. *Oncology*. 1999;13(1):47-59.

3. Dousay L, Mu C, Giarratana MC, et al. Amifostine improves the antileukemic therapeutic index of mafosfamide: Implications for marrow purging. *Blood*. 1995; 88:2849-2855.

4. Kemp G, Rose P, Lurain J, et al. Amifostine pretreatment for protection against cyclophosphamide-induced and cisplatin-induced toxicities: results of a randomized control trial in patients with advanced ovarian cancer. *J Clin Oncol*. 1996;14:2101-2112.

5. Kligerman M, Glover D, Turrisi A, Simone CB, et al. Toxicity of WR-2721 administered in single and multiple doses. *Int J Radiat Oncol Biol Phys*. 1984; 10:1773-76.

6. Schein, P. Results of chemotherapy and radiation therapy protection trials with WR-2721. *Cancer Investigation*. 1992; 10(1):24-26.

7. Schiller JH, Storer B, Berlin J, et al. Amifostine, cisplatin and vinblastine in metastatic non-small cell lung cancer: A report of high response rates and prolonged survival. *J Clin Oncol*. 1996; 14:1913-1921.

8. Tannehill SP, Mehta MP. Amifostine and radiation therapy: past, present, and future. *Semin Oncol*. 1996; 23:69-77.

9. Wasserman TH, Brizel DM. The role of amifostine as a radioprotector. *Oncology*. 2001; 15(10):1349-1354.

DEXRAZOXANE (ICRF-187)

10. Carlson, R. Reducing the cardiotoxicity of the anthracyclincs. *Oncology*. 1992; 6(6):95-108.

11. Hellmann K. Anthracycline cardiotoxicity prevention by dexrazoxane: Break-

through of a barrier-sharpens antitumor profile and therapeutic index. *J Clin Oncol.* 1996;14(2): 332-333.

12.   Klein P, Muggio FM. Cytoprotection: Shelter from the storm. *The Oncologist.* 1999; 4:112-121.

13.   Swain SM, Whaley FS, Gerber MC, Ewer MS, et al. Delayed administration of dexrazoxane provides cardio-protection for patients with advanced breast cancer treated doxorubicin-containing therapy. *J Clin Oncol.* 1997; 15:1333-1340.

IRON INTERMEDIATE

14.   Myers C, Gianni L, Simone CB, Klecker R, Greene R. Oxidative destruction of erythrocyte ghost membranes catalysed by the doxorubicin-iron complex. *Biochemistry.* 1982;21(8):1707-1713.

15.   Carmine TC, Evans P, Bruchelt G, et al. Presence of iron catalyst for free radical reactions in patients undergoing chemotherapy: implications for therapeutic management. *Cancer Lett.* 1995;94:219-226.

16.   Gordeuk VR, Brittenham GM. Bleomycin-reactive iron in patients with acute nonlymphocytic leukemia. *FEBS lett.* 1992;308:4-6.

17.   Halliwell B, Aruoma OI, Mufti G, Bomford A. Bleomycin-detectable iron in serum from leukaemic patients before and after chemotherapy. Therapeutic implications for treatment with oxidant-generating drugs. *FEBS Lett.* 1988;241:202-204.

ERRONEOUS INFORMATION THAT ANTIOXIDANTS INTERFERE WITH TREATMENT

18.   Brody J quoting Larry Norton, M.D. of Memorial Sloan Kettering, NYC. Vitamin Mania, Millions Take a Gamble on Health. New York Times. October 26, 1997. Front page.

19.   Labriola D, Livingston R. Possible interactions between dietary antioxidants and chemotherapy. *Oncology.* 1999; 13:1003-11.

20.   Agus DB, Vera JC, Golde DW: Stromal cell oxidation: A mechanism by which tumors obtain vitamin C. *Cancer Res.*1999; 59:4555-58.

21.   Gottlieb N. Cancer treatment and vitamin C: the debate lingers. *JNCI.* 1999; 91(24):2073-2075.

22.   American Cancer Society Workgroup on Nutrition and Physical Activity for Cancer Survivors. Brown J, Byers T, Thompson K, Eldridge B, Doyle C, Williams AM. Nutrition during and after cancer treatment: a guide for informed choices by cancer survivors. *CA: Cancer J Clinicians.* 2001;51(3):153-87.

23.   The American Cancer Society. Chemotherapy Principles: An Indepth Discussion Of The Techniques And Its Role In Cancer Treatment. July 26, 2001.

THERAPY REDUCES SERUM ANTIOXIDANTS

24.   Basu TK. Significance of vitamins in cancer. *Oncology.* 1976; 33:183-186.

25.   Bhuvarahamurthy V, et al. Effect of radiotherapy and chemoradiotherapy on the circulating antioxidant system of human uterine cervical carcinoma. *Mol Cell Biochem.* 1996; 158:17-23.

26.   Clemens MR. Vitamins and therapy of malignancies. *Ther Umsch.* 1994; 51:483-488.

27.   Erhola M, Kellokumpu et al. Effects of anthracyclin chemotherapy on plasma antioxidant capacity in small cell lung cancer patients. *Free Radic Biol Med.*1996; 21(3): 383-390.

28.   Faber M, Coudray C, et al. Lipid peroxidation products, and vitamin and trace element status in patients with cancer before and after chemotherapy, including adriamycin. *Biol Trace Elem Res.* 1995; 47: 117-123.

29.   Look MP, Musch E. Lipid peroxides in the polychemotherapy of cancer patients. *Chemotherapy.* 1994. 40:8-15.

30.   Sangeetha P, Das UN, et al. Increase in free radical generation and lipid-peroxidation following chemotherapy for patients with cancer. *Free Radic Biol Med.* 1990; 8:15-19.

***In Vitro* Cellular Studies**

31.   Anderson D, Basaran N, Blowers SD, Edwards AJ. The effect of antioxidants on bleomycin treatment in in vitro and in vivo genootoxicity assays. *Mutat Res.* 1995; 329:37-47.

32.   Bump EA, Braunhut SJ, et al. Novel concepts in modification of radiation sensitivity. *Int J Radiat Oncol Biol Phys.* 1994; 29: 249-253.

33.   Chiang CD, Song EJ, et al. Ascorbic acid increases accumulation and reverses vincristine resistance of human non-small cell lung cancer cells. *Biochem J.* 1994; 301:759-64.

34.   DeLoecker W, et al. Effects of vitamin C treatment on human tumor cell growth in vitro. Synergism with combined chemotherapy action. *Anticancer Res* 1993; 13:103-106.

35.   Miura T, Muraoka S, Ogiso T. Effect of ascorbate on adriamycin-Fe induced lipid peroxidation and DNA damage. *Pharmacol Toxicol.* 1994; 74:89-94.

36.   Prasad KN, Hernandez C, et al. Modification of the effect of tamoxifen, cisplatin, DTIC, and interferon-alpha 2b on human melanoma cells in culture by a mixture of vitamins. *Nutrition and Cancer.* 1994; 22:233-45.

37.   Prasad KN, Rama BN. Modification of the effect of pharmacological agents, ionizing radiation and hyperthermia on tumor cells by vi-

tamin E. In: Vitamin, Nutrition and Cancer. Prasad KN ed. Karger, Basel. Pp 76. 1984.

38. Vadgama JV, Wu Y, Shen D, et al. Effect of selenium in combination with adriamycin or taxol on several different cancer cells. Anticancer Res. 2000; 20:1391-1414.

39. Zucali JR. Mechanisms of protection of hematopoietic stem cells from irradiation. *Leuk Lymphoma.* 1994; 13: 27-32.

Animal Studies

40. Baldew GS, Mol JG, et al. The mechanism of interaction between cisplatin and selenite. *Biochem. Pharmacol.* 1991; 41:1429-37.

41. Ben-Amotz A, et al. Natural beta-carotene and whole body irradiation in rats. *Radiat Environ Biophys.* 1996; 35: 285-88.

42. Bogin E, Marom M, Levi. Changes in serum, liver and kidneys of cisplatin treated rats; effects of antioxidants. *Eur J Clin Chem Clin Biochem.* 1994; 32: 843-851.

43. Crary EJ, McCarty MF. Potential clinical applications for high-dose nutritional antioxidants. *Medical Hypothesis* 1984; 13:77-98.

44. El-Nahas SM, Mattar FE, Mohamed. Radioprotective effect of vitamins C and E. *Mutat Res.* 1993; 301:143-147.

45. Kilinc C, Ozcan O, et al. Vitamin E reduces bleomycin-induced lung fibrosis in mice. *J Basci Clin Physiol Pharmacol.* 1993; 4:249-269.

46. Nakamura T, Pinnell SR, et al. Vitamin C abrogates the deleterious effects of UVB radiation on cutaneous immunity by a mechanism that does not depend on TNF-alpha. *J Invest Dermatol.* 1997; 109:20-24.

47. Ravi R, Somani SM, Rybak LP. Mechanism of cisplatin ototoxicity: antioxidant system. Pharmacol Toxicol. 1995;76:386-394.

48. Riabchenko NI, Ivannik BP, et al. The molecular, cellular and systemic mechanisms of the radioprotective action of multivitamin antioxidant complexes. *Radiats Biol Radioecol.* 1996; 36:895-99.

49. Sminia P, van der Kracht, et al. Hyperthermia, radiation carcinogenesis and the protective potential of vitamin A and N-acetylcysteine. *J Cancer Res Clin Oncol.* 1996; 122: 343-350.

50. Srinivasan V, Weiss JF. Radioprotection by vitamin E: injectable vitamin E administered alone or with WR-3689 enhances the survival of irradiated mice. *Int J Radiat Oncol Biol Phys.* 1992; 23: 841-845.

51. Vinitha R, et al. Effect of administering cyclophosphamide and vitamin E on the levels of tumor-marker enzymes in rats with experi-mentally induced fibrosarcoma. *Jpn J Med Sci Biol.* 1995; 48:145-156.

52. Wiseman JS, Senagore, Chaudry. Methods to prevent colonic injury in pelvic radiation. *Dis Colon Rectum.* 1994; 37:1090-94.

HUMAN STUDIES – VITAMIN A

53. Israel L, Hajji O, Grefft-Alami A, Desmoulins D, et al. Vitamin A augmentation of the effects of chemotherapy in metastatic breast cancers after menopause. Randomized trial in 100 patients. *Annnles De Medecine Interne.* 1985;136(7):551-554.

54. Komiyama S, Kudoh S, Yanagita T, Kuwano M. Synergistic combination of 5FU, vitamin A, and cobalt-60 radiation for head and neck tumors – antitumor combination therapy with vitamin A. *Auris, Nasus, Larynx.* 1985;12 S2:S239-S243.

55. Meyskens FL, Kopecky KJ. Phase III randomized trial of the treatment of chronic stage CML with pulse, intermittent busulfan therapy (SWOG 7984): improved survival with the addition of oral vitamin A (50,000 IU/day). *Seventh International Conference on the Adjuvant Therapy of Cancer.* Tucson, Arizona. March 10-13, 1993. Pg. 35.

56. Recchia F, de Filippos S, Rea S, Corrao G, Frati L. Cisplatin, vindesine, 5FU, beta-interferon and retinyl palmitate in advanced non-small cell lung cancer. A phase II study. *Proc Annu Meet Am Soc Clin Oncol.* 1993;12:A1144.

57. Recchia F, Lelli S, DiMatteo G, Rea S, Frati L. 5FU, cisplatin and retinol palmitate in the management of advanced cancer of the oral cavity. Phase II study. *Clin Ter.* 1993;142(5):403-409.

58. Recchia F, Rea S, Pompili P, Casucci D, Rea MJ, Rizzo F, Gulino A, Frati L. Beta-interferon, retinoids and tamoxifen as maintenance therapy in metastatic breast cancer. A pilot study. *Clin Ter.* 1995;146(10):603-610.

59. Recchia F, Serafini F, Rea S, Frati L. Phase II study of 5FU, folinic acid, epirubicin, mitomycin-C, beta-interferon and retinol palmitate in patients with unresectable pancreatic carcinoma. *Proc Annu Meet Am Assoc Cancer Res.* 1992;33:A1296.

60. Recchia F, Sica G, de Filippos S, Discepoli S, Rea S, Torchio P, Frati L. Interferon-beta, retinoids, and tamoxifen in the treatment of metastatic breast cancer: a phase II study. *J Interferon Cytokine Res.* 1995;15(7):605-610.

HUMAN STUDIES – BETA-CAROTENE

61. Mills EED. The modifying effect of beta-carotene on radiation and chemotherapy induced oral mucositis. *Br J Cancer.* 1988;57:416-417.

62. Santamaria L, Bianchi-Santamaria A, dell'Orti M. Carotenoids in cancer, mastalgia, and AIDS: prevention and treatment—an overview. *J Envirn Path, Tox & Oncol.* 1996;15(2-4):89-95.

HUMAN STUDIES – VITAMIN E

63. Besa EC, Abraham IL, Bartholomew MJ, Hysninski M, Nowell PC. Treatment with 13 cis-retinoic acid in transfusion-dependent patients with myelodysplastic syndromes and decreased toxicity with addition of alpha-tocopherol. *Am J Med.* 1990;89:739-747.

64. Dimery I, Shirinian M, Heyne K, Lippman S, et al. Reduction in toxicity of high dose 13 cis-retinoic acid with alpha-tocopherol. *Proc Annu Meet Am Soc Clin Oncol.* 1992;11:A399.

65. Ganser A, Mauer A, Contzen C, Seipelt G, et al. Improved multilineage response of hematopoiesis in patients with myelodysplastic syndromes to a combination therapy with all-trans-retinoic acid, granulocyte colony-stimulating factor, erythropoietin and alpha-tocopherol. *Ann Hematol.* 1996;72(4):237-244.

66. Gottlober P, Krahn G, Korting HC, Stock W, Peter RU. The treatment of cutaneous radiation-induced fibrosis with pentoxifylline and vitamin E. *Strahlenther Onkol.* 1996;172(1):34-38.

67. Legha SS, Wang YM, Mackay B, et al. Clinical and pharmacological investigation of the effects of alpha-tocopherol on adriamycin cardiotoxicity. Ann N Y Acad Sci. 1982; 393:411-418.

68. Lenzhofer R, Ganzinger U, Rameis H, Moser K. Acute cardiac toxicity in patients after doxorubicin treatment and the effect of combined tocopherol and nifedipine pretreatment. J Cancer Res Clin Oncol. 1983;106:143-147.

69. Lopez I, Goudou C, Ribrag V, Sauvage C, Hazebroucq, Dreyfus F. Treatment of mucositis with vitamin E during administration of neutropenic antineoplastic agents. *Ann Med Interne.* 1994;145(6):405-408.

70. Wadleigh RG, Redman RS, Graham ML, Krasnow SH, Anderson A, Cohen M. Vitamin E in the treatment of chemotherapy induced mucositis. *Am J Med.* 1992;92(5):481-484.

71. Weitzman SA, Lorell E, Carey RW, Kaufman S, Stossi TP. Prospective study of tocopherol prophylaxis for anthracycline cardiac toxicity. *Curr Ther Res.* 1980;28:682-686.

72. Wood LA. Possible prevention of adriamycin-induced alopecia by tocopherol. *NEJM.* 1985;312(16):1060.

HUMAN – ANTIOXIDANT COMBINATIONS

73. Copeland EM 3rd, MacFadyen BV Jr, Lanzotti VJ, Dudrick SJ. Intravenous hyperalimentation as an adjunct to cancer chemotherapy. *Am J Surg.* 1975;129(2):167-73.

74. Filler RM, Dietz W, Suskind RM, Jaffe N, Cassady JR. Parenteral feeding in the management of children with cancer. *Cancer.* 1979;43(5 S):2117-20.

75. Jaakkola K, Lahteenmaki P, Laaksa J, Harju E, et al. Treatment with antioxidant and other nutrients in combination with chemotherapy, irradiation in patients with small cell lung cancer. *Anticancer Res.* 1992;12(3):599-606.

76. Lockwood K, Moesgaard S, Hanioka T, Folkers K. Apparent partial remission of breast cancer in 'high risk' patients supplemented with nutritional antioxidants, essential fatty acids and coenzyme Q10. *Mol Aspects Med.* 1994;15 Suppl:231-240.

77. Osaki T, Ueta E, Yoneda K, Hirota J, Yamamoto T. Prophylaxis of oral mucositis associated with chemoradiotherapy for oral carcinoma by Azelastine with other antioxidants. *Head Neck.* 1994;16(4):331-339.

78. Pyrhonen S, Kuitunen T, Nyandoto P, Kouri M. Randomized comparison of fluorouracil, epidoxorubicin and methotrexate (FEMTX) plus supportive care with supportive care alone in patients with nonresectable gastric cancer. *Br J Cancer.* 1995;71(3):587-591.

79. Rougereau A, Sallerin T, Chapet J, Robin JC, Rougereau G. Adjuvant treatment of patients with neoplastic lesions using the combination of a vitamin complex and an amino acid. Apropos of a series of 17 cases of epidermoid carcinoma of the upper aerodigestive tract. *Ann Gastroenterol Hepatol.* 1993;29(2):99-102.

80. Sakamoto A, Chougule PB, Prasad KN. Retrospective analysis of the effect of vitamin A, C, and E in human neoplasms. In: Medulation and Mediation of Cancer by Vitamins. Karger, Basel. 1983. Pg. 330-333.

81. Thiruvengadam R, Kaneshiro C, Iyer P, Slater L, Kurosaki T. Effect of antioxidant vitamins and mineral on chemotherapy induced cytopenia. *Proc Annu Meet Am Soc Clin Oncol.* 1996;15:A1793.

82. Wagdi P, Rouvinez G, Fluri M, Aeschbacher B, Thoni A, Schefer H, Meier B. Cardioprotection in chemo- and radiotherapy for malignant diseases – an echocardiographic pilot. *Schweiz Rundsch Med Prax.* 1995;84(43):1220-1223.

HUMAN STUDIES – B VITAMINS

83. Kim JH, He SQ, Dragovic J, et al. Use of vitamins as adjunct to conventional cancer therapy. In: Nutrients in Cancer Prevention and Treatment. Prasad KN, Santamaria L, Williams RM, eds. Humana Press. 1995. Pg. 363-372.

84. Ladner HA, Salkeld RM. Vitamin B6 status in cancer patients: effects of tumour site, irradiation, hormones and chemotherapy. In: Nutrition, Growth, and Cancer. Alan R. Liss, Inc. 1988. Pg. 273-281.

85. Wiernik PH, Yeap B, Vogl SE, Kaplan BH, Comis RL, et al. Hexamethylmelamine and low or moderate dose cisplatin with or without pyridoxine for the treatment of advanced ovarian carcinoma: a study of the Eastern Cooperative Oncology Group. *Cancer Invest.* 1992;10(1):1-9.

HUMAN STUDIES – VITAMIN D_3

86. DeRosa L, Montuoro A, DeLaurenzi A. Therapy of 'high risk' myelodysplastic syndromes with an association of low dose Ara-C, retinoic acid and 1,25 dihydroxyvitamin D3. *Biomed Pharmacoth.* 1992;46(5-7):211-217.

HUMAN STUDIES – VITAMIN K_3

87. Margolin KA, Akman SA, Leong LA, Morgan RJ, Somlo G, et al. Phase I study of mitomycin C and menadione in advanced solid tumors. *Cancer Chemother Pharmacol.* 1995;36(4):293-298.

88. Nagoumey, et al. Menadiol in combination with cytotoxic chemotherapies: feasibility for resistance modification. *Proc Ann Meet Am Soc Clin Oncol.* 1987;6:A132.

HUMAN STUDIES – GLUTATHIONE

89. Bohm S, Oriana S, Spatti G, et al. Dose intensification of platinum compounds with glutathione protection as induction chemotherapy for advanced ovarian carcinoma. *Oncology.* 1999;57(2):115-20.

90. Bohm S, Battista Spatti G, Di Re F, Oriana S, Pilotti S, Tedeschi M, Tognella S, Zunino F. A feasibility study of cisplatin administration with low-volume hydration and glutathione protection in the treatment of ovarian carcinoma. *Anticancer Res.* 1991; 11(4):1613-6.

91. Cascinu S, Cordella L, Del Ferro E, Fronzoni M, Catalano G. Neuroprotective effect of reduced glutathione on cisplatin-based chemotherapy in advanced gastric cancer: a randomized double-blind placebo-controlled trial. *J Clin Oncol.* 1995;13(1):26-32.

92. Cozzaglio L, Doci R, Colella G, et al. A feasibility study of high-dose cisplatin and 5-fluorouracil with glutathione protection in the treatment of advanced colorectal cancer. *Tumori.* 1990;76(6):590-4.

93. Di Re F, Bohm S, Oriana S, Spatti GB, Pirovano C, Tedeschi M, Zunino F. High-dose cisplatin and cyclophosphamide with glutathione in the treatment of advanced ovarian cancer. *Ann Oncol.* 1993;4(1):55-61.

94. Di Re F, Bohm S, Oriana S, Spatti GB, Zunino F. Efficacy and safety of high-dose cisplatin and cyclophosphamide with glutathione protection in the treatment of bulky advanced epithelial ovarian cancer. *Cancer Chemother Pharmacol.* 1990;25(5):355-60.

95. Fontanelli R, Spatti G, Raspagliesi F, Zunino F, Di Re F. A preoperative single course of high-dose cisplatin and bleomycin with glutathione protection in bulky stage IB/II carcinoma of the cervix. *Ann Oncol.* 1992;3(2):117-21.

96. Leone R, Fracasso ME, Soresi E, et al. Influence of glutathione administration on the disposition of free and total platinum in patients after administration of cisplatin. *Cancer Chemother Pharma.* 1992;29(5):385-90.

97. Locatelli MC, D'Antona A, Labianca R, et al. A phase II study of combination chemotherapy in advanced ovarian carcinoma with cisplatin and cyclophosphamide plus reduced glutathione as potential protective agent against cisplatin toxicity. *Tumori.* 1993;79(1):37-9.

98. Nobile MT, Vidili MG, Benasso M, et al. A preliminary clinical study of cyclophosphamide with reduced glutathione as uroprotector. *Tumori.* 1989;75(3):257-8.

99. Oriana S, Bohm S, Spatti G, Zunino F, Di Re F. A clinical experience with reduced glutathione as protector against cisplatin-toxicity. *Tumori.* 1987; 73: 337-40.

100. Parnis FX, Coleman RE, Harper PG, et al. A randomised double-blind placebo controlled clinical trial assessing the tolerability and efficacy of glutathione as an adjuvant to escalating doses of cisplatin in the treatment of advanced ovarian cancer. *Eur J Cancer.* 1995;31A(10):1721.

101. Plaxe S, Freddo J, Kim S, et al. Phase I trial of cisplatin in combination with glutathione. *Gynecol Oncol.* 1994;55(1):82-6.

102. Smyth JF, Bowman A, Perren T, et al. Glutathione reduces the toxicity and im-

proves quality of life of women diagnosed with ovarian cancer treated with cisplatin: results of a double-blind, randomised trial. *Ann Oncol.* 1997;8(6):569-73.

OBSERVATIONAL V. RANDOMIZED STUDY

103. Benson K, Hartz AJ. A comparison of observational studies and randomized, controlled trials. *NEJM.* 2000;342(25):1878-86.

104. Ottenbacher K. Impact of random assignment on study outcome: an empirical examination. *Controlled Clinical Trials.* 1992;13(1):50-61.

105. Concato J, Shah N, Horwitz RI. Randomized, controlled trials, observational studies, and hierarchy of research designs. *NEJM.* 2000;342(25):1887-92.

FOLIC ACID

106. Leeb BF. Folic acid and cyanocobalamin levels in serum and erythrocytes during low-dose methotrexate therapy of rheumatoid arthritis and psoriatic arthritis patients. *Clin Exp Rheum.* 1995; 13:459-463.

107. Morgan SL, Baggott JE, Vaughn WH, Austin JS, Veitch TA, Lee JY, et al. Supplementation with folic acid during methotrexate therapy for rheumatoid arthritis. A double blind, placebo-controlled trial. *Ann Intern Med.* 1994; 121(11):833-841.

108. Hunt PG, Rose CD, McIlvain-Simpson G, Tejani S. The effects of daily intake of folic acid on the efficacy of methotrexate therapy in children with juvenile rheumatoid arthritis. A controlled study. *J Rheumatology.* 1997; 24(11):2230-2.

LIFESTYLE

109. Simone CB. Use of therapeutic levels of nutrients to augment oncology care. In: Adjuvant Nutrition in Cancer Treatment. Quillin P, and Williams M, eds. Academic Press, Tulsa, OK, p. 72. 1992.

110. Simone CB. Cancer and Nutrition, A Ten Point Plan to Decrease Your Risk of Getting Cancer. New York, McGraw-Hill 1981; revised, Garden City Park, Avery 1992.

111. Wynder E, Kajitani T, et al. A comparison of survival rates between American and Japanese patients with breast cancer. *Surg Gyn Obstet.* 1963;196-200.

112. Nemoto T, Tominago, et al. Differences in breast cancer between Japan and the U.S. *JNCI* 1977;58:193-197.

113. Sakamoto G, Sugano, Hartmann. Comparative clinicopathological study of breast cancer among Japanese and American females. *Jpn J Cancer Clin* 1979; 25:161-70.

114. Ward-Hinds M, Kolonel, Nomura, Lee. Stage-specific breast cancer incidence rates by age among Japanese and Caucasian women in Hawaii. *Br J Cancer* 1982; 45:118-123.

115. Kolonel L, Hankin, Lee, et al. Nutrient intakes in relation to cancer incidence in Hawaii. *Br J Cancer* 1981; 44:332-339.

116. Armstrong and Doll. Environmental factors and cancer incidenceand mortality in different countries with special reference to dietary practices. *Int J Cancer* 1975; 15:617-631.

117. Morrison AS, Lowe CR, et al. Some international differences in treatment and survival in breast cancer. *Int J Cancer.* 1976; 18:269-273.

118. Morrison AS, Lowe CR, MacMahon, et al. Incidence, risk factors and survival in breast cancer: report on five years of follow-up observation. *Europ J Cancer.*1977; 13:209-214.

119. Donegan WL, Hartz AJ, Rimm. The association of body weight with recurrent cancer of the breast. *Cancer* 1978; 41:1590-1594.

120. Abe R, Kumagai, et al. Biological characteristics of breast cancer in obesity. *Tohoku J Exp Med* 1976; 120:351-359.

121. Donegan WL, Rimm. The prognostic implications of obesity for surgical cure of breast cancer. *Breast* 1978; 4:14-17.

122. Sohrabi A, Sandoz J, et al. Recurrence of breast cancer. Obesity, tumor size, and axillary lymph node metatstases. *JAMA* 1980; 244:261-265.

123. Boyd NF, Campbell JE, et al. Body weight and prognosis in breast cancer. *JNCI* 1981; 67:785-789.

124. Tartter PI, Papapestas AE, et al. Cholesterol and obesity as prognostic factors in breast cancer. *Cancer.* 1981; 47:2222-27.

125. Buchwald, H. Cholesterol inhibition, cancer, chemotherapy. *Lancet* 1992; 339: 1154-56.

126. Hoffer A and Pauling L. Hardin Jones biostatistical analysis of mortality data for cohorts of cancer patients with a large surviving fraction surviving at the termination of the study using vitamin C and other nutrients. *J Orthomolecular Med* 1990; 5:143.

127. Goodman MT, Kolonel LN, et al. Dietary factors in lung cancer prognosis. *European J Cancer* 1992; 28:495-501.

128. Foster, H.D. Lifestyle influences on spontaneous cancer regression. *Intl J Biosocial Research* 1988; 10:17-20.

129. Carter JP. Macrobiotic diet and cancer survival. *J Am College Nutr* 1993; 12:209-15.

130. Sakamoto G, Hartmann. et al. In: Modulation and Mediation of Cancer by Vitamins. Karger, Basel. 1983; p. 330.

131. Lamm DL. Megadose vitamins in bladder cancer: a double blind clinical trial. *J Urol.* 1994; 151:21-26.

132. Saxe GA, Rock CL, Wicha MS, et al. Diet and risk for breast cancer recurrence and survival. *Breast Can Res Treat.* 1999; 53(3):241-253.

133. Agus DB, Vera JC, Golde DW: Stromal cell oxidation: A mechanism by which tumors obtain vitamin C. *Cancer Res..*1999; 59:4555-58.

CONCLUSION

134. Gopalakrishna R, Gundimeda U, and Chen Z. Vitamin E succinate inhibits protein kinase C: correlation with its unique inhibitory effects on cell growth and transformation. In: Nutrients in Cancer Prevention and Treatment. Prasad KN, Santamaria L and Williams RM, eds. Humana Press: NJ. 1995. Pg. 21-37.

135. Prasad KN, Cohrs RJ, Sharma OK. Decreased expression of c-myc and H-ras oncogenes in vitamin E succinate induced differentiation murine B-16 melanoma cells in culture. *Biochem Cell Biol.* 1990;68:1250-1255.

136. Cohrs RJ, Torelli S, Prasad KN, Edwards-Prasad J, *et al.* Effect of vitamin E succinate and a Camp stimulating agent on the expression of c-myc and H-ras in murine neuroblastoma. *Int J Dev Biol Neurosci.* 1991; 9:187-194.

137. Kline K, Yu W, Zhao B. Vitamin E succinate: Mechanisms of action as tumor cell growth inhibitor. In: Nutrients in Cancer Prevention and Treatment. Prasad, Santamaria, eds. Humana Press:NJ. 1995. Pg. 39-55.

Chapter 7
Free Radicals

1. Cross, et al. Oxygen radicals and human disease. *Ann Int Med.* 1987; 107:526-45.

2. Southorn P, Powis. Free radicals in medicine, chemical nature and biological reactions. *Mayo Clin Proc.* 1988; 63:381-389.

3. Aruoma Okezie I, et al. Oxygen free radicals and human diseases. *J Roy Soc Health.* 1991; 111:172-177.

4. Saul, et al. Free radicals, DNA damage, and aging. In Annals: Modern biological theories of aging. 1987. N Y: Raven Press, 113-29.

5. Cerutti. Pro-oxidant states and tumor promotion. *Science.* 1985; 227:375-82.

6. Rubanyi. Vascular effects of oxygen-derived free radicals. *Free Rad Bio Med.* 1988; 4:107-20.

7. Hennig and Chow. Lipid peroxidation and endothelial cell injury: Implications in atherosclerosis. *Free Rad Bio Med.* 1988; 4:99-106.

8. Re-profusion injury after thrombolytic therapy for acute myocardial infarction. *Lancet.* 1989; Sept:655-57.

9. McCord. Oxygen derived free radicals in post ischemic tissue injury.*NEJM.*1985; 312:159-63.

Chapter 8
Nutritional Factors

1. Wynder E, Gori P. Contribution of the environment to cancer incidence: An epidemiologic exercise. *JNCI.* 1977; 58:825.

2. The National Academy of Sciences. Nutrition, Diet, and Cancer. 1983.

3. Simone CB. Cancer and Nutrition: A Ten-Point Plan to Reduce Your Chances of Getting Cancer. 1982. NY: McGraw-Hill Book Co

4. Moody. Aboriginal Health. 1983. Canberra, Australia: Australian National University Press, p. 92.

5. Truswell and Hansen. Medical research among the Kung. In Hunter-Gatherers. Lee and DeVore Ed S. Kalahari. Cambridge, Mass: Harvard University Press 1976.

6. Eaton, Konner. Paleolithic nutrition. *NEJM.* 1985; 312:283-89.

7. Howe, et al. Dietary factors and risk of breast cancer; combined analysis of 12 case-control studies. *JNCI.* 1990; 82:561-569.

8. Graham S, et al. Diet in the epidemiology of breast cancer. *Am J Epidemiol.* 1982; 116:68-75.

9. Ewertz M,Caroline. Dietary factors and breast cancer risk in Denmark. *Inst J Epidemiol.* 1990; 46:779-784.

10. Van't Veer P, et al. Dietary fat and the risk of breast cancer. *Int J Epidem.* 1990; 19:12-18.

11. Graham S, et al. Nutritional epidemiology of postmenopausal breast cancer in Western New York. *Am J Epidemiol.* 1991; 34:552-566.

12. Frisch R. Dietary fat and the risk of breast cancer. *NEJM.* 1987; 317:165.

13. Lee H, et al. Dietary effects on breast cancer risk in Singapore.*Lancet.*1991;337:1197-1200.

14. Kritchevsky D. Diet and cancer. *CA- Cancer J Clin.* 1991;41(6):328-33.

15. Weinhouse S, et al. ACS Guidelines on diet, nutrition, and cancer. *CA- Cancer J Clin.* 1991; 41:334-38.

16. Boyle P, et al. Trends in diet related cancers in Japan: A conundrum? *Lancet.* 1993; 342:752.

17. Golden B, et al. Estrogen excretion patterns and plasma levels in vegetarian and omnivorous women. *NEJM.* 1982; 307:1542-47.

18. Wydner EL, et al. Environmental factors of cancer of the colon and rectum. II. Japanese epidemiological data. *Cancer.* 1969; 32:1210.

19. Phillips R. Role of life-style and dietary habits in risk of cancer among Seventh-Day Adventists. *Cancer Res.* 1975; 35:3513.

20. Lyon J, Gardner, Klauber, Smart. Low cancer incidence and mortality in Utah. *Cancer.*1977; 39:2608.

21.   Rosen P, Hellerstein, Horwitz. The low incidence of colorectal cancer in a high-risk population. *Cancer*. 1981; 48:2692.

22.   Baptista J, Bruce, et al. On distribution of fecapentaenes, the fecal mutagens, in the human population. *Cancer Lett*. 1984; 22:299.

23.   Bruce W, Varghese, Farrer. A mutagen in the feces of normal humans. In:Origins of Human Cancer. ed. H Hiatt, Watson, Winsten, Cold Spring Harbor Lab, Cold Spring Harbor, NY. 1977; pps. 1641-44.

24.   Jones D, et al. Dietary fat and breast cancer in the National Health and Nutrition Examination Survey I: epidemiologic follow-up study. *JNCI*. 1987; 79:465-471.

25.   Knekt P, et al. Dietary fat and risk of breast cancer. *Am J Clin Nutr*. 1990; 52:903-908.

26.   Howe G, et al. A study of fat intake and risk of breast cancer. *JNCI*. 1991; 83:336-340.

27.   Kushi L, et al. Dietary fat, breast cancer, adjustment for energy intake and categorization of risk. *Am J Epidemiol*. 1991; 134:714.

28.   Ganz P, Schag. Nutrition and breast cancer. *Oncology*. 1993; 7:71-76.

29.   Report of the Council on Scientific Affairs. Diet and Cancer: Where do matters stand? *Arch Intern Med*. 1993;153:50-56.

30.   Toniolo P, et al. Calorie providing nutrients and risk of breast cancer. *JNCI*. 1989; 81:278.

31.   LaVeccia C, et al. Comparative cancer epidemiology in the U.S. and Italy. *Cancer Res*. 1988; Dec 15: 1202-07.

32.   Willett W, Hunter, et al. Dietary fat and fiber in relation to risk of breast cancer. *JAMA*. 1992; 268:203744.

33.   Giovannucci E, et al. A comparison of prospective and retrospective assessments of diet in the study of breast cancer. *Am J Epidemiol*. 1991;134:714.

34.   Marshall E. Search for a killer: shift from fat to hormones. *Science*. 1993; 259:618-621.

35.   Petrakis N, Gruenke, Craig. Cholesterol and cholesterol epoxide in nipple aspirate of human breast fluid. *Cancer Res*. 1981; 41:2563.

36.   Wu AH, Ziegler RG, Nomura, et al. Soy intake and risk of breast cancer in Asians and Asian Americans. *Am J Clin Nutr*. 1998; 68:1437S-1443S.

37.   Swain S, Santen R, Burger H, Pritchard K, eds. Treatment of Estrogen Deficiency Symptoms in Women Surviving Breast Cancer: Prevention of Osteoporosis and CV Effects of Estrogens and Antiestrogens. *Oncology*. 1999; 13:397-432.

38.   Hsieh CY, Santell RC, et al. Estrogenic effects of genistein on the growth of estrogen receptor positive human breast cancer (MCF-

7) cells *in vitro* and *in vivo*. *Cancer Res*. 1998; 58:3833-38.

39.   McMichael-Phillips DF, Harding C, et al. Effects of soy protein supplementation on epithelial proliferation in the histologically normal human breast. *Am J Clin Nutr*. 1998; 68: 1431S-36S.

40.   Eagon PK, Tress NB, Ayer, et al. Medicinal botanicals with hormonal activity. *Am Assoc for Cancer Res*. April 1999. 1073.

41.   Hargreaves DF, Potten CS, Harding C, et al. Two-week dietary soy supplementation has an estrogenic effect on normal premenopausal breast. *J Clin Endocrin Metab*. 1999; 84:4017-24.

42.   Dees C, Foster JS, Ahamed S, Wimalasena J. Dietary estrogens stimulate human breast cells to enter the cell cycle. *Environ Health Perspect*. 1997;105:633-6.

43.   Welshons WV, Murphy CS, et al. Stimulation of breast cancer cells in vitro by the environmental estrogen enterolactone and the phytoestrogen equal. *Breast Cancer Res Treat*. 1987;10:169-75.

44.   Collins-Burow BM, Burow ME, et al. Estrogenic and antiestrogenic activities of flavonoid phytochemicals through estrogen receptor binding-dependent and -independent mechanisms. *Nutr Cancer*. 2000;38(2):229-44.

45.   Allred CD, Ju YH, Allred KF, et al.. Dietary genistin stimulates growth of estrogen-dependent breast cancer tumors similar to that observed with genistein. *Carcinogenesis*. 2001; 22:1667-73.

46.   Allred CD, Allred KF, Ju YH, et al. Soy diets containing varying amounts of genistein stimulate growth of estrogen-dependent (MCF-7) tumors in a dose-dependent manner. *Cancer Res*. 2001;61:5045-50.

47.   Ju YH, Allred CD, Allred KF, et al. Physiological concentrations of dietary genistein dose-dependently stimulate growth of estrogen-dependent human breast cancer (MCF-7) tumors implanted in athymic nude mice. *J Nutr*. 2001;131:2957-62.

48.   Santell RC, Kieu N, Helferich WG. Genistein inhibits growth of estrogen-independent human breast cancer cells in culture but not in athymic mice. *J Nutr*. 2000; 130:1665-9.

49.   Willard ST, Frawley LS. Phytoestrogens have agonistic and combinatorial effects on estrogen-responsive gene expression in MCF-7 human breast cancer cells. *Endocrine*. 1998;8:117-21.

50.   Ju YH, Doerge DR, Allred KF, et al. Dietary genistein negates the inhibitory effect of tamoxifen on growth of estrogen-dependent

human breast cancer (MCF-7) cells implanted in athymic mice. *Cancer Res.* 2002;62:2474-7.

51. Maggiolini M, Bonofiglio D, et al. Estrogen receptor alpha mediates the proliferative but not the cytotoxic dose-dependent effects of two major phytoestrogens on human breast cancer cells. *Mol Pharmacol.* 2001;60:595-602.

52. Zava DT, Duwe G. Estrogenic and anti-proliferative properties of genistein and other flavonoids in human breast cancer cells in vitro. *Nutr Cancer.* 1997;27(1):31-40.

53. Zava DT, Blen M, Duwe G. Estrogenic activity of natural and synthetic estrogens in human breast cancer cells in culture. *Environ Health Perspect.* 1997;105:637-45.

54. Nakagawa H, Yamamoto D, et al. Effects of genistein and synergistic action in combination with eicosapentaenoic acid on the growth of breast cancer cell lines. *J Cancer Res Clin Oncol.* 2000;126:448-54.

55. Ju YH, Carlson KE, Sun J, et al. Estrogenic effects of extracts from cabbage, fermented cabbage, and acidified brussels sprouts on growth and gene expression of estrogen-dependent human breast cancer (MCF-7) cells. *J Agric Food Chem.* 2000;48:4628-34.

56. Dowsett M, Archer C, et al. Clinical studies of apoptosis and proliferation in breast cancer. *Endocr Relat Cancer.* 1999;6:25-8. Review.

57. Peterson TG, Ji GP, et al. Metabolism of the isoflavones genistein and biochanin A in human breast cancer cell lines. *Am J Clin Nutr.* 1998 Dec;68(6 Suppl):1505S-1511S.

58. Wang TT, et al. Molecular effects of genistein on estrogen receptor mediated pathways. *Carcinogenesis.* 1996;17:271-5.

59. Balabhadrapathruni S, et al. Effects of genistein and structurally related phytoestrogens on cell cycle kinetics and apoptosis in MDA-MB-468 human breast cancer cells. *Oncol Rep.* 2000;7:3-12.

60. Tanji M, Carpenter DO. A steroid-binding protein mediates estrogen-dependent inhibition of growth of MCF-7 breast cancer cells. *Anticancer Res.* 2000; 20:2785-9.

61. Jain PT, Pento JT, et al. Antiproliferative activity of a series of novel cyclopropyl anti-estrogens on MCF-7 human breast cancer cells in culture. *Anticancer Drugs.* 1991;2:487-93.

62. Davidson NE, Bronzert DA, et al. Use of two MCF-7 cell variants to evaluate the growth regulatory potential of estrogen-induced products. *Cancer Res.* 1986;46:1904-8.

63. Selcer KW, Jagannathan S, et al. Inhibition of placental estrone sulfatase activity and MCF-7 breast cancer cell proliferation by es-trone-3-amino derivatives. *J Steroid Biochem Mol Biol.* 1996;59:83-91.

64. Leveque J, Foucher F, et al. Benefits of complete polyamine deprivation in hormone responsive and hormone resistant MCF-7 human breast adenocarcinoma in vivo. *Anticancer Res.* 2000;20:97-101.

65. You L, Casanova M, et al. Combined effects of dietary phytoestrogen and synthetic endocrine-active compound on reproductive development in Sprague-Dawley rats: genistein and methoxychlor. *Toxicol Sci.* 2002;66:91-104.

66. Tannenbaum A. The genesis and growth of tumors. Effects of a high-fat diet. *Cancer Res.* 1942; 2:468.

67. Woutersen RA, Appel MJ, et al. Dietary fat and carcinogenesis: A Review. *Mutat Res.* 1999; 443:111-27.

68. Newman LA, Kuerer HM, et al. Special considerations in breast cancer risk and survival. *J Surg Oncol.* 1999;71:250-60.

69. Lewis CJ, Yetley EA. Health claims and observational human data: relation between dietary fat and cancer. *Am J Clin Nutr.* 1999;69:1357S-1364S.

70. Hilakivi CL, Clarke R. Influence of maternal diet on breast cancer risk among female offspring. *Nutrition.* 1999;15:392-401.

71. Wu AH, Pike MC, Stram. Meta-analysis: dietary fat intake, serum estrogen, and the risk of breast cancer. *JNCI.* 1999;91:529-34.

72. Eichholzer M. Nutrition and cancer. *Ther Umsch* 2000; 57:146-51.

73. Blair SN, Brodney S. Effects of physical inactivity and obesity on morbidity and mortality: current evidence and research issues. *Med Sci Sports Exerc* 1999;31:S646-62.

74. McCarty MF. Vegan proteins may reduce risk of cancer, obesity, and cardiovascular disease by promoting increased glucagon activity. *Med Hypotheses* 1999;53:459-85.

75. Saxe GA, Rock CL, Wicha MS. Diet and risk for breast cancer recurrence and survival. *Breast Cancer Res Treat* 1999; 53:241-53.

76. Bingham SA. High-meat diets and cancer risk. *Proc Nutr Soc* 1999; 58:243-8.

77. Bartsch H, Nair J, Owen RW. Dietary polyunsaturated fats and cancers of the breast and colorectum: evidence for their role as risk modifiers. *Carcinogenesis* 1999; 20:2209-18.

78. Kant AK, Schatzkin A, et al. A prospective study of diet quality and mortality in women. *JAMA* 2000;283:2109-15.

79. Wynder EL, Gori GB. Contribution of the environment to cancer incidence: An epidemiologic exercise. *JNCI.* 1977; 58:825.

80. Nutrition and Cancer, ed. W.D. DeWys. 1983. *Seminars in Oncol.* 1983; 10:1-367.

81. Workshop: Nutrition-Cancer Causation and Prevention. *Cancer Res.* 1983. 43:2386-2519.

82. Diet and Human Carcinogenesis Proceedings. *Nutrition and Cancer.* 1986; 8:1-71.

83. Executive Summary. Diet, Nutrition, and Cancer. *Cancer Res.* 1983; 43:3018-23.

84. Cohen L. Diet and cancer. *Scientific American.* 1987; 257:42-48.

85. Reddy B. Dietary fat and colon cancer. *Prev Med.* 1987; 16:460-467.

86. Proceeding Workshop. Dietary fat, fiber in carcinogenesis. *Prev Med.* 1987; 16:449-527.

87. National Research Council. Diet, Nutrition and Cancer. 1982. Washington, D.C.: National Academy Press.

88. Paptestas A, et al. Fecal steroid metabolites and breast cancer risk. *Cancer.* 1982;49:1201.

89. Brammer S, DeFelice. Dietary advice in regard to risk for colon and breast cancer. *Prev Med.* 1980; 9:544.

90. Vonderhaar BK. Prolactin in breast cancer. *Endocr Relat Cancer.* 1999;6:389-404.

91. Proceedings of the First International Conference on Chemoprevention of Prostate Cancer. *J Urol.* 2004; 171(2): Part 2 of 2.

92. Hebert JR, Hurley TG, Olendzki BC, et al. Nutritional and socioeconomic factors in relation to prostate cancer mortality: a cross-national study. *JNCI* 1998; 90: 1637-1647.

93. Barnard RJ, Ngo TH, et al. A low-fat diet and/or strenuous exercise reduce prostate cancer growth. *Prostate.* 2003; 56:201-206.

94. West DW, Slattery ML, Robison LM, et al. Adult dietary intake and prostate cancer risk with emphasis on aggressive tumors. *Cancer Causes Control.* 1991; 2:85-94.

95. Giovannucci E, Rimm EB, et al. A prospective study of dietary fat and risk of prostate cancer. *JNCI.* 1993; 85:1571-79.

96. Wynder El, Rose DP, Cohen LA. Nutrition and prostate cancer: A proposal for dietary intervention. *Nutr and Cancer.* 1994; 22:1-10.

97. Alcantara E, Speckman. Diet, nutrition, and cancer. *Am J Clin Nutr.* 1976; 29:1035.

98. Carroll K. Experimental evidence of dietary factors and hormone dependent cancers. *Cancer Res.* 1975; 35:3374.

99. Kolonel L, Hankin, et al. Nutrient intakes in relation to cancer incidence in Hawaii. *Br J Cancer.* 1981; 44:332.

100. Simone CB II, Simone N, Simone, CB. Consumption of fiber reduces the risk of cancer: A review. *J Orthomol Med.* 2000; 15:96-102.

101. Goldin, BR, Adlercreutz, et al. Estrogen excretion patterns and plasma levels in vegetarian and omnivorous women. *NEJM.* 1982; 307: 1542-47

102. Knox EG. Foods and diseases. *Br J Prev Soc Med.* 1977; 31:71-80.

103. Armstrong and Doll. Environmental factors, cancer incidence, mortalities in countries.

104. Jain, M., et al. A case control study of diet and colo-rectal cancer.

105. Hill MJ, Caygill CP. Sugar intake and the risk of colorectal cancer. *Eur J Cancer Prev* 1999;8:465-8.

106. Hems G. The contribution of diet and childbearing to breast cancer rates. *Br J Cancer.* 1978; 37:974-982.

107. DominoF, et al. The nicotine content of common vegetables. *NEJM.* 1993; 329:437.

108. Castro, Monji. Dietary nicotine and its significance in studies on tobacco smoking. *Biochem Arch.* 1986; 2:91-97.

109. Davis RA, et al. Dietary nicotine: a source of urinary cotinine. *J Food Chem Toxicol.* 1991; 29:821-827.

110. Domino EF, et al. Current experience with HPLC and GC-MS analyses of nicotine and cotinine. *Med Sci Res.* 1992; 20:859-860.

111. Ames BN. Dietary carcinogens and anticarcinogens: A Review. *Science.* 1983; 221:1256.

112. Browner WS, et al. What if Americans ate less fat? *JAMA.* 1998; 265:3285-3291.

113. Burr, et al. Effects of changes in fat, fish, and fiber intakes on death and heart attack. *Lancet.* 1989;757-61.

114. Ferraro C. Why is high-fat food marketed? Customers demand it, that's why. *Investor's Daily* Sept 6, 1990:15.

115. Woodbury R. The great fast-food pig-out. *Time.* June 28, 1993:51.

116. O'Neill M. Eat, drink, and be merry' may be the next trend. *New York Times.* Jan. 2, 1994, front page.

117. Eating in America. Natural Foods. June 1994:20. (Survey conducted by MRCA for the National Livestock and Meat Board.)

Chapter 9
Obesity

1. The Lancet. Who pays in the obesity war. *Lancet.* 2004; 363:339.

2. Calle E, Rodriguez C, Walker-Thurmond, Thun. Overweight, obesity, and mortality from cancer in a prospectively studied cohort of US adults. *NEJM.* 2003; 348:1625-38.

3. Freedland SJ, Aronson WJ, Kane CJ,et al. Impact of obesity on biochemical control after radical prostatectomy for clinically localized prostate cancer: a report by the Shared Equal

Access Regional Cancer Hospital database study group. *J Clin Oncol.* 2004; 22:446-53.

4. Amling CL, Riffenburgh RH, Sun L, et al. Pathologic variables and recurrence rates as related to obesity and race in men with prostate cancer undergoing radical prostatectomy. *J Clin Oncol.* 2004; 22:439-45.

5. Amling CL, Kane CJ, Riffenburgh RH, et al. Relationship between obesity and race in predicting adverse pathologic variables in patients undergoing radical prostatectomy. *Urology.* 2001; 58:723-8.

6. Albanes D. Caloric intake, body weight, and cancer. *Nutr Cancer.* 1987; 9:199-217.

7. Huang Z, Hankinson SE, et al. Dual effects of weight and weight gain on breast cancer risk. *JAMA.* 1997; 278:1407-11.

8. Kelsey JL, Baron J. Weight and risk for breast cancer. *JAMA.* 1997; 278:1448.

9. Bonn D. How weight gain affects breast cancer risk clarified. *Lancet.* 1997; 350:1371.

10. Armstrong B, Doll R. Environmental factors and cancer incidence and mortalities in different countries with special reference to dietary practices. *Int J Cancer.* 1975; 15:616.

11. Mirra AP, Cole P, et al. Breast cancer in an area of high parity, Sao Paolo, Brazil. *Cancer Res* 1971; 31:77-83.

12. Kumar NB, Lyman, et al. Timing of weight gain and breast cancer risk. *Cancer* 1995; 76:243-9.

13. Michels KB, Trichopoulos D, et al. Birthweight as a risk factor for breast cancer. *Lancet.* 1996; 348:1542-46.

14. London, et al. Prospective study of relative weight, height, and risk of breast cancer. *JAMA.* 1989; 262:2853-2858.

15. Schapira, et al. Abdominal obesity and breast cancer risk. *Ann Intern Med.* 1990; 112:182-186.

16. Ballard-Barbesh, et al. Body fat distribution and breast cancer in the Framingham study. *JNCI.* 1990; 82:286-290.

17. Folsom, et al. Increased incidence of breast cancer associated with abdominal adiposity in postmenopausal women. *Am J Epidemiol.* 1990; 131:794-803.

18. LeMarchand, et al. Body size at different periods of life and breast cancer risk. *Am J Epidemiol.* 1990;128:137-152.

19. Sellers, et al. Effect of family history, body-fat distribution, and reproductive factors on the risk of postmenopausal breast cancer. *NEJM* 1992; 326:1323-1329.

20. Gaskill SP, McGuire WL, et al. Breast cancer mortality and diet in the United States. *Cancer Res.* 1979; 39:3628.45.

21. MacDonald PC, et al. Effect of obesity on conversion of plasma androstenedione to estrone in postmenopausal women with and without endometrial cancer. *Am J Obstet Gynecol.* 1978; 130:448-455.

22. Marshall E. Breast cancer. *Science.* 1993; 259:618-21.

23. Grodin, et al. Source of estrogen production in postmenopausal women. *J Clin Endocrinol Metab.* 1973; 36:207-214.

24. Sitteri, et al. Role of extraglandular estrogen in human endocrinology. In: Handbook of physiology, ed. Greep, Astwood. 1973; vol 2, pp. 15-629. Wash, DC: Am Physiol Soc.

25. Rose P, et al. Low-fat diet in fibrocystic disease of the breast with cyclical mastalgia: a feasibility study. *Am J Clin Nutr.* 1985; 42:856.

26. Schapira, et al. Estimate of breast cancer risk reduction with weight loss. *Cancer.* 1991; 67:2622-2625.

27. Wynder and Hill. Prolactin, estrogens, and lipids in breast fluid. *Lancet.* 1977; 2:840..

28. Rose P, et al. Serum and breast duct fluid prolactin and estrogen levels in Finnish and American women and patients with fibrocystic breast disease. *Cancer.* 1986; 57:1550-54.

29. Lee-Han, et al. Compliance in a randomized clinical trial of dietary fat reduction in patients with breast dysplasia. *Am J Clin Nutr.* 1988; 48:575-586.

30. Insuli, et al. Results of a randomized feasibility study of a low fat diet. *Arch Intern Med.* 1990; 150:421-427.

31. Heber, et al. Reduction in serum estradiol in postmenopausal women given free access to a low fat high carbohydrate diet. *Nutrition.* 1991; 7:137-139.

32. Prentice, et al. Dietary fat reduction and plasma estradiol in healthy postmenopausal women. *JNCI.* 1990; 82:129-134.

33. Manson, et al. Body weight and longevity: A review. *JAMA.* 1987; 257:353-358.

Chapter 10

Food Additives, Contaminants, Pesticides

1. Munro EC, Moodie C, et al. A carcinogenicity study of commercial saccharin in the rat. *Toxicol Appl Pharmacol.* 1975; 32:513.

2. Kessler I. Non-nutritive sweeteners and human bladder cancer: Preliminary findings. *J Urol.* 1976; 115:143.

3. Shubik P. Food additives. *Cancer.* 1979; 43:1982.

4. Sen NP. The evidence for the presence of dimethylnitrosamine in meat products. *Food Cosmet Toxicol.* 1972; 10:219.

5. Newberne PM. Nitrite promotes lymphoma incidence in rats. *Science.* 1979; 204:1079.

6. Toth B, Nagel D. Tumors induced in mice by N-methyl-N-formylhydrazine of the false moral *Gyromitra esculenta. J Nat Cancer Inst.* 1978; 60:201.

7. Lijinsky W, Shubik P. Benzo(a)pyrene and other polynuclear hydrocarbons in charcoal broiled meats. *Science.* 1964; 145:53.

8. Jeyaratnam J. Health problems of pesticide usage in the Third World. *Br J Indust Med.* 1985; 42:505-6.

9. Pimentel D, Perkins J. *Pest Control: Cultural and Environmental Aspects.* 1980; Boulder, Colorado: Westview Press.

10. Wong K., et al. Potent induction of human placental mono-oxygenase activity by previous dietary exposure to polychlorinated biphenyls and their thermal degradation products. *Lancet.* 1985 (March 30): 721-724.

11. Ramamoorthy K, Wang F, et al. Potency of combined estrogenic pesticides. *Science.* 1997; 275:405.

12. Alavanja MC, Samanic C, Dosemeci M,et al. Use of agricultural pesticides and prostate cancer risk in the Agricultural Health Study cohort. *Am J Epidemiol.* 2003; 157:800-14.

13. Dich J, Wiklund K. Prostate cancer in pesticide applicators in Swedish agriculture. *Prostate.*1998;34:100-12.

14. Mills PK, Yang R. Prostate cancer risk in California farm workers. *J Occup Environ Med.* 2003;45:249-58.

15. Borzsonyi M, et al. Agriculturally related carcinogen at risk. International Agency for Research on Cancer. *Science Publication.* 1984; 56:465-486.

16. National Toxicology Program. Fourth Annual Report on Carcinogens: Summary. U.S. Department of Health and Human Services. 1985; Publication NTP 85-002.

17. Vainio H, et al. Data on the carcinogenicity of chemicals in the IARC monographs programme. *Carcinogenesis.* 1985; 6:1653-1665.

18. Environmental Protection Agency. Carcinogens. Federal Register. 1986; (September 24).

19. Watterson A. Pesticide user's health and safety handbook: An international guide. 1988; New York: Van Nostrand Reinhold, 420.

20. Eriksson M, et al. Exposure to dioxins as a risk factor for soft tissue sarcoma.

21. Hardell L, et al. The association between soft tissue sarcomas and exposure to phenoxyacetic acids: A new case-referent study. *Cancer.* 1988; 62:652-56.

22. Hardell L., et al. Epidemiologic study of socioeconomic factors and clinical findings in Hodgkin's disease, and reanalysis of previous data regarding chemical exposure. *Br J Cancer.* 1983; 48:217-25.

23. Hardell L, et al. Malignant lymphoma and exposure to chemicals, especially organic solvents, chlorophenols and phenoxy acids: A case-control study. *Br J Cancer.* 1981; 43:169-76.

24. Woods JS, et al. Soft tissue sarcoma and non-Hodgkin's lymphoma in relation to phenoxyherbicide and chlorinated phenol exposure in western Washington. *JNCI.* 1987; 78:899-910.

25. Persson B, et al. Malignant lymphomas and occupational exposures. *Br J Ind Med.* 1989; 46:516-20.

26. Axelson O, et al. Herbicide exposure and tumor mortality: An updated epidemiologic investigation on Swedish railroad car workers. *Scand J Work Environ Health.* 1980; 6:73-9.

27. Thiess AM, et al. 1982. Mortality study of persons exposed to dioxin in a trichlorophenol-process accident that occurred in the BASF AG on Nov 17, 1953. *Am J Ind Med.* 1982; 3:179-89.

28. Hardell L, et al. Epidemiological study of nasal and nasopharyngeal cancer and their relation to phenoxy acid or chlorophenol exposure. *Am J Ind Med.* 1982; 3:247-57.

29. Kociba R, et al. Results of a two-year chronic toxicity and oncogenicity study of 2, 3, 7, 8-tetrachlorodibenzo-p-dioxin in rats. *Toxicol Appl Pharmacol.* 1982; 46:279-303.

30. National Toxicology Program. Carcinogenesis bioassay of 2, 3, 7, 8-tetrachlorodibenzo-p-dioxin in Osborne-Mendel rats and B6C3F1 mice. 1982. Washington, D.C.: Government Printing Office, NIH 82-1765.)

31. Menegon A, Board PG, et al. Parkinson's disease, pesticides and polymorphisms. *Lancet.* 1998; 352:1344-46.

32. Stephenson J. Exposure to home pesticides linked to Parkinson disease. *JAMA.* 2000; 283:3055-56.

33. Fingerhut, et al. Cancer death in workers exposed to dioxin. *NEJM.* 1991; 324:212-18.

34. Bailer JC. How dangerous is dioxin? *NEJM.* 1991; 324:260-262.

35. Handbook on Pest Management in Agriculture. 1991. Boca Raton, FL: CRC Press.

Chapter 11
Smoking

1. Glantz SA, Barnes DE, et al. Looking through a keyhole at the tobacco industry: the Brown and Williamson documents. *JAMA.* 1995; 274:219-224.

2. Mackay J. The global tobacco epidemic. *Public Health Rep.* 1998; 113:14-21.

3. Conference on Smoking and Health. *Lancet.* 1990; 28:1026.

4. Brown P. WHO agrees on measures to stop global spread of tobacco use. *BMJ.* 1999; 318:1437.

5. Yang G, Fan L, et al. Smoking in China: the 1996 National Prevalence Survey. *JAMA.* 1999; 282:1247-53.

6. Public Health Service. Smoking and health, a report of the surgeon general. U.S. Dept. of HEW. 1979.

7. Henningfield J, Fant R, et al. Tobacco dependence: Scientific and public health basis of treatment. *TEN.* 2000; 2:42-46.

8. Neugut A, et al. New warning for breast cancer patients who smoke. *Oncology Times.* 1993; 15:1.

9. Plaskon LA, Penson DF, Thomas L. Vaughan TL, Stanford JL. Cigarette smoking and risk of prostate cancer in middle-aged men. *Cancer Epidemiol Biomarkers Prev* 2003; 12: 604-609.

10. Hayes RB, Pottern LM, Swanson GM,et al. Tobacco use and prostate cancer in blacks and whites in the United States. *Cancer Causes Control.* 1994; 5:221-6.

11. Hiatt RA, Armstrong MA, Klatsky AL, Sidney S. Alcohol consumption, smoking, and other risk factors and prostate cancer in a large health plan cohort in California. *Cancer Causes Control.* 1994; 5:66-72.

12. Rodriguez C, Tatham LM, Thun MJ, et al. Smoking and fatal prostate cancer in a large cohort of adult men. *Am J Epidemiol.* 1997;145:466-75.

13. Giovannucci, Rimm E, Ascherio A, et al. Smoking and risk of total and fatal prostate cancer in United States Health Professionals. *Canc Epidem Bio Prev.* 1999; 8: 277-282.

14. Ambrosone CB, Freudenheim JL, et al. Cigarette smoking, N-acetyltransferase 2 genetic polymorphisms, and breast cancer risk. *JAMA;* 1996; 276:1494-1501.

15. Brinton LA, Schairer C, et al. Cigarette smoking and breast cancer. *Am J Epidemiol.* 1986; 123:614-622.

16. Brownson RC, Blackwell CW, et al. Risk of breast cancer in relation to cigarette smoking. *Arch Intern Med.* 1988; 148:140-144.

17. Chu SY, Stroup NE, et al. Cigarette smoking and the risk of breast cancer. *Am J Epidemiol.* 1990; 131:244-253.

18. Meara J, McPherson K, Roberts M, et al. Alcohol, cigarette smoking and breast cancer. *Br J Cancer.*1989; 60:70-73.

19. Morabia A, Bernstein M, et al. Relation of breast cancer to passive and active exposure tobacco smoke. *Am J Epidemiol.* 1996; 143:918-928.

20. Palmer JR, Rosenberg L, et al. Breast cancer and cigarette smoking. *Am J Epidemiol.* 1991; 134:1-13.

21. Rohan TE, Baron JA. Cigarette smoking and breast cancer. *Am J Epidemiol.* 1989; 129:36-42.

22. Stockwell HG, Lyman GH. Cigarette smoking and the risk of female reproductive cancers. *Am J Obstet Gynecol.* 1987; 157:35-40.

23. Slattery M, et al. Cigarette smoking and exposure to passive smoke are risk factors for cervical cancer. *JAMA.* 1989; 261:1593-1598.

24. Trevathan E, et al. Cigarette smoking, dysplasia, carcinoma *in situ* of the uterine cervix. *JAMA.*1984; 250:499-502.

25. Hoff, et al. Relationship between tobacco smoking and colorectal polyps. *Scand J Gastroenterol.* 1987; 22: 13-16.

26. Kikendall, et al. Cigarettes and alcohol as risk factors for colonic adenomas. *Gastroenterology* 1989; 97:660-664.

27. Fenoglio, et al. Colorectal adenomas and cancer. *Cancer.* 1982; 50:2601-2608

28. Ricker, et al. Adenomatous lesions of the large bowel. *Cancer.* 1979; 43:1847-1857.

29. Zahm, et al. Tobacco smoking as a risk factor for colon polyps. *Am J Public Health.* 1991; 81:846-849.

30. Winn DM, Blot W, et al. Snuff dipping and oral cancer among women in the southern United States. *NEJM.* 1981; 304:745.19.

31. Pic A. Heavy smoking and exercise can trigger MI. *Int Med News.* 1981; 14:3.

32. Abbott, et al. Risk of stroke in male cigarette smokers. *NEJM.* 1986; 315:717-720.

33. Wolf, et al. Cigarette smoking, risk factor for stroke. *JAMA.* 1988; 259:1025-29.

34. Colditz, et al. Cigarette smoking and risk of stroke in middle-aged women. *NEJM.* 1988; 318:937-941.

35. Rogers, et al. Abstention from cigarette smoking improves cerebral perfusion among the elderly chronic smokers. *JAMA*. 1985; 253:2970-2974.

36. Baron JA. Smoking and estrogen-related disease. *Am J Epidemiol*. 1984; 119:9-22.

37. Baird, et al. Cigarette smoking associated with delayed conception. *JAMA*. 1985; 253:2979-2983.

38. Stjernfeldt, et al. Maternal smoking during pregnancy and risk of childhood cancer. *Lancet*. 1986; June 14:1350-1352.

39. Hopkin JM, Evans. Cigarette smoke induced DNA damage and lung cancer risks. *Nature*. 1980; 283:388.

40. Evans H, et al. Sperm abnormalities and cigarette smoking. *Lancet*. 1981; (March):627.

41. Hersey, et al. Effects of cigarette smoking on the immune system. *Med J Aust*. 1983; 2:425-9.

42. Burrows, et al. Interactions of smoking and immunologic factors in relation to airway obstruction. *Chest*. 1983; 84(6):657-61.

43. McSharry, et al. Effect of cigarette smoking on antibody response to inhaled antigens. *Clin Allergy*. 1985; 15:487-96.

44. Fielding and Phenow. Health effects of involuntary smoking. *NEJM*. 1988; 319:1452-1460.

45. Department of Health and Human Services. Health consequences of smoking: Chronic obstructive lung disease: A report of the surgeon general. Washington, D.C.: Government Printing Office. 1984; PHS 84-50205.

46. Department of Health and Human Services. Health consequences of involuntary smoking: A report of the surgeon general. Washington, D.C.: GPO. 1987; Pub No.87-8398.

47. National Research Council, Committee on passive smoking. Environmental tobacco smoke: Measuring exposures and assessing health effects. Washington, D.C.: 1987; GPO.

48. Johnson K, Hu, Mao. The Canadian Cancer Registries Epidemiology Research Group. Passive and active smoking and breast cancer risk in Canada. *Cancer Causes Control*. 2000; 11:211-21.

49. Jee S, Ohrr H, Kim. Effects of husbands smoking on the incidence of cancer in Korean women. *Int J epidemiol*. 1999; 28:824-8.

50. Lash TL, et al. Active and passive cigarette smoking on the occurrence of breast cancer. *Am J Epidemiol*. 1999; 149:5-12.

51. Wells AJ. Breast cancer, cigarette smoking and passive smoking. *Am J Epidemiol*. 1991; 133:208-10.

52. Morabia A, Bernstein M, et al. Relation of breast cancer with passive and active exposure to tobacco smoke. *Am J Epidemiol*. 1996; 143:918-28.

53. Smith S, Deacon J, Chilvers. The UK National case control study. Alcohol, smoking, passive smoking, and caffeine in relation to breast cancer risk in young women. *Br J Cancer*. 1994; 70:112-9.

54. Sandler D, Everson, Wilcox. Passive smoking in adulthood and cancer risk. *Am J Epidemiol*. 1985; 121:37-48.

55. Sandler, Wilcox, Everson. Cumulative effects of lifetime passive smoking on cancer risk. *Lancet*. 1985; 1:312-5.

56. Hirayama T. Cancer mortality in nonsmoking women and smoking husbands in a large cohort study in Japan. *Prev Med*. 1984; 13:680-90.

57. Uberla. Lung cancer from passive smoking: Hypothesis or convincing evidence? *Ant Arch Occupa Environ Health*. 1987; 59:421-37.

58. Janerich D, et al. Lung cancer and exposure to tobacco smoke in the household. *NEJM*. 1990; 323(10):632-636.

59. Stjernfeldt, et al. Maternal smoking during pregnancy and risk of childhood cancer.MI 57.

60. Klonoff-Cohen H, Edelstein S, et al. The effect of passive smoking and tobacco exposure through breast milk on sudden infant death syndrome. *JAMA*. 1995; 273:795-798.

61. Slattery M, et al. Cigarette smoking and exposure to passive smoke are risk factors for cervical cancer. *JAMA*.1989; 261:1593-1598.

62. Kabat GC, et al. Bladder cancer in nonsmokers. *Cancer*. 1986; 57:362-367.

63. Hermanson B, et al. Beneficial six year outcome of smoking cessation in older men and women with coronary heart disease: Results from the CASS registry. *NEJM*. 1988; 319:1365-9.

64. LaCroix A, et al. Smoking and mortality of older men and women in three communities. *NEJM*. 1991; 324:1619-25.

65. Williamson D, et al. Smoking cessation and weight gain in a national cohort. *NEJM*. 1991; 324:739-45.

66. Sharfstein and Sharfstein. Campaign contributions from the AMA Political Action Committee to members of Congress. *NEJM.* 1994; 330:32-37.

Chapter 12
Alcohol and Caffeine
1. Sesso HD, Paffenbarger RS Jr, Lee IM. Alcohol consumption and risk of prostate cancer: The Harvard Alumni Health Study. *Int J Epidemiol.* 2001 Aug;30(4):749-55.
2. Hayes RB, Brown LM, Schoenberg JB et al. Alcohol use and prostate cancer risk in US blacks and whites. *Am J Epidemiol.* 1996 1;143(7):692-7.
3. Sharpe CR, Siemiatycki J. Case-control study of alcohol consumption and prostate cancer risk in Montreal, Canada. *Cancer Causes Control.* 2001; 12(7):589-98.
4. Friend T. Alcohol may speed up cancer. Society for Neuroscience meeting. *USA Today.* Oct. 1992; 28:1.
5. Stampfer, et al. A prospective study of moderate alcohol consumption and the risk of coronary heart disease and stroke in women. *NEJM.* 1988; 319:267-273.
6. Gill, et al. Stroke and alcohol consumption. *NEJM* 1986; 315:1041-1046.
7. Liu RS, Lemieux L, Shorvon SD. Association between brain size and abstinence from alcohol. *Lancet.* 2000; 355:1969-70.
8. Vatten LJ, et al. Coffee consumption and risk of breast cancer: A prospective study of 14,593 Norweigen women. *Br J Cancer.*1999; 62:267-70.
9. Posner J, et al. Association of coffee intake in women with breast cancer. *Surg.* 1986; 100:482-88.
10. Simon D, Yen D, Cole P. Coffee drinking and cancer of the lower urinary tract system. *JNCI.* 1975; 54(3):587.
11. Cnattingius S, Signorelli L, et al. Coffee intake and the risk of first trimester spontaneous abortion. *NEJM.* 2000; 343:1839-45.
12. Soyka LF. Effects of methylxanthines on the fetus. *Clinics in Perinatol.* 1979; 6:37.
13. Weathersbee P, Olsen L, Lodge. Caffeine and pregnancy. *Postgrad Med.* 1977; 62:64.
14. Mulvihill J. Caffeine as teratogen and mutagen. *Teratology* 1973; 8:69.
15. Weinstein, Mauer, Solomon. Effects of caffeine on chromosomes of human lymphocytes. *Mutat Res.* 1992; 16:391.
16. LaCroix A, et al. Coffee consumption and the incidence of coronary heart disease. *NEJM.* 1986; 315:977-982.

17. Barrett-Connor E, et al. Coffee-associated osteoporosis offset by daily milk consumption. *JAMA.* 1994; 271:280-283.

Chapter 13
Hormonal and Sexual-Social Factors
1. Gann PH, Hennekens CH, Ma J, et al. Prospective study of sex hormone levels and risk of prostate cancer. *JNCI.* 1996; 88:1118-26.
2. Stattin P, Lumme S, Tenkanen L, et al. High levels of circulating testosterone are not associated with increased prostate cancer risk: a pooled prospective study. *Int J Cancer.* 2004; 108:418-24.
3. Swerdloff RS, Wang C. Three-year follow-up of androgen treatment in hypogonadal men: preliminary report with testosterone gel. *Aging Male.* 2003;6(3):207-11.
4. Hwang JJ, Dharmawardana PG, Uchio EM, et al. Prostate cancer in Klinefelter syndrome during hormonal replacement therapy. *Urology.* 2003; 62:941.
5. Kaufman JM. The effect of androgen supplementation therapy on the prostate. *Aging Male.* 2003; 6:166-74.
6. Swerdlow A, Stavola B, et al. Risks of breast and testicular cancers in young adult twins in England and Wales: evidence on prenatal and genetic aetiology. *Lancet.* 1997; 350:1723-28.
7. Trichopoulos D. Hypothesis: does breast cancer originate in utero? *Lancet.* 1990; 335:939-940.
8. Conley, et al. Seminoma and epididymal cysts in a young man with known DES exposure in utero. *JAMA.* 1983; 249:1325-26.
9. Loizzo, et al. Italian baby food containing DES: 3 years later. *Lancet.*1984;May:1013-14.
10. Symmers WS. Carcinoma of the breast in transsexuals. *Br Med J.* 1968;1:83.
11. Ozasa K, Nakao M, Watanabe Y, et al. Serum phytoestrogens and prostate cancer risk in a nested case-control study among Japanese men. *Cancer Sci.* 2004; 95(1):65-71.
12. Colebunders, et al. Breast feeding and transmission of HIV. *Lancet* 1988;Dec: 1487.
13. Goldberg, et al. HIV and oral-genital transmission. *Lancet* 1988; Dec: 1363.
14. Rozenbaum, et al. HIV transmission by oral sex. *Lancet* 1988 June: 1395.
15. Haverkos, and Edelman. The epidemiology of acquired immunodeficiency syndrome among heterosexuals. *JAMA* 1988; 260:1922-29.

16. Donahue, et al. Transmission of HIV by transfusion of screened blood. *NEJM* 1997; 323:1709.

17. Greenhouse. Female to female transmission of HIV. *Lancet* 1987; Aug: 401.

18. Transmission of HIV by human bite. *Lancet* 1987; Aug: 522.

19. Blaser, M. Insect-borne transmission of Aids. *JAMA* 1986; 255:463-464.

20. Vittecoq, et al. Acute HIV after acupuncture treatments. *NEJM* 1989; 320: 250-51.

21. Conacher. AIDS, condoms, and prisons. *Lancet* 1988; July: 41-42.

22. Wahn, et al. Horizontal transmission of HIV infection between two siblings. *Lancet* 1986; Sept: 694.

23. Quinn, A.G., et al. Long-lasting viability of HIV after patient death. *Lancet* 1991; 338:63.

Chapter 14
Air and Water

1. Buell P. Relative impact of smoking and air pollution on lung cancer. *Arch Environ Health.* 1967; 15:291-297.

2. Cederlof R, et al. The relationship of smoking and social covariables to mortality and cancer mortality, a ten year follow up in Sweden. 1975; Stockholm: Depart of Environmental Hygiene, Karolinska Institute.

3. Dean G. Lung cancer and bronchitis in Northern Ireland. *Br Med J.* 1966; 1:1506.

4. Lee ML, Novotny N, Bartle. Gas chromatography mass spectometric and nuclear magnetic resonance determination of polynuclear aromatic hydrocarbons in airborne particulates. *Anal Chem.* 1976; 48:1566.

5. Ware J. Particulate air pollution and mortality. *NEJM.* 2000; 343:1798-99.

6. Samet JM, Dominici F, et al. Fine particulate air pollution and mortality in 20 US cities. *NEJM.* 2000; 343:1742-9.

7. Dockery DW, et al. An association between air pollution and mortality in six U.S. cities. *NEJM* 1993; 329:1753-1759.

8. Hoffmann D, Schmeltz, Hecht, et al. Volatile carcinogens. Occurence, formation, and analysis. In: *Prevention and detection of cancer.* 1996. Part 1. Prevention. Vol. 2. Etiology, prevention methods, ed. H.E. Nieburgs. New York and Basel: Marcel Dekker, Inc., pps. 1943-59.

9. National Research Council. Vapor-phase organic pollutants. Committee on medical and biological effects of environmental pollutants. Washington, D.C.: National Academy of Sciences; 1976.

10. U.S. Department of Health and Human Services, National Institute for Occupational Safety and Health. 1988. Carcinogenic effects of exposure to diesel exhaust. Washington, D.C.: Government Printing Office. Bulletin No. 50. August.

11. Hocking M. Paper versus polystyrene: A complex choice. *Science.* 1991; 251:504-505.

12. Blumthaler and Ambach. How well do sunglasses protect against ultraviolet radiation? *Lancet.* 1991; 337:1284.

13. World Health Organization. Indoor air pollutants: Exposure and health effects assessment. 1983. Report No. 78. Nordlingen Copenhagen: WHO.

14. Nero AV. Indoor radon exposures from radon and its daughters. *Health Physics.* 1983; 45:277-88.

15. Abelson P. Uncertainties about health effects of radon. *Science* 1990; 250:353.

16. BEIR IV. Health risks of radon and other internally deposited alpha emitters. Wash DC: National Academy Press,1988.

17. Repace JL. Consistency of research data on passive smoking and lung cancer. *Lancet.* 1984; i:506.

18. US Environmental Protection Agency. Preliminary assessment of suspected carcinogens in drinking water. 1975. Washington, D.C.: Government Printing Office.

19. Harris RH, T Page. Carcinogenic hazards of organic chemicals in drinking water. In: Book A. Incidence of Cancer in Humans. 1975. ed. HH Hiatt, JD Watson, and JA Winsten. Cold Spring Harbor, NY: Cold Spring Harbor Laboratory.

20. Hogan MD et al. Association between chloroform and various site-specific cancer mortality rates. *J Environ Pathol Toxicol.* 1979; 2:873.

21. Cantor KP, et al. Associations of cancer mortality with halomethanes in drinking water. *JNCI.* 1978; 61:979.

22. National Research Council. 1978. Chloroform, carbon tetrachloride, and other halomethanes: An environmental assessment. Washington, D.C.: National Academy of Sciences.

23. Rafferty PJ. 1978. Public health aspects of drinking water quality in North Carolina. Master's thesis, Department of Environmental Sciences and Engineering, School of Public Health, University of North Carolina, Chapel Hill, NC.

24. Spivey GH, et al. 1977. Cancer and chlorinated drinking water. Final report. EPA

No. CA-6-99-3349-J. Cincinnati, Ohio: U.S. EPA.

25. US Atomic Energy Commission. 1974. Plutonium and other transuranium elements; Sources, environmental distribution and biomedical effects. Wash DC: Govt Print Office.

Chapter 15
Electromagnetic Radiation

1. Land, et al. Breast cancer risk from low dose exposures to ionizing radiation. *JNCI.* 1980; 65:353-376.

2. Miller, et al. Mortality for breast cancer after radiation during fluoroscopic examinations in patients being treated for tuberculosis. *NEJM.* 1989; 321:1285-1289.

3. Paterson A, Frush D, Donnelly. Helical CT of the body are settings adjusted for pediatric patients? *AJR* 2001; 176: 297-301.

4. Donnelly LF, Emery K, et al. Minimizing radiation dose for pediatric body applications of single-detector helical CT at a large children's hospital. *AJR* 2001; 176: 303-306.

5. deGonzalez A, Darby. Risk of cancer from diagnostic X-rays: estimates for the UK and 14 other countries. *Lancet.* 2004; 363:345-51.

6. Roberts T. Women radiated for Hodgkin's have high breast cancer risk. *Radiology Today.* 1992; (Sept):12-13.

7. Hall EJ, WuuCS. Radiation-induced second cancers: the impact of 3D-CRT and IMRT. *Int J Radiat Oncol Biol Phys.* 2003; 56:83-88.

8. Boice JD, Harvey EB, et al. Cancer in the contralateral breast after radiation for breast cancer. *NEJM.* 1992; 326:781-785.

9. Storm H, O Jensen. Risk of contralateral breast cancer in Denmark. *Br J Cancer.* 1986; 54:483-492.

10. Storm H, Anderson H, et al. Adjuvant radiation therapy and risk of contralateral breast cancer. *JNCI.* 1992; 84:1245-1250.

11. Basco V, Coldman AJ. Radiation dose and second breast cancer. *Br J Cancer.* 1985; 52:319-325.

12. Bernstein J, Thompson WD, Risch N, et al. Risk factors predicting the incidence of second primary breast cancers. *Am J Epidemiol.* 1992; 136:925-936.

13. Fisher B, et al. Ten year results of a randomized clinical trial comparing radical mastectomy and total mastectomy with or without radiation. *NEJM.* 1985; 312:674-681.

14. McCredie J, et al. Consecutive primary carcinomas of the breast. *Cancer.* 1975; 35:1472-1477.

15. Schell S, et al. Bilateral breast cancer in patients with initial stage I and II. *Cancer.* 1982; 50:1191-1194.

16. Burns P. Bilateral breast cancer in northern Alberta. *Can Med Assoc Journal.* 1984; 130:881-886.

17. Horn P, W Thompson. Risk of contralateral breast cancer. *Cancer.* 1988; 62:412-424.

18. Parker R, et al. Contralateral breast cancers following treatment for initial breast cancer in women. *Am J Clin Oncol.*1989; 12:213-216.

19. Jacobson JA, Danforth, et al. Ten-year results of a comparison of conservation with mastectomy in the treatment for breast cancer. *NEJM.* 1995; 332:907-911.

20. Arriagada R, Le MG, et al. Conservative treatment vs mastectomy in early stage breast cancer. *J Clin Oncol.*1996; 14:1558-1564.

21. Sarrazin D, Le M, et al. Ten-year results of a randomized trial comparing conservative treatment to mastectomy. *Radiotherap Oncol.*1989; 14:177-184.

22. Zucali R, Luini, et al. Contralateral breast cancer after limited breast surgery plus radiotherapy of early mammary tumors. *Eur J Surg Oncol.* 1987; 13:413-417.

23. Neugut AI, Weinburg M, et al. Carcinogenic effects of radiotherapy for breast cancer. *Oncology.* 1999; 13:1245-1256.

24. Bonnell JA. Effects of electric fields near power transmission plant. *J Roy Soc Med.* 1982; 75:933-44.

25. Pool R. Electromagnetic fields: The biological evidence. *JAMA.* 1990; 249:1378-1381.

26. Vena JE, et al. Use of electric blankets and risk of postmenopausal breast cancer. *Am J Epidemiol.*1992; 134:180-185.

27. Wertheimer, Leeper. Electrical wiring configurations in childhood cancer. *Am J Epidemiol.* 1979; 109:273-84.

28. Wertheimer, Leeper. Adult cancer related to electrical wires near the home. *Int J Epidemiol.* 1982; 11:354-55.

29. Gauger JR. Household appliance magnetic field survey. IEEE Trans PAS-104, No. 9. In: Epidemiological studies relating human health to electric and magnetic fields; criteria for evaluation, June 1988. Intl Electricity Res. Exchange.

30. Milham. Mortality from leukemia in workers exposed to electrical and magnetic fields. *NEJM.* 1982; 307:249.

31.   Wright, et al. 1982. Leukemia in workers exposed to electrical and magnetic fields. *Lancet.* 1982; ii: 1160-61.

32.   McDowall. Leukemia mortality in electrical workers in England and Wales. *Lancet.* 1983; 246.

33.   Tynes, Anderson. Electromagnetic fields and male breast cancer. *Lancet.* 1990; 336:1596.

34.   Demers PA, et al. Occupational exposure to electromagnetic fields and breast cancer in men. *Am J Epidemiol.* 1991; 134:340-347.

35.   Ozonoff DM. Fields of controversy. *Lancet.* 1997; 349:74.

36.   Worries about radiation continue, as do studies. *The New York Times.* July 8, 1990.

37.   Rothman KJ. Epidemiological evidence on health risks of cellular phones. *Lancet.* 2000; 356:1837-40.

38.   Hyland GJ. Physics and biology of mobile telephony. *Lancet.* 2000; 356:1833-36.

39.   Blettner M, Schlehofer B. Is there an increased risk of leukemia, brain tumors or breast cancer after exposure to high-frequency radiation? Review of methods and results of epidemiologic studies. *Abteilung Epidemiologie, Deutsches Krebsforschungszentrum. Med Klin* 1999; 94:150-8.

40.   Galeev AL. Effects of the microwave radiation from the cellular phones on humans and animals. Russian Acad. Sci., Moscow, Russia. *Ross Fiziol Zhlm IM Sechenova.* 1998; 84:1293-302.

41.   Juutilainen J, de Seze R. Biological effects of amplitude-modulated radiofrequency radiation. *Scand J Work Environ Health.* 1998; 24(4):245-54.

42.   Senior K. Mobile phones: are they safe? *Lancet.* 2000. 355:1793.

43.   *Immunol Lett.* 1986. 13:295-299.

Chapter 16
Sedentary Lifestyle

1. Olivera S, Christos P. The epidemiology of physical activity and cancer. *Ann NY Acad Sci.* 1997; 833:79-80.

2. Hoffman-Goetz L, Apter D, et al. Possible mechanisms mediating an association between physical activity and breast cancer. *Cancer.* 1998; 83:621-628.

3. Nieman DC, Henson DA. Role of endurance exercise in immune senescence. *Med Sci Sports Exerc.* 1994; 26:172-81.

4. Tomasi, et al. Immune parameters in athletes before and after strenuous exercise. *J Clin Immunol.* 1982; 2:173-178.

5. Soppi, et al. Effect of strenuous physical stress on circulating lymphocyte number and function before and after training. *J Clin Lab Immunol.* 1982; 8:43-46.

6. Robertson, et al. The effect of strenuous physical exercise on circulating blood lymphocytes and serum cortisol levels. *J Clin Lab Immunol* 1981; 5:53-57.

7. Hanson, et al. Immunological responses to training in conditioned runners. *Clin Soc.* 1981; 60:225-228.

8. Green, et al.. Immune function in marathon runners. *Ann Allergy.* 1983; 47:73-75.

9. Busse WW, et al. The effect of exercise on the granulocyte response to isoproterenol in the trained athlete and unconditioned individual. *J Allergy Clin Immunol .* 1980; 65:358-364.

10.   Eskola, et al. Effect of sport stress on lymphocytes and antibody formation. *Clin Exp Immunol.* 1978; 32:339-345.

11.   Yu, et al. Effect of corticosteroid on exercise induced lymphocytosis. *Clin Exp Immunol.* 1977; 28:326-331.

12.   Hedfors, et al. Variations of blood lymphocytes during work studied by cell surface markers, DNA synthesis and cytotoxicity. *Clin Exp Immunol.* 1976; 24:328-335.

13.   Cannon and Kluger. Endogenous pyrogen activity in human plasma after exercise. *Science.* 1983; 220:617-619.

14.   Dinarello and Wolff. Molecular basis of fever in humans. *Am J Med.* 1982; 72:799-819.

15.   Gershbein LL, et al. An influence of stress on lesion growth and on survival of animals bearing parental and intracerebral leukemia. *Oncology* 1974; 30:429.

16.   DeRosa G, NR Suarez. Effect of exercise on tumor growth and body composition of the host. *Fed Am Soc Exp Biol.* 1980; 1118.

17.   Proceedings of the First International Conference on Chemoprevention of Prostate Cancer. *J Urol.* 2004; 171(2): Part 2 of 2.

18.   Willer A. Reduction of the individual cancer risk by physical exercise. *Onkologie.* 2003; 26:283-9.

19.   Moyad MA. The use of complementary/preventive medicine to prevent prostate cancer recurrence/progression following definitive therapy: part I--lifestyle changes. *Curr Opin Urol.* 2003;13:137-45.

20.   Barnard RJ, Ngo TH, Leung PS, et al. A low-fat diet and/or strenuous exercise alters the IGF axis in vivo and reduces prostate tumor cell growth in vitro. *Prostate.* 2003; 56:201-6.

21. Monga U, Garber SL, Thornby J, et al. Role of exercise to prevent fatigue and improve quality of life in localized prostate cancer patients undergoing radiation therapy. *Int J Radiat Oncol Biol Phys.* 2003 Oct 1; 57:S445.

22. Demark-Wahnefried W, Morey MC, Clipp EC, et al. Leading the Way in Exercise and Diet (Project LEAD): intervening to improve function among older breast and prostate cancer survivors. *Control Clin Trials.* 2003; 24:206-23.

23. McTiernan A, Kooperberg C, White E, et al. Recreational physical activity and the risk of breast cancer in postmenopausal women. *JAMA.* 2003; 290:1331-1336.

24. Albanes D, Blair A, et al. Physical activity and risk of breast cancer in NHANES I population. *Am J Pub Health.* 1989; 79:744-750.

25. Bernstein L, Henderson BE, et al. Physical exercise and reduced risk of breast cancer in young women. *JNCI.* 1994; 86:1403-1408.

26. D'Avanzo B, Nanni O, et al. Physical activity and breast cancer risk. *Cancer Epidemiol Biomarkers Prev.* 1996; 5:155-160.

27. Fredenreich CM, Rohan TE. Physical activity and risk of breast cancer. *Eur J Cancer Prev.* 1995; 4:145-151.

28. Mittendorf R, Longnecker MP, et al. Strenuous physical activity in young adulthood and risk of breast cancer. *Cancer Causes Control.* 1995; 6:347-353.

29. Thune I, Brenn T, Lund E, Gaard M. Physical activity and the risk of breast cancer. *NEJM.* 1997; 336:1269-1275.

30. Rockhill B, Willett WC, Hunter DJ, et al. A prospective study of recreational physical activity and breast cancer risk. *Arch Intern Med.* 1999; 159:2290-2296.

31. Garabrant, D.H., et al. Job activity and colon cancer risk. *Am J Epidemiol.* 1984; 119(6): 1005-1014.

32. Vena, J.E., et al. Lifetime occupational exercise and colon cancer. *Am J Epidemiol.* 1985; 122: 357-365.

33. Gerhardsson, M., et al. Sedentary jobs and colon cancer. Am J Epidemiol. 1986; 123(5):775-780.

34. Manson JE, Hu FB, Rich-Edwards JW, et al. A prospective study of walking as compared with vigorous exercise in the prevention of coronary heart disease in women. *NEJM.* 1999; 341:650-658.

35. Lee IM. Physical activity in women. How much is good? *JAMA.* 2003; 290:1377.

36. Dunn AL, Marcus BH, et al. Comparison of lifestyle and structured intervention to increase physical activity and cardiorespiratory fitness: a randomized trial. *JAMA.* 1999; 281:327-34.

37. Andersen RE, Wadden TA, Bartlett SJ, et al. Effects of lifestyle activity vs structured aerobic exercise in obese women: a randomized trial. *JAMA.* 1999; 281:335-340.

38. Mittleman M, Maclure M, et al. Triggering of acute myocardial infarction by heavy physical exertion. *NEJM.* 1993; 329:1677-83.

39. Willich S, Lewis M, et al. Physical exertion as a trigger of acute myocardial infarction. *NEJM.* 1993; 329:1684-90.

40. Manson JE, Greenland P, LaCroix A, et al. Walking compared with vigorous exercise for prevention of cardiovascular events in women. *NEJM.* 2002; 347:716-25.

41. Erikssen G, Liestol K, et al. Changes in physical fitness and changes in mortality. *Lancet.* 1998; 352:759-62.

42. Somers VK, et al. Effects of endurance training on baroreflex sensitivity and blood pressure in borderline hypertension. *Lancet.* 1991; 337:1363-68.

43. Kraus W, Houmard J, Duscha B, et al. Effects of amount and intensity of exercise on lipoproteins. *NEJM.* 2002; 347: 1483-92

44. Louis Harris and Associates, Inc. Perrier survey of fitness in America. 1978. Study No. S 2813. New York, NY.

45. Paffenbarger R, et al. Physical activity, all cause mortality, and longevity of college alumni. *NEJM.* 1986; 314:605-613.

46. Harris SS, et al. Physical activity counseling for healthy adults as a primary preventive intervention in the clinical setting report for the U.S. Preventive Services Task Force. *JAMA.* 1989; 261:3590-3598.

47. Medical News and Perspectives. Exercise, health links need hard proof, say researchers. *JAMA.* 1991; 265:2928.

48. Horton E. Exercise and decreased risk of NIDDM. *NEJM.* 1991; 325(3):196-97.

49. Helmrich S, et al. Physical activity and reduced occurrence of non-insulin-dependent diabetes mellitus. *NEJM.* 1991; 325:147-52.

50. Winningham ML, et al. Exercise for cancer patients: Guidelines and precautions. *Physician and Sports Medicine.* 1986; 14(10):125-134.

51. Petty BG, et al. Physical activity and longevity of college alumni, letter. *NEJM.* 1986; 315(6):399.

Chapter 17
Stress

1. LeShan LL. Psychological states as factors in the development of malignant disease: A critical review. *JNCI.* 1959; 22:1-18.

2. Angeletti R, Hickey W. A neuroendocrine marker in tissues of the immune system. *Science.* 1985; 230:89-90.

3. Bulloch K. Neuralmodulation of Immunity.1985. New York: Raven Press, 111.

4. Riley V. Psychoneuroendocrine influences on immunocompetence and neoplasia. *Science.*1985; 212:1100-09.

5. Berczi I. The stress concept and neuroimmunoregulation in modern biology. *Ann N Y Acad Sci.* 1998; 85:3-12.

6. Cohen F, Kearney KA, et al. Differential immune system changes with acute and persistent stress for optimists vs pessimists. *Brain Behav Immun.* 1999; Jun;13:155-74.

7. Davis SL. Environmental modulation of immune system via the endocrine system. *Domest Anim Endocrinol.* 1998;15:283-9.

8. Hiramoto RN, Solvason HB, et al. Psychoneuroendocrine immunology: perception of stress can alter body temperature and natural killer cell activity. *Int J Neurosci* 1999; 98:95-129.

9. Kemeny ME, Gruenewald TL Psychoneuroimmunology update. *Semin Gastrointest.* 1999;10:20-9.

10. Miller AH. Neuroendocrine and immune system interactions in stress and depression. *Psychiatr Clin North Am.* 1998; 21:443-63.

11. Nieman DC. Nutrition, exercise, and immune system function. *Clin Sports Med* 1999; 18:537-48.

12. Peters ML, Godaert GL, et al. Immune responses to experimental stress: effects of mental effort and uncontrollability. *Psychosom Med.* 1999;61:513-24.

13. R~aberg L, Grahn M, et al. On the adaptive significance of stress-induced immunosuppression. *Proc R Soc Lond B Biol Sci.* 1998; 265:1637-41.

14. Rozlog LA, Kiecolt-Glaser JK, et al.Stress and immunity: implications for viral disease and wound healing. *J Periodontol.* 1999; 70:786-92.

15. Bartrop R, et al. Depressed lymphocyte function after bereavement. *Lancet.* 1977; i:834-836.

16. Schleifer SJ, et al. Suppression of lymphocyte stimulation following bereavement. *JAMA.* 1983; 250:374-377.

17. Kronfol Z, et al. Impaired lymphocyte function in depressive illness. *Life Science.* 1983; 33:241-247.

18. Schleifer SJ, et al. Lymphocyte function in major depressive disorder. *Arch J Psychiatry.*1984; 41:484-486.

19. Schleifer SJ, et al. Lymphocyte function in ambulatory depressed patients, hospitalized schizophrenic patients, and patients hospitalized for herniorrhaphy. *Arch Jen Psychiatry.* 1985; 42:129-133.

20. Locke S, et al. Life change, stress, psychiatric symptoms, and natural killer cell activity. *Psychosomatic Med.*1984; 46:441-53.

21. Heisel JS, et al. Natural killer cell activity and MMPI scores of college students. *Am J Psychiatry.* 1984; 143:1382-86.

22. Jemmott JB, et al. Academic stress, power motivation and decrease in secretion rate of salivary secretory immunoglobulin A. *Lancet.* 1983; ii:1400-02.

23. Ader R, N Cohen. Behaviorally conditioned immunosuppressant. *Psychosomatic Medicine* 1985; 37:333-340.

24. Black S, et al. Inhibition of mantoux reaction by direct suggestion under hypnosis. *Br Med J.* 1963; 1:1649-1652.

25. Smith GR, et al. Psychological modulation of human immune response to varicella zoster. *Arch Intern Med.*1985; 145:2110-12.

26. Horne RL, RS Picard. Psychosocial risk factors for lung cancer. *Psychosomatic Medicine.* 1979; 41:503-514.

27. Jacobs TJ, E Charles. Life events and the occurrence of cancer in children. *Psychosomatic Medicine.* 1980; 42:11-24.

28. Bloom BL, et al. Marital disruption as a stressor: A review and analysis. *Psychological Bulletin.* 1978; 85:867-894.

29. Fox BH. Premorbid psychological factors as related to cancer incidence. *J Behavioral Medicine.* 1978; 1:45-133.

30. Bloom BL, et al. Marital disruption as a stressor: A review and analysis. *Psychological Bulletin.* 1978; 85:867-894.

31. LeShan LL. An emotion and life history pattern associated with neoplastic disease. *Ann NY Acad Sci.*1966; 125:780-793.

32. Ernster BL, et al. Cancer incidence by marital status: U.S. third national cancer survey. *JNCI.* 1979; 63:567-585.

33. Mastrovito RC, et al. Personality characteristics of women with gynecological cancer. *Cancer Detection and Prevention.* 1979; 2:281-287.

34. Stavraky KC, et al. Psychological factors in the outcome of human cancer. *J Psychosomatiegc Res.* 1968; 12:251-259.

35. Bacon CL, et al. A psychosomatic survey of cancer of the breast. *Psychosomatic Medicine.* 1952; 14:453-560.

36. Greer S, T Morris. Psychological attributes of women who develop breast cancer: A controlled study. *J Psychosomatic Res.* 1975; 19:147-153.

37. Horne RL, RS Picard. Psychosocial risk factors for lung cancer. *Psychosomatic Medicine.* 1979; 41:503-514.

38. Paykel ES. Recent life events in the development of depressive disorders. In: *The Psychobiology of the Depressive Disorders.* 1979; ed. R.A. Depue. New York: Academic Press.

39. Schmale A, et al. The psychological setting of the uterine cervical cancer. *Ann NY Acad Sci.* 1966; 125:807-813.

40. Editorial. Stress and colorectal cancer. *Epidemiol.* 1993; Sept 37.

41. Rogentine G, et al. Psychological factors in prognosis of malignant melanoma. *Psychosomatic Med.* 1979; 41:647-655.

42. Newcomer JW, Selke G, Melson AK, et al. Decreased memory performance in healthy humans induced by stress-level cortisol treatment. *Arch Gen Psychiatry.* 1999;56:527-533

43. Kiecolt-Glaser J, Marucha PT et al. Slowing of wound healing by psychological stress. *Lancet.* 1995; 346:1194-96.

44. Hansen D, Lou, Olsen. Serious life events and congential malformations: a national study with complete follow-up. *Lancet.* 2000; 356:875-80.

45. Cox DJ, Gonder-Frederick LA. The role of stress in diabetes mellitus. In *Stress, coping and disease*, Hillsdale, NJ: Erlbaum. 1991:119-134.

46. Halford WK, Cuddihy, Mortimer. Psychological stress and blood glucose regulation in Type I diabetic patients. *Health Psychology* 1990;9:516-528.

47. Bieliauskas LA. *Stress and its relationship to health and illness.* Boulder, CO: Westview. 1982..

48. Maunsell E. Better survival in patients with confidants. *Oncology News International.* 1993; December:16.

49. Phillips et al. Psychology and survival. *Lancet.* 1993; 342:1142-45.

50. Urbani D. Can regular sex ward off colds and flu? *New Scientist.* April 19, 1999. Study by Drs. Charnetski and Brennan at Wilkes University. The effect of sexual behavior on the immune system.

51. Nunn C, Gittleman, Antonovics. Promiscuity and the primate immune system. *Science.* 2000; 290:1168-1170.

52. Kinsey AC, Pomeroy WB, et al. Sexual behavior in the human female. Philadelphia, Saunders. 1953.

53. Wellings K, Field J, et al. Sexual behaviour in Britain. Harmondsworth: Penquin B. 1994.

Chapter 18
Lack of Spirituality

1. Van Biema D. Does heaven exist? *Time.* March 1, 1997: 70-8.

2. Kaplan M. Ambushed by spirituality. *Time.* June 24, 1996:62.

3. McNichol T. The new faith in medicine. *USA Today.* April 7, 1996:4.

4. Matthews DA. Prayer and spirituality. *Rheum Dis Clin North Am.* 2000; 26:177-87.

5. Koenig HG, et al. The relationship between religious activities and blood pressure in older adults. *Intl J Psych In Medicine.* 1998; 28:189-213.

6. Baider L, Russak SM, et al. The role of religious and spiritual beliefs in coping with malignant melanoma: An Israeli sample. *Psycho-Oncology.* 1999; 8: 27-35.

7. Gioiella ME, Berkman B, Robinson M. Spirituality and quality of life in gynecology patients. *Cancer Pract.* 1998; 6:333-8.

8. Holland JC, Passik S, et al. The role of religious and spiritual beliefs in coping with malignant melanoma. *Psycho-Oncology* 1999; 8:14-26.

9. Mytko JJ, Knight SJ. Body, mind, and spirit: towards the integration of religiousity and spirituality in cancer quality of life research. *Psychooncology.* 1999; 8:439-50.

10. Roberts JA, Brown, Elkins, Larson. Factors influencing views of patients with gynecological cancer about end-of-life decisions. *Am J Obstet Gyn.* 1997; 176:166-172.

11. Taylor EJ, Outlaw FH, Bernardo TR, Roy A. Spiritual conflicts associated with praying about cancer. *Psychooncology.* 1999; 8:386-94.

12. Bliss JR, McSherry E, Fassett J. NIH Conference on Spirituality and Health Care. 1995.

13. Byrd RC. Positive therapeutic effects of intercessory prayer in a coronary care unit population. *Southern Med Journal.* 1988; 81:826-829.

14. Harris RC, et. al. The role of religion in heart transplant recipients long-term health and well-being. *J Religion and Health.* 1995; 34:17-32.

15. Harris WS, et al. A randomized controlled trial of the effects of remote intercessory prayer on outcomes in patients admitted to the coronary care unit. *Arch Int Med.* 1999; 159;2273-78.

16. McSherry E, Ciulla, et al. *Social Compass.* 1987; 35:515-37.

17. Azhar MZ, Varma SL, Dharap. Acta Psychiatrica Scandinavica. 1994; 90:1-3.

18. Ardelt M. Wisdom and life satisfaction in old age. *J Gerontology, Psychological Sciences.* 1997; 52:15-27.

19. Chu CC, Klein HE. *JAMA.* 1985; 77:793-796.

20. Kendler KS, Gardner CO, Prescott. Religion, psychopathology, and substance use and abuse: A multimeasure, genetic-epidemiologic study. *Am J Psychiatry.* 1997; 154:322-329.

21. Koenig HG, Larson DB, Weaver AJ. Research on religion and mental illness. In: Spirituality and Religion in Recovery from Mental Illness, ed., Roger Fallott. New Directions for Mental Health Services 1998.

22. Koenig HG, George LK, Peterson. Religiosity and remission of depression in medically ill older adults. *Am J Psychiatry.* 1998; 155:536-542.

23. Koenig HG, Pargament KI, Nielson J. *J Nervous and Mental Diseases.* 1998; 186:513-521.

24. McCullough ME, Larson DB. Religion and depression: a review of the literature. *Twin Research.* 1999; 2:126-136.

25. McCullough ME. Research on religion-accommodative counseling: review and meta-analysis. *J Counseling Psychology.* 1999; 46:1-7.

26. Miller L, et al. Religiosity and depression: Ten-year follow-up of depressed mothers and offspring. *J Am Acad Child Adolescent Psychiatry.* 1997; 36:1416-25.

27. Myers DG, Diener E. Who is happy? *Psychological Science.* 1995; 6:10-19.

28. Pfeiefer S, Waelty. Psychopathology and religious commitment: A controlled study. *Psychopathology.* 1995; 28:70-77.

29. Pressman P, Lyons JS, et al. *Am J Psychiatry.* 1990; 147:758-59.

30. Propst LR, et al. *J Consulting and Clin Psychology.* 1992; 60:94-103.

31. Strawbridge WJ. et al. Religiosity buffers effects of some stressors on depression but exacerbates others. *J Gerontology, Social Sciences.* 1995; 53:5115-26.

32. Weaver AJ, et al. An analysis of research on religious and spiritual variables in three major mental health nursing journals. *Issues in Mental Health Nursing.* 1998; 19:263-276.

33. Weaver AJ, Samford, Larson JA, et al. A systematic review of research on religion in four major psychiatric journals: 1991-1995. *J of Nervous and Mental Disease.* 1998; 186:187-189.

34. Weaver AJ, Kline AE, et al. Is religion taboo in psychology? A systematic analysis of research on religion in seven major American psychological association journals: 1991-1994. *J of Psychology and Christianity.* 1998;17:220-32.

35. Koenig HK, Cohen HJ, et al. Attendance at religious services, Interleukin-6, and other biological parameters of immune function in older adults. *Intl J Psychiatry in Medicine.* 1997; 27:233-250.

36. Bradley DE. Religious involvement and social resources: Evidence from the data set "Americans' Changing Lives." *Journal for the Scientific Study of Religion.* 1995; 34:259-267.

37. Daaleman, TP, Frey B. Prevalence and patterns of physician referral to clergy and pastoral care providers. *Archives of Family Med* 1998; 7: 548-553.

38. Florell JL Bulletin of the American Protestant Hospital Association. 1997; 37:29-36.

39. Fryback PB, Reinert BR. Spirituality and people with potentially fatal diagnosis. *Nurs Forum.* 1999; 34:13-22.

40. Goldman N, Korenman S, Weinstein R. Marital status and health among the elderly. *Social Science and Medicine.* 1995; 40: 1717-30.

41. Hill PC, Butter EM. The role of religion in promoting physical health. *J Psychology and Christianity.* 1995; 14:141-155.

42. Hummer RA, Rogers RG, Nam CB. Religious involvement and U.S. adult mortality. *Demography.* 1999; 36: 1-13

43. Kaldjian LC, et al. End-of-life decisions in HIV-positive patients: The role of spiritual beliefs. *AIDS.*1998; 12:103-107.

44. Kark JD, et al. *Am J Public Health.* 1996; 86:341-346.

45. Koenig HG, Pargament KL, Nielson J. Religious coping and health status in medically ill hospitalized older adults. *J of Nervous and Mental Disease* 1998; 186:513-521.

46. Koenig HG, et al. *J Gerontology.* 2000; 7:321-328.

47. Koenig HG, Larson DB. Use of hospital services, religious attendance, and religious

affiliation. *Southern Medical Journal.* 1998; 91:925-932.

48. Koenig HG. *Intl J Geriatric Psychiatry.* 1998; 13:213-224.

49. Levin JS, Lyons JS, Larson DB. Prayer and health during pregnancy: Findings from the Galveston Low Birthweight Survey. *Southern Med J* 1993; 86:1022-27.

50. McBride JL, Arthur G, et al. The relationship between a patient's spirituality and health experiences. *Family Medicine* 1998; 30:122-126.

51. McDowell D, Galanter M, et al. Spirituality and the treatment of the dually diagnosed: An investigation of patient and staff attitudes. *J Addictive Diseases.* 1996; 15:55-68.

52. Oman D, Reed D. Religion and mortality among the community-dwelling elderly. *Am J Public Health.* 1998; 88:1469-75.

53. Oxman TE, Freeman DH, Manheimer ED. Lack of social participation or religious strength or comfort as risk factors for death after cardiac surgery in the elderly. *Psychosomatic Medicine.* 1995; 57:5-15.

54. Smith BW. Coping as a predictor of outcomes following the 1993 Midwest flood. *J Social Behavior Personality.* 1996; 11: 225-39.

55. Strawbridge W, et al. *Am J Public Health.* 1997; 87:957-961.

56. Bjarnason T. Parents, religion and perceived social coherence: A Durkheimian framework of adolescent anomie. *J of Scientific Study of Religion.* 1998; 37:742-54.

57. Daaleman TP, Frey B. Spiritual and religious beliefs and practices of family physicians: A National Survey. *J Family Practice.* 1999; 48: 98-104.

58. Ebrahim S, Wannamethee, et al. Marital status, change in marital status, and mortality in middle-aged British men. *Am J of Epidemiology.* 1995; 142: 834-842.

59. Idler EL, Kasl SV. *J Gerontology.* 1997; 52B: S307-S316.

60. Koenig HG, Larson DB, Hays JC, et al. Religion and the survival of 1010 hospitalized veterans. *J Religion and Health.* 1999; 37: 15-29.

61. Levin JS, Chatters LM. Religion, health, and psychological well-being in older adults: Findings from three national surveys. *J of Aging and Health.* 1998; 10: 504-531.

62. Liu QA, Ryan, et al. The influence of local church participation on rural community attachment. *Rural Sociology.* 1998; 63:432-450.

63. Nathanson IG. Divorce and women's spirituality." *J of Divorce and Remarriage.* 1995; 22:179-188.

64. Wilson J, Musick M. Personal autonomy in religion and marriage: Is there a link? *Review of Religious Res.* 1995; 37:3-18.

65. Koenig HG, et al. *J Gerontology.* 1998; 53(A).

66. Miller WR. Researching the spiritual dimensions of alcohol and other drug problems. *Addiction.* 1998; 93:979-90.

Chapter 19
Genetics

1. Lichtenstein P, Holm N, et al. Environmental and heritable factors in the causation of cancer. *NEJM.* 2000; 343:78-85.

2. Ferguson-Smith, et al. Genomic imprinting and cancer. *Cancer Survive.* 1990; 9:487-503.

3. Reik W. 1989. Genomic imprinting and genetic disorders in man. *Trends Genet.* 1989; 5:331-336.

4. Karp J, et al. Oncology. *JAMA.* 1993; 270:237-239.

5. Culotta E, Koshland. p53 sweeps through cancer research. *Science.* 1994; 262:1958-61.

6. Hollstein M, et al. 1991. p53 mutations in human cancers. *Science.* 1991; 253:49-52.

7. Harris C. p53: at the crossroads of molecular carcinogenesis and risk assessment. *Science.* 1993; 262:1980-81.

Chapter 20
Cancer Angiogenesis

1. Folkman J. Tumor angiogenesis: therapeutic implications. *NEJM.* 1971; 285:1182.

2. Folkman J. et al. Isolation of a tumor factor responsible for angiogenesis. *J Exp Med.* 1971; 133:286-7.

3. Folkman J. The vascularization of tumors. *Scientific American.* 1976; 234:59-68.

4. Liotta L, Stetler-Stevenson W. Tumor invasion and metastasis: an imbalance of positive and negative regulation. *Canc Research.* 1991; 51:5054S-59S.

5. Ingber D E. Extracellular matrix as a solid-state regulator in angiogenesis: identification of new targets for anti-cancer therapy. *Seminars in Cancer Biol.* 1992; 3:57-63.

6. Liotta L, et al. Quantitative relationships of intravascular tumor cells, tumor vessels, and pulmonary metastases following tumor implantation. *Cancer Res.* 1974; 34:997.

7. Fidler I J, Hart I. Biologic diversity in metastatic neoplasms origins and implications. *Science.* 1982; 217:998-1001.

8. Weidner N, et al. Tumor angiogenesis and metastasis correlation in invasive breast carcinoma. *NEJM.* 1991;324:1.

9. Toi M, et al. Tumor angiogenesis is an independent prognostic indicator in primary breast carcinoma. *Int J Cancer*. 1993;55:371.

10. Srivastava A, et al. The prognostic significance of tumor vascularity in intermediate thickness skin melanoma. *Am J Pathol.*1988; 133:419.

11. Macchiarini P, et al. Relation of neovascularization to metastasis on non small cell lung cancer. *Lancet.*1992; 340:145.

12. Weidner N, et al. Tumor angiogenesis correlates with metastasis in invasive prostate carcinoma. *Am J Pathol* 1993; 143:401.

13. Bouch N. Understanding tumor angiogenesis. *Contemporary Onc.* 1994. April:14-23.

14. Pili R, et al. Altered angiogenesis underlying age-dependent changes in tumor growth. *JNCI.* 1994; 86:1303-14.

15. Guo J, Stolina M, et al. Stimulatory effects of B7-related protein-1 on cellular and humoral and humoral immune responses in mice. *J Immunol* 2001; 166: 5578-84.

16. Folkman J, Klagsbrun M. Angiogenic factors. *Science.*1987; 235:445-446.

17. Jackson D. et al. Stimulation and inhibition of angiogenesis by placental proliferin and proliferin-related protein. *Science.* 1994; 266:1581-84.

Chapter 21
Prostate Cancer Detection

1. Chodak GW, Keller P, Schoenberg HW. Assessment of screening for prostate cancer using the digital rectal examination. *J Urol.* 1989; 141: 1136-8.

2. AJCC Cancer Staging Manual. 5th ed. Philadelphia, PA: Lippincott-Raven; 1997.

3. Thompson IM, Zeidman EJ. Presentation and clinical course of patients ultimately succumbing to carcinoma of the prostate. *Scand J Urol Nephrol.* 1991; 25: 111-4.

4. Richert-Boe KE, Humphrey LL, Glass AG, et al.. Screening digital rectal examination and prostate cancer mortality: a case-control study. *J Med Screen.* 1998; 5: 99-103.

5. Screening for prostate cancer: an update of the evidence. *Ann Internal Med.* 2002; 137:919.

6. Osterling JE, Jacobsen SJ, Chute CG, et al. Serum prostate-specific antigen in a community based population of healthy men. Establishment of age specific reference ranges. *JAMA* 1993; 270:860-4.

7. Morgan TO, Jacobsen SJ, McCarthy WF, et al. Age-specific reference ranges for prostate-specific antigen in black men. *NEJM* 1996; 335:304-310.

8. Mettlin C, Littrup PJ, Kane RA, et al. Relative sensitivity and specificity of serum PSA level compared with age-referenced PSA, PSA density, and PSA change. Data from the American Cancer Society National Prostate Cancer Detection Project. *Cancer.* 1994; 74:1615-20

9. Smith DS, Catalona WJ. Rate of change in serum prostate specific antigen levels as a method for prostate cancer detection. *J Urol.* 1994; 152:1163-7.

10. Stenman UH, Hakama M, Knekt P, et al. Serum concentrations of prostate specific antigen and its complex with alpha-1-antichymotrypsin before diagnosis of prostate cancer. *Lancet.* 1994; 344:1594-8.

11. Catalona WJ, Partin AW, Slawin KM, et al. Use of the percentage of free prostate-specific antigen to enhance differentiation of prostate cancer from benign prostatic disease: a prospective multicenter clinical trial. *JAMA* 1998; 279: 1542-7.

12. Kratz A, Lewandrowski KB, Siegel AJ, et al. Effect of marathon running on total and free serum prostate-specific antigen concentrations. *Arch Pathol Lab Med.* 2003; 127:345-8.

13. Gormley GJ, Ng J, Cook T, et al. Effect of finasteride on prostate specific antigen density. *Urology.* 1994:43;53-59.

14. Petricoin EF, Ardekani, Hitt B, Levine P, Steinberg S, Mills G, Simone CB, et al. Use of proteomic patterns in serum to identify ovarian cancer. *Lancet.* 2002; 359: 572-577.

15. Petricoin EF, Ornstein D, Paweletz C, Ardekani A, Simone CB, et al. Serum proteomic patterns for detection of prostate cancer. *JNCI.* 2002; 94:1576-1578.

Chapter 22
Establishing the Diagnosis and Stage

1. Harisinghani MG, Barentsz J, Hahn P, et al. Noninvasive detection of clinically occult lymph node metastases in prostate cancer. *NEJM.* 2003; 348:2491-9.

2. Sakr WA, Partin AW. Histological markers of risk and the role of high-grade PIN. *Urology.* 2001; 57:115-20.

3. Wills ML, Hamper UM, et al. Incidence of high grade PIN in sextant needle biopsy specimens. *Urology.* 1997; 49:367-73.

4. Bostwick DG, Amin MB, et al. Architectural patterns of high-grade prostatic intraepithelial neoplasia. *Hum Pathol.* 1993; 24:298-310.

5. Bostwick DG, Foster CS. Predictive factors in prostate cancer: current concepts from the

1999 College of American Pathologists Conference on Solid Tumor Prognostic Factors. *Semin Urol Oncol.* 1999; 17:222-272.

6. Baisden BL, Kahane H, et al. Perinerual invasion, mucinous fibroplasias and glomerulations: diagnostic features of limited cancer on prstate needle biopsy. *Am J Surg Pathol.* 1999; 23:918-24.

Chapter 23
Localized Treatment Options for Prostate Cancer

1. Moul JW. Treatment options for prostate cancer: Part I – Stage, grade, PSA, and changes in the 1990s. *Am J Managed Care.* 1998; 4:1031-1036.

2. Middleton RG, Thompson IM, Austenfield MS et al. Prostate cancer clinical guidelines panel summary report on the management of clinically localized prostate cancer. *J Urol.* 1995; 154:2144-2148.

3. Bumpus HC. Carcinoma of the prostate: A comparative study of modes of treatment. *J Urol.* 1940; 44:169.

4. Barnes R, Hirst A, Rosenquist R. Early carcinoma of the prostate: Comparison of stages A and B. *J Urol.* 1976; 115:404-405.

5. Madsen PO, Graverson PH, Gasser TC, et al. Treatment of localized prostate cancer: Radical prostatectomy vs. placebo – a 15 year follow-up. *Scand J Urol Nephrol.* 1988; 110:95-100.

6. Chodak GW, Thisted RA, Gerber GS, et al. Results of conservative management of clinically localized prostate cancer. *NEJM.* 1994; 330:242-248.

7. Adolfsson J. Deferred treatment of low-grade stage T3 prostate cancer without distant metastases. *J Urol.* 1993; 149: 326-329.

8. Johansson JE, Holmberg L, Johansson S, et al. Fifteen-year survival in prostate cancer. A prospective, population-based study in Sweden. *JAMA.* 12997; 277:467-471.

9. Albertsen PC, Hanley JA, Gleason DF, et al. Competing risk analysis of men aged 55-74 years at diagnosis managed conservatively for clinically localized prostate cancer. *JAMA.* 1998; 280:975-980.

10. Fleming C, Wasson JH, Albertsen PC, et al. A decision analysis of alternative treatment strategies for clinically localized prostate cancer. *JAMA.* 1993; 269:2650-58.

11. Yoshimura N, Takami N, Ogawa O, et al. Decision analysis for treatment of early stage prostate cancer. *JPN J Cancer Res.* 1998; 89:681-689.

12. Wasson JH, Cushman CC, Bruskewitz RC, et al. A structured literature review of treatment for localized prostate cancer. Prostate Disease Patient Outcome Research Team. *Arch Fam Med.* 1993; 2:487-493.

13. Graversen PH, Nielsen KT, Gasser TC, et al. Radical prostatectomy versus expectant primary treatment in stages I and II prostate cancer: A fifteen year follow-up. *Urol.* 1990; 36:493-498.

14. Iversen P, Madsen PO, and Corle DK: Radical prostatectomy versus expectant treatment for early carcinoma of the prostate. Twenty-three year follow-up of a prospective randomized trial. *Scand J Urol Nephrol*, 1995, Jan 1;172:65-72.

15. Holmberg L, Bill-Axelson A, Helgesen F, et al. A randomized trial comparing radical prostatectomy with watchful waiting in early prostate cancer. *NEJM.* 2002; 347(11):781-9.

16. Steineck G, Helgesen F, Adolfsson J, et al. Quality of life after radical prostatectomy or watchful waiting. *NEJM.* 2002; 347(11):790-6.

17. Lu-Yao GL, Yao S-L. Population-based study of long-term survival in patients with clinically localized prostate cancer. *Lancet.* 1997; 349: 906-810.

18. Catalona WJ, Smith DS. Cancer recurrence and survival rates after anatomic radical retropubic prostatectomy for prostate cancer. *J Urol.* 1998; 160:2428-2434.

19. Pound CR, Partin AW, Epstein JI, et al. Prostate-specific antigen after anatomic radical retropubic prostatectomy: patterns of recurrence and control. *Urol Clin North Am.* 1997; 24:395-406.

20. Zincke H, Oesterling JE, Blute MI, et al. Long-term (15 years) results after radical prostatectomy for clinically localized prostate cancer. *J Urol.* 1994; 152:1850-1857.

21. Mettlin CJ, Murphy GP, Sylvester J, et al. Results of hospital cancer registry surveys by the American College of Surgeons: Outcomes of prostate cancer treatment by radical prostatectomy. *Cancer.* 1997; 80:1875-81.

22. Eschwege P, Dumas F, Blanchet P, et al. Haematogenous dissemination of prostatic epithelial cells during radical prostatectomies. *Lancet.* 1995; 346:1528-30.

23. Tefilli MV, Gheiler EL, Tiguert R, et al. Role of radical prostatectomy in patients with prostate cancer of high Gleason score. *Prostate.* 1999; 39:60-66.

24. Begg CB, Riedel ER, Bach P, et al. Variations in morbidity after radical prostatectomy. *NEJM.* 2002; 346:1138-44.

25.   Beyer DC. Salvage Brachytherapy after external beam irradiation for prostate cancer. *Oncology.* 2004; 18:151-158.

26.   D'Amico, et al. Pretreatment nomogram for prostate-specific antigen recurrence after radical prostatectomy or external beam radiation for clinically localized prostate cancer. *J Clin Oncol.* 1999; 17: 168-72.

27.   Zelefsky MJ, Wallner KE, Ling CC, et al. Comparison of the 5-year outcome and morbidity of three-dimensional conformal radiation versus transperineal permanent iodine-125 implantation for early stage prostate cancer. *J Clin Oncol.* 1999; 17:517-22.

28.   D'Amico, et al. Biochemical outcome after radical prostatectomy, external beam radiation therapy, or interstitial radiation for clinically localized prostate cancer. *JAMA.* 1998; 280:969-74.

29.   Cohen JK. Editorial: cryotherapy comes of age. *J Urol.* 2003; 170:1131.

30.   Han KR, Cohen JK, Miller RJ, et al. Treatment of organ confined prostate cancer with third generation cryosurgery: preliminary multicenter experience. *J Urol.* 2003; 170:1126-30.

31.   Chen BT, Wood DP. Salvage prostatectomy in patients who have failed radiation therapy or cryotherapy as primary treatment for prostate cancer. *Urol.* 2003; 62 Suppl 1:69-78.

32.   Shinohara K. Prostate cancer: cryotherapy. *Urol Clin North Am.* 2003; 30:725-36.

33.   Han KR, Belldegrun AS. Third-generation cryosurgery for primary and recurrent prostate cancer. *BJU Int.* 2004 Jan; 93(1):14-8.

34.   Schmidt JD, Doyle J, Larison S. Prostate cryoablation: update 1998. *CA – A Can J Clin.* 1998; 48:239-253.

35.   Fradet Y. The role of neoadjuvant androgen deprivation prior to radical prostatectomy. *Urol Clin North Am.* 1996; 23:575-585.

36.   Soloway MS, Sharifi R, Wajsman Z, et al. Randomized prospective study comparing radical prostatectomy alone versus radical prostatectomy preceded by androgen blockade in stage B2 prostate cancer. *J Urol.* 1995; 154:424-28.

37.   Prostate Cancer Trialists' Collaborative Group. Maximum androgen blockage in advanced prostate cancer: an overview of the randomized trials. *Lancet.* 2000; 355:1491-98.

38.   Pound CR, Partin AW, Eisenberger MA, et al. Natural history of progression after PSA elevation following radical prostatectomy. *JAMA.* 1999; 281:1591-1597.

39.   Link P, Freiha FS. Radical prostatectomy after definitive radiation therapy for prostate cancer. *Urol.* 1991; 37:189-192.

40.   Pontes JE, Montie J, Klein E, et al. Salvage surgery for radiation failure. *Cancer.* 1993; 71:976-980.

Chapter 24
Conventional Systemic Treatment for Prostate Cancer

1. Denis L, Murphy GP. Overview of phase III trials on combined androgen treatment in patients with metastatic prostate cancer. *Cancer.* 1993; 72:3888-3895.

2. The Veterans Administration Cooperative Urological Research Group. Carcinoma of the prostate: Treatment comparisons. *J Urol.* 1967; 98:516-22.

3. The Veterans Administration Cooperative Urological Research Group. Treatment and survival of patients with cancer of the prostate. *Surg Gynecol Obstet.* 1967; 124:1011-17.

4. Bailer JD, Byar DP. Estrogen treatment for cancer of the prostate. Early results with 3 doses of DES and placebo. *Cancer.* 1970; 26:257-261.

5. Byar JD. Proceeding: The Veterans Administration Cooperative Urological Research Group's studies of cancer of the prostate. *Cancer.* 1973; 32:1126-30.

6. Maatman TJ, Gupta MK, Montie JE. Effectiveness of castration versus intravenous estrogen therapy in producing rapid endocrine control of metastatic cancer of the prostate. *J Urol.* 1985; 133:620-621.

7. Blackard CE, Byar DP, Jordan WP. Orchiectomy for advanced prostatic carcinoma: A reevaluation. *Urol.* 1973; 1:553-560.

8. Chadwick DJ, Gillatt DA, Gingell JC. Medical or surgical orchiectomy: The patient's choice. *BMJ.* 1991; 302:572.

9. Potosky AL, Knopf K, Clegg LX, et al. Quality of life outcomes after primary androgen deprivation therapy: Results from the Prostate Cancer Outcomes Study. *J Clin Oncol.* 2001; 17:3750-3757.

10.   Robinson MR, Smith PH, Richards B, et al. The final analysis of the EORTC Genito-Urinary Tract Cancer Cooperative Group phase III clinical trial comparing orchiectomy, orchiectomy plus cyproterone acetate and low dose stilboestrol in the management of metatstatic carcinoma of the prostate. *Eur Urol.* 1995; 28:273-283.

11.   Emtage LA, Trethowan C, Kelly K, et al. A phase III open randomized study of Zoladex 3.6 mg depot versus DES 3 mg in untreated

advanced prostate cancer. *Prog Clin Biol Res.* 1989; 303:47-52.

12. Peeling WB. Phase III studies to compare goserelin with orchiectomy and with DES. *Urol.* 1989; 33:45-52.

13. Citrin DL, Resnick MI et al. A comparison of Zoladex and DES in the treatment of advanced prostate cancer. Results of a randomized multicenter trial. *Prostate.* 1991; 18:139-146.

14. Waymont B, Lynch TH, et al. Phase III randomized study of Zoladex versus DES. *Br J Urol.* 1992; 69:614-20.

15. Leuprolide Study Group. Leuprolide versus DES for metastatic prostate cancer. *NEJM.* 1984; 311:1281-1286.

16. Chang A, Yeap B, et al. Double-blind randomized study of primary hormonal treatment of stage D2 prostate cancer: Flutamide versus DES. *J Clin Oncol.* 1996; 14:2250-2257.

17. Smith PH, Suciu S, et al. A comparison of the effect of DES with low-dose estramustine in the treatment of advanced prostate cancer. Final analysis of a Phase III trial of the European Organization for Research on Treatment of Cancer. *J Urol.* 1986; 136:619-623.

18. Pavone-Macaluso M, et al. Comparison of DES, cyproterone and medroxyprogesterone in the treatment of advanced prostate cancer. Final analysis of a Phase III trial of the European Organization for Research on Treatment of Cancer. *J Urol.* 1986; 136:624-31.

19. Denis L. European Organization for Research and Treatment of Cancer (EORTC) prostate cancer trials, 1976-1996. *Urol.* 1998; 51:50-57.

20. Chodak G, Sharifi R, et al. Single-agent therapy with bicalutamide: A comparison of medical or surgical castration in the treatment of advanced prostate cancer. *Urol.* 1995; 46:849-855.

21. Ho SM. Estrogens and anti-estrogens: Key mediators of prostate carcinogenesis and new therapeutic candidates. *J Cell Biochem.* 2004; 91:491-503.

22. Guns ES, Goldenberg SL, Brown PN. Mass spectral analysis of PC-SPES confirms the presence of diethylstilbestrol. *Can J Urol.* 2002; 9:1684-8.

23. Sovak M, Seligson A, et al. PC-SPES in prostate cancer: an herbal mixture currently containing warfarin and previously diethylstilbesterol and indomethacin. Annual Meeting of Am Assoc Cancer Res, San Francisco. 2002; abstr LB152.

24. Pandha HS, Kirby RS. PC-SPES: phytotherapy for prostate cancer. *Lancet.* 2002; 359:2213-2214.

25. Das P, Kaplan I. The role of PC-SPES, selenium, and vitamin E in prostate cancer. *Oncology.* 2002; 16:285-291.

26. Smith DC, Redman BG, et al. A phase II tiral of DES as a second-line hormonal agent. *Urol.* 1998; 52:257-60.

27. Small EJ, Vogelzang NJ. Second-line hormonal therapy for advanced prostate cancer: a shifting paradigm. *J Clin Oncol.* 1997; 15:382-88.

28. Prostate Cancer Trialists' Collaborative Group. Maximum androgen blockade in advanced prostate cancer: an overview of the randomized trials. *Lancet.* 2000; 355:1491-98.

29. Bales GT, Sinner MD, Kim JH, et al. Impact of intermittent androgen deprivation on quality of life. *J Urol.* 1996; 155:1069.

30. Tannock IF, Gospodarowicz M, et al. Treatment of metastatic prostate cancer patients with low dose prednisone: evaluation of pain and quality of life as indices of response. *J Clin Oncol.* 1989; 7:590-597.

31. Nisjimura K, Nonomura N, Yasunaga Y, et al. Low dose oral dexamethasone for hormone-refractory prostate cancer. *Cancer.* 2000; 89:2570-2576.

32. Tannock IF, Osoba D, et al. Chemotherapy with mitoxantrone plus prednisone or prednisone alone for symptomatic hormone-resistant prostate cancer: a Canadian randomized trial with palliative end points. *J Clin Oncol.* 1996; 14:1756-64.

33. Catalona WJ. Management of cancer of the prostate. *NEJM.* 1994; 15:996-1004.

34. Dawson NA. Treatment of progressive metastatic prostate cancer. *Oncology.* 1993; 7:17-24.

35. Scher HI. Cytotoxic chemotherapy for advanced prostate cancer: does it work, and if no, how do we prove it? In: Perry MC, ed. Educational Book, 34th Annual Meeting ASCO; May 16-19, 1998. Los Angeles. 356-367.

36. Eisenberger MA, Abrams JS. Chemotherapy for prostatic cancer. *Semin Urol.* 1988; 6:303-310.

37. Bayoumi AM, Brown AD, Garber AM. Cost-Effectiveness of Androgen Suppression Therapies in Advanced Prostate Ca. *JNCI.* 2000; 92:1731-1739.

38. Gunawardana DH, Lichtenstein M, Better N, Rosenthal M. Results of strontium-89 therapy in patients with prostate cancer resistant to chemotherapy. *Clin Nucl Med.* 2004; 29:81-5.

39. Serafini AN, Houston SJ, Resche I, et al. Palliation of pain associated with metastatic bone cancer using samarium-153 lexidronam: a double blind study. *J Clin Oncol.* 1998; 16:1574-1581.

40.   Body JJ. Clinical research update: Zoledronate. *Cancer*. 1997; 80:1699-1701.

41.   Holland JF. Karnofsky Memorial Lecture: Breaking the cure barrier. *J Clin Oncol*. 1983; 1:74-90.

42.   Cassileth, B., et al. Survival and quality of life among patients receiving unproven as compared with conventional cancer therapy. *NEJM*. 1991; 324:1180-85.

43.   Dodwell D. Adjuvant chemotherapy for early breast cancer: doubts and decisions. *Lancet*. 1998; 351:1506-07.

44.   Rajagopal S, Goodman, Tannock. Adjuvant chemotherapy for breast cancer: discordance between physicians' perception of benefit and the results of clinical trials. *Lancet*. 1998;351:1506-07.

45.   Richards M, Ramirez A, et al. Offering choice of treatment to patients with cancers: a review. *Eur J Cancer*. 1995; 31A:112-16.

Chapter 25
Quality of Life and Ethics

1. *Cancer Treat Rep*. 1985. 69:1155-57.

2. Hurny C, et al. Quality of life studies in international groups. *Eur J Cancer*. 1992; 28:118-24.

3. Kurtzman S, et al. Rehabilitation of the cancer patient. *Am J Surg*. 1988; 155:791-803.

4. Bullard DG, et al. Sexual health care and cancer. *Front Radiat Ther Oncol*. 1980; 14:55-58.

5. Masters and Johnson. Human Sexual Response. 1966; Boston: Little, Brown.

6. Steinhauser K, Christakis N, et al. Factors considered important at the end of life by patients, family, physicians, and other care providers. *JAMA*. 2000; 284:2476-82.

7. President's Commission for the Study of Ethical Problems in Medicine. *Making Health Care Decisions*. 1982; **2**: 245-246.

8. Arato v. Avedon. 5 Cal 4th 1172, 23 Cal Rptr. 1993. 2D. 131, 858P. 2D 598.

9. Smith TJ. Editorial. *JAMA*. 1998; 279:1746-48.

10.   Peppercorn JM, Weeks JC, Cook E, Joffe S. Comparison of outcomes in cancer patients treated within and outside clinical trials: conceptual framework and structured review. *Lancet*. 2004; 363:263-70.

11.   Moertel CG. Off-label drug use for cancer therapy and National Health Care Priorities. *JAMA*. 1991; 266:3031-32.

1. Enas, AE. Triglycerides and small, dense low-density lipoprotein. *JAMA*. 1998; 280:1990.

Chapter 26
The Simone Ten Point Plan

Glossary of Medical Terms

Adjuvant treatment. Treatment given in addition to the primary one.

Adrenal glands. Located on top of the kidneys, the adrenal glands produce a small amount of the male hormone, testosterone.

Aspiration. Removal of liquids or solids from a lump using a needle and syringe.

Autosomal dominant trait. A single gene, acting alone, to produce an outcome.

Benign prostatic hyperplasia (BPH). Enlarged prostate that is not cancer. This enlargement constricts the urethra making it difficult to unrinate.

Biopsy. The gross and microscopic examination of tissues removed from the body to make a medical diagnosis; excisional biopsy is the removal of the entire breast lump, whereas incisional biopsy is the removal of a small piece of the breast mass.

Brachytherapy. See Implant radiation.

Cancer. A malignant uncontrollable growth that invades surrounding tissues and spreads to other organs as well.

Carcinoma. A cancer that begins in the lining or coverings of organs.

Chemotherapy. Chemical drugs used to treat an illness.

Computed tomography (CT). A computerized X-ray study that details the cross-sectional anatomy of a part of a body.

Digital rectal examination (DRE). Physical examination of the prostate using a gloved finger into the rectum to feel one surface of it.

Dribbling. Dripping of urine at the conclusion of, or during, urination.

Estrogen. A hormone produced mainly in the ovaries responsible for the development of female characteristics and the menstrual cycle. It is used to treat prostate cancer.

External radiation. Radiation from a machine outside the body delivered to a site in the body. See also Implant radiation; Radiation therapy.

Frequency. A need to urinate very often.

Genotype. The hereditary make-up of someone as determined by genes.

Hesitancy. Unable to start the urine stream for some time.

Hormone therapy. Adding or removing hormones to treat cancer.

Hormones. Steroid chemicals produced by various organs for different purposes.

Implant radiation (also known as brachytherapy). A radioactive substance is placed directly into the tissue in the body that needs treatment. See also External radiation; Radiation therapy.

Impotence. The inability to have an erection.

Incontinence. Loss of urinary control.

Intermittency The stopping and starting of urine flow.

LH-RH analogs. Human-made compounds similar to the natural leutinizing releasing hormone that helps produce of testosterone.

Local-regional therapy. Treatment directed to the tumor bed and its adjacent surrounding tissues.

Lymph nodes. Oval or round bodies located along the lymphatic vessels that remove bacteria or foreign particles from the lymph. Cancers can spread to lymph nodes causing the lymph nodes' size to increase.

Lymphedema. Fluid that sometimes collects in the tissues of extremities as a result of removing lymph vessels or lymph nodes.

Malignant. A cancerous tumor that is growing and spreading.

Mendelian inheritance. Classical genetics that has two genes operating to produce a single outcome.

Metastasis. The spread of cancer from the primary organ, like breast, to another more distant organ, like bone.

Nocturia. Being awakened during the night by need to urinate.

Oncologist. Physician who treats cancer.

Orchiectomy: Surgical removal of the testicles.

Palpation. Examining organ by feeling to detect abnormalities.

Pathologist. Physician who reads prepared microscopic slides containing biopsied tissue in order to determine a diagnosis.

Pathology. The study and classification of tissue specimens with the use of a microscope.

Prostate gland. A gland about the size of a walnut located between the urinary bladder and the rectum. It produces nourishing fluid to transport the sperm out during ejaculation.

Prostate specific antigen (PSA). A protein that made only by the prostate gland.

Prostatitis. An inflammation of the prostate.

Prosthesis. The artificial replacement of a body part, as with a breast that is worn underneath clothing.

Radiation therapy. Treatment of cancer using high energy radiation from X-ray or other sources. See also External or Implant radiation.

Prostatectomy. Surgical removal of the prostate.

Rectum. The last few inches of the colon that leads outside the body.

Semen. A thick, white fluid secreted by the prostate to carry sperm.

Screening. Tests used to find disease when a person has no symptoms of an illness.

Staging. Determining where the cancer is located in the body.

Systemic therapy. Treatment that travels to all parts of the body, usually by way of the bloodstream.

Testosterone. A male sex hormone produced mostly by the testicles with a small amount produced by the adrenal glands. Testosterone stimulates a man's sexual activity and growth of other sex organs, including the prostate.

Transurethral resection of the prostate (TURP) The removal of part of the prostate by inserting an instrument through the urethra and scraping away the prostate tissue.

Tumor. The Latin word that means growth or swelling; today's usage refers to an abnormal growth of tissue; it does not imply, however, that the mass is a cancer.

Tumor marker. Something detectable in the body that may suggest a cancer is growing, for instance, Prostate Specific Antigen (PSA).

Ultrasound. A diagnostic test that bounces sound waves off body tissues, a process that can differentiate solid from liquid. This is most useful to distinguish the contents of a mass in a breast. A solid mass needs further investigation, but a liquid-filled mass may not.

Urethra. Urine passes through this tube from the bladder to outside the body, via the penis. Semen also passes through the urethra.

Urgency. The necessity to urinate quickly.

Urologist. A specialized physician who treats the organs of the urinary tract.

Sources of Information

National Cancer Institute (NCI), Cancer Information Service – call 800-4-CANCER for your questions and booklets on topics.

NCI Comprehensive and Clinical Cancer Centers around the country – call 301-496-4000 to find the Center near you.

> National Cancer Institute　Building 31, Room 10A24
> 9000 Rockville Pike　　　Bethesda, MD 20892

The Health Insurance Association of America (HIAA) will answer your questions concerning insurance coverage.

> Fulfillment Department　PO Box 41455
> Washington, DC 20018　202-866-6244

PDQ (Physicians Data Query) – NCI database provides prognostic, stage, treatment information, and protocol summaries. A computer modem is needed. For information, call the NCI at 310- 496-7403.

National Organizations

4-Cancer　800-4-CANCER　A service of the National Cancer Institute. Supplies information about cancer prevention, symptoms, kinds of cancer, clinical trials, second opinions, and referrals to support groups.

US-TOO International, Inc.: Prostate Cancer Survivor Support Groups. 800-808-7866

About the Author (DrSimone.com)

During your life, there are people you would like to meet....and there are people you should meet. Meet now Charles B. Simone, Masters of Medical Sciences, Medical Doctor, **Internist** (trained at the Cleveland Clinic 1975-1977), **Medical Oncologist** (National Cancer Institute 1977-1982), **Tumor Immunologist** (National Cancer Institute 1977-1982), and **Radiation Oncologist** (Univ of Pennsylvania 1982-1985).

At the National Cancer Institute, Dr Simone discovered how white blood cells kill, showed how complement proteins kill, showed how adriamycin operates at the cellular level, and conceived and developed the idea of splicing monoclonal antibodies to killing cells that seek out cancer. He later helped in the proteomic pattern research for early cancer detection.

While thoroughly engrossed in basic science at the NCI, Dr Simone found new direction as a result of his patients. Vice President Humphrey died not of his cancer but of malnutrition and a young man with cancer was dying because he lacked certain vitamins. Newly interested in nutrition and cancer his research led to the landmark book, *Cancer and Nutrition* (1980) thrusting him into the alternative medicine arena. In 1992 he was asked to help organize the Office of Alternative Medicine, National Institutes of Health. He later received FDA approval to investigate the use of shark cartilage to treat advanced cancers.

Because of his expertise in treating malnourished dehydrated patients who experience muscle wasting, he was asked to formulate a nutritional drink that can prevent dehydration and cramping. In 1990, the formula was tested and proven successful in the harsh conditions of the North African desert in Cairo, Egypt. It is successfully used by World Class, Professional, and amateur athletes, as well as people in everyday activities.

In 1993 he was called upon to write the language that led to the compromise in the US Congress ensuring that all Americans have free access to information and food supplements – the Dietary, Health and Education Act of 1994 (DSHEA).

Then he helped win landmark cases against the Food and Drug Administration [*Pearson v. Shalala*] in which the FDA was found to violate the First and Fifth Amendment rights of American citizens. For all this patriotic work in behalf of the American people, he was bestowed the first **Bulwark of Liberty Award** in 2001 and the **James Lind Scientific Achievement Award** in 2004 by the American Preventive Medical Association and the Foundation for Alternative Medicine for "outstanding contributions to nutrition science and to public understanding of the role of nutrients in reducing disease risk."

He has authored more than 60 peer-reviewed articles and many books.

Dr. Simone consults for heads of state of the US and other countries, celebrities, and advises many governments. He testifies for the US Congress regarding health, cancer, disease prevention, children's health programs, FDA reform, alternative medicine, and the dissemination of truth to patients. He appears on 60 MINUTES, Prime Time Live, MS NBC, Fox, and others.

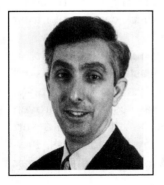

"What is needed is some person, some institution, some inescapable "force" that captures the imagination of our citizens and demonstrates that cancer and other diseases will be eliminated only when each of us comes to understand that this can only occur as part of a lifelong process of sanity, balance, moderation, and self-respect."

About Charles B. Simone, M.D. ....

"Nancy joins me in sending you our best wishes for the success of your vital work."
Ronald Reagan, President

"Dr. Charles B. Simone, an expert in the field of cancer research and treatment, is an individual for whom I have the highest respect."
Peter W. Rodino, Jr., Former Chairman, Judiciary

"If everyone would follow Dr. Simone's plan, we would make major strides toward putting the cancer doctors out of work."
Robert A. Good, MD, PhD, Frm Chairman, Memorial Cancer, NYC

"I congratulate Dr. Simone on innovative work."
Dr. Linus Pauling, two-time Nobel Laureate

"Valuable and timely. Should prove beneficial to the public."
George E. Stringfellow, American Cancer Society

"Thank you for having the courage to come forward. Your testimony is a powerful indicator of the great need for change in America's system of health care and the importance of an individual's freedom of choice when treating illness."
Dan Burton, Chairman Committee Government Reform and Oversight

"Thank you for all your work on behalf of alternative therapies."
Tom Harkin, US Senator

"I agree with you that we need to focus not just on treatment but also on prevention."
Henry Waxman, US House

"Excellent work." **Dr. Denis Burkitt**

"Your work will reduce cancer." **William Bennett, Frm Sec Education**

Index